THE TRAIN IN THE NIGHT

A Story of Music and Loss

NICK COLEMAN

JONATHAN CAPE
LONDON

Published by Jonathan Cape 2012

2 4 6 8 10 9 7 5 3

First published in Great Britain in 2012 by
Jonathan Cape
Random House, 20 Vauxhall Bridge Road,
London SW1V 2SA

www.vintage-books.co.uk

Addresses for companies within The Random House Group Limited can be found at:
www.randomhouse.co.uk/offices.htm

The Random House Group Limited Reg. No. 954009

A CIP catalogue record for this book is available from the British Library

ISBN 9780224093576

The Random House Group Limited supports The Forest Stewardship Council (FSC®), the
leading international forest certification organisation. Our books carrying the FSC label are
printed on FSC® certified paper. FSC is the only forest certification scheme endorsed by
the leading environmental organisations, including Greenpeace. Our paper procurement
policy can be found at: www.randomhouse.co.uk/environment

Typeset in Adobe Garamond by Palimpsest Book Production Limited,
Falkirk, Stirlingshire

Printed and bound in Great Britain by
Clays Ltd, St Ives plc

For Roger and Mary

THE TRAIN IN THE NIGHT

1

Silence descended suddenly and without warning. I put two mugs of tea on the bedside table, sat down, passed one to my wife, hoicked my legs into bed, lowered my head and . . . *pfffff.*

One ear gone.

The silence did not descend silently, however. It made a small sound. You might compare it to the sound of a kitten dropping on to a pillow – a soft sonic dimple, barely there; a dimple gathering scope to itself, widening like a pool. After an hour, the *pffff* had developed a pulse. Then the pulse smoothed itself out and I started to throw up. Eventually I went to hospital.

After a few days in hospital and a number of unexciting pharmacological adventures, the *pffff* evolved into a wild humming and the inside of my head began to resound like the inside of an old fridge hooked up to a half-blown amplifier. The alphabet involved modulated from Ps and Fs, to Rs and As and GHs and protracted MNs – torquey skeins of sound punctuated every now and then by clanks, zizzes and whistles. Some of the clanks I chose to interpret as holes in the fabric of the torquey skeins. These were cause for little outbursts of optimism and I greeted them with gasps. It appeared that something good was happening. It was as if a plug had been pulled.

And then the plug would go back in. *Pfffff-zzzzzz-mmmmmnnnn.* Such are the excitements of tinnitus.

Soon, every outside-world sound that went in the one good

ear produced a balancing, then overwhelming noise response in the other one, on top of the basic fridge noises. It was deafening in there. A fight. A riot. I began to be frightened of any sort of ambient sound and of people who threatened to make it by scraping chair legs or laughing or handling paper bags. I began to treasure the thought as well as the actuality of silence. It became the best thing imaginable. Both literally and metaphorically, I'd spend the day with pillows wrapped around my head to keep sound out, while, on the inside, my head felt ready to explode with pressure, as if my brains were pushing like a slowly inflating balloon against the inner surface of my skull. And then new detail began to manifest within the lagging. In the still of the night I was lullabied by a tiny monkey playing a tiny pipe organ.

I quite liked him. His noise was at least semi-musical, in the sense that he was fiddling with keys on a tuned instrument rather than whacking the central heating with a wrench. His playing was somehow suggestive of order, even if his melodic sense deviated from the conventions of Western tonality. *Needle-weedle*, he went. *Needle-weedle-woodle* – half tones, quarter tones, eighth tones, teeny-tiny tones slipping and sliding into and around one another like eels in a bucket. It seemed lovely somehow. Dreamy. In due course the monkey was joined by the singing of a drowning choir.

I floated for days on steroids and sedatives and anti-vertigo drugs and oxygen and eel music, when it was quiet enough in the ward to hear the monkey play it. I thought great thoughts and a few unpleasant ones, all of them dreamy. I ate fruit intently (that was the steroids: I normally eat fruit diffidently) and smiled bravely at long-faced sympathisers; scowled at them too. I did not move a muscle, apart from those which enable hand to move to mouth.

One night, after lying immobile on my back in Bart's for what seemed like weeks but was in fact three days, I began to think

I might like some fresh air. I hadn't thrown up for thirty-six hours. I had a pair of my late father-in-law's walking sticks and I had the anti-wobble medication to mitigate, at least theoretically, the sensation that I was no longer a reasonably vital middle-aged man but a half-blind centenarian with a balloon in his head, lately descended on shaky legs from a big dipper. I narrowed my eyes to slits and shuffled very slowly down the stairs and out into the eighteenth-century courtyard which remains the hub of the Bart's experience. The world pitched and yawed. I hung on to whatever presented itself to hang on to. There, among heaving shoals of consultant-owned Audis and Alfa Romeos, where a mighty fountain still plays to soothe the invalid breast, I sat on a bench with the sticks between my knees like a proper invalid and chatted to a wheelchair-bound inmate from my ward. He'd just had a tumour removed from his armpit and had come out for a fag. His voice was tiny. I couldn't hear a word he said over the noise of the fountain, so I nodded and smiled until his carer took him back inside and I was left to myself.

The night was orange. The fountain did not soothe me with the tinkle of healing water music. It crashed like corrugated iron lashed with chicken wire. It hurt like a bastard. It was then that I registered how different things were.

What to do? How to respond?

As I considered these questions I made myself small on the bench. Huddled inwards – and kept on going. Shrank and shrank. The shrinking became a falling, then a separation. For the first time in my life I felt all my internal linkages begin to stretch, then sag . . . then detach. Quite quickly I came apart right there on the bench in the car park, quietly but without any control over what was happening, sitting still, staring at nothing much at all like a baby. I imagined a clock ticking inside my head, but instead of a ticking sound I heard a dull *duh-duh-duh-duh* pulsating through the uproar of white noise. I began to consider myself in the third person, not as a ramped-up sportsman might but as any man might when he can't bear being inside himself any more.

Who is he? What is he doing here? Is this how it's going to go on? Why is everything orange?

The world tipping.

I rang my wife. I pressed the mobile to my good ear and heard her voice clearly, but was not clear in my mind about what she was saying. I felt sick again. I shuffled back to the ward and drew the curtains around my bed, expecting to cry.

Nothing came. But then it wouldn't. Weeping makes noise.

*

After five days they let me out, undiagnosed. A scan had revealed neither a tumour nor a bleed; straightforward labyrinthine infection of the inner ear had been discounted, as had Ménières disease. Endless audiograms showed only that I was as deaf as a post in my right ear. 'You're off the scale,' said the audiologist, smiling kindly and blowing out her cheeks. The audiograms had nothing to say about the racket inside my head.

My balance had not improved at all. In fact, it had got worse. I could neither stand nor sit up unsupported; the world was a vibrating blur; I teetered continuously on the brink of throwing up the food that the steroids encouraged me to scoff like a starving man. Words like 'stroke of the inner ear', 'nerve damage', 'vascular event' and 'auto-immune disease' had been bellowed over my head, while tuning forks had been applied to the back of it, behind my ear, as proof that the junior doctor was not as authoritative in these matters as the surgeon. If further proof were needed, the surgeon also had demonstratively the loudest voice.

'You'll just have to wait and see,' they said to me repeatedly. 'Sit tight.'

'But am I going to get it back? My hearing is my most important sense. Well, to me it is. I need both ears for work. Music is my greatest passion in life. I do it a bit too. I'd rather lose an eye, a foot . . .'

'We don't guarantee that hearing will return. We never do that. But don't worry. It may come back.' The surgeon then sidestepped his own sidestep. 'Anyway, lots of people live perfectly normal lives with only one ear. And hey, at least the scan shows there's nothing scary in there.'

*

No one has written better or more songs than Bob Dylan about what it is to step outside time – the necessity of doing so as a survival mechanism as well as the mechanical inevitability of it as a part of life: the need to, as it were, let yourself be seized by the moment and held close by it while time flows on by, doing its thing. It's an awkward theme for all kinds of reasons but it is one of Dylan's favourites. For Bob, time is a current out of which you may step pretty much whenever you feel like it. You might say that the invented figure of Bob Dylan is what allows the real man Robert Zimmerman to pull off the trick. You'd be guessing, of course.

Possibly my favourite *extra-tempore* song of his is one of the simpler ones: 'Watching the River Flow'. It's not a major song, not by any means. It's a cranky blues from 1971 when nothing much was working for him. It finds Bob stuck fast in the small hours in an all-night café with nothing much to say; then on a sandbank by the side of a river in the middle of nowhere, far from the city and people who know him. Far from people, out of time. Dylan's singing is as transporting as the water he watches from his spit of sand. It is a compelling, unsentimental blues, unlike any other white man's blues I can think of. The arrangement has a joke false ending in it, near the beginning. It's the song I listened to repeatedly in the hospital with one ear, while struggling to ignore an engulfing tide of concrete mixers in the other. In the face of the tide, the song got smaller and smaller and more and more distorted until it was drowned in the uproar. It did not comfort me. It only confirmed that for me music was never going to be the same again.

This is a hard idea for me to get my head round. How can music no longer be the same thing? Music is just music. It doesn't change. People change. But I haven't changed. My body has. I haven't. At least, I hope not. I can't have changed that much because I still love music. The problem is that I can't hear it any more.

Still, I can look at it, I suppose.

Almost half the living room in our house is taken up by my record and CD collection. I don't like to think of it as a collection – the word 'collection' implies system and scholarliness, bourgeois acquisitiveness and, of course, anality. I don't like to identify myself with any of those things. But that's what it is, I suppose: a collection. It is certainly the collected material of a life's commitment to music. It fills two walls, floor to ceiling. An edifice. When you enter the house, you can't get to the kitchen without walking past the door into the living room, and I've always enjoyed the corner-of-the-eye glimpse you get of it all as you go by. My dark star. It looms on its railway-sleeper shelves. The spines of the record sleeves glimmer faintly in the gloom; the CD jewel cases glint. The sheer weight of all that vinyl, cardboard and plastic bears down and down, gravity's big, fat bastard of a henchman forever plunging south. My poor wife Jane, who has twice had to move house with the thing, has always worried that one day we're going to disappear with all our children, books and furniture into the sewers. My record collection is monumental.

Monumental?

A monument to what?

On the day I got out of hospital I did not shoot a sideways glance at the record-stacks as I shuffled down the hall; wouldn't have been a good idea, as I would have fallen over. Sidelong glances are no longer advisable. And when I went into the living room for the first time I kept my eyes fixed on my destination, the sofa in front of the television. *Ker-flump.* Gently, gently. Cushions, please, up my back and round my head, to support it and lag it. There, that's better. *Ooof.* The world may now steady itself in the stately compass of my vision and I may watch the news for five minutes till the racket in my head gets unbearable, and I can go upstairs, drop some Temazepam and fuck off to la-la land.

One thing I shall not be doing is glancing at my record collection as I go. I won't be considering its absurd bulk, its tumescence, its weight, its scope, its depth, its pregnancy, its volume of contained emotion. I shan't think about it at all. I intend to ignore it, pretend it isn't there. After all, what is the use of it now? It might be both tumescent and pregnant; it may well have scope and reach; it may enshrine in its accumulation of grooves and digital bytes a realm of feeling unfelt by any single mortal creature, apart from me; it might well be the single most concentrated mass of beauty in the world. But what use is it if I don't have access to it any more? If all it amounts to is chicken wire and iron?

Well, of course, it does have one application. It stands as a monument to a life I once had.

I am uneasy with this thought, as one ought to be. A monument? A *what*? Monuments are meant to commemorate something – something worthwhile; something more valuable than one individual's selfhood. Nevertheless, isn't this what we're doing when we accumulate stuff that we can't let go of: creating monuments to ourselves?

Here's another thing: I can't help but reflect that the best monuments always look like containers.

Perhaps this is because containers make the best monuments. I'm thinking here about buildings like the pyramids and earthworks like Sutton Hoo – their primary function, as containers of human remains, invests them with a mystique which no pristine column of marble or steel or light can ever aspire to. We mark graves because it is absolutely necessary to, not because it's convenient or polite or decorative. It's because graves have contents.

But I'm also thinking about the monument which rises to a weird height above the battlefield at Waterloo. It's an artificial mound with a lion on top; a rather severe, unreadable topographical hump, like an exaggerated tumulus, heaped together from the sanguinary topsoil scraped off the foreslopes of Wellington's ridge. You're meant to climb to the top of it and look in wonder at the extraordinary expanse of the battlefield; to map the battle's narrative in your mind as you do so. But as you climb the steps, you can't help but register the hump's barrow-ishness, as well as its proportional similarity to a pyramid, and you can't shake off the thought that were you to pile 40,000 dismembered corpses one on top of another, then cover them with topsoil and crown the heap with a gunmetal lion, the end result would be pretty much like this. The Waterloo monument is not in reality a container of dead bodies but, by all that's uneasy, it feels like one when you're standing on it.

Similarly, my record collection does not contain the remains of anything material: it is just a mound of vinyl, cardboard and plastic. But it feels like it does, especially when you're looking at it for the first time after losing your hearing.

I over-dramatise, I suppose. Monuments are meant to be seen by everyone and reverenced accordingly. My record collection isn't meant to be seen by anyone, or reverenced. In fact I'd rather it wasn't seen at all – the thing embarrasses me slightly (one view you might take is that it is a monument to my adolescence and therefore an emblem of my unwillingness to grow up – but with that you'd only be scratching the surface, I'm afraid). All I want is for it to be used by me. Listened to. Lived with. I may have written the thing into my will, so that after my death my children can benefit from its catacombed inscriptions of the better urges of the human spirit, but that doesn't mean I want queues of mourners straggling round the block to finger my original West 63rd Street pressing of Jackie McLean's *New Soil*, in order that they might finger my soul. Not while I'm still sitting here. I'm not that narcissistic.

Nevertheless, I am forced to consider the possibility that my record collection now performs for me the function of the high-end container-monument. It is by no means a heroic container-monument. It does not, as the Simpsons would say, embiggen me. It isn't, objectively, a solemn thing. But it is a heavy thing.

Perhaps it's better to think of it as a container-monument in a more abstract way: its contents *are* substanceless ciphers of my selfhood. Yes, that's it. Somehow, my wounded, deafened, self-pitying psyche regards my record collection as a sort of reliquary of the old, lost me; maybe as a *narratable* version of me. Me through time. It tells my story over the thirty-four years' passage since I was thirteen, in 1973, which was when I bought the first record and plunged, half-knowingly, half-not, into a dialogue involving myself and the world; one I imagined would go on forever and which now, quite clearly, isn't going to.

What I don't fully understand is how it does that, and why.

I do not own this music, any more than I own the prose contained in the books on the bookshelves in the rest of the house. Not really. I can touch the music's casing, but I can't finger the music itself. The music is a thing which exists completely independently of me. It has no corporeality as such.

It is not mine. I cannot, in all reasonableness, claim it. Yet it is me. I am it. I cannot be divided from it. I identify so deeply with it, with its pulsations and its throbs, its gasps, wails, mutterings, idle chat and screaming abdabs, its measlinesses and its triumphs, its flights and burrowings, its colours and shapes, its matrix of references and its abstractions, its cadences, its circulatory swirls, its ducts, its veins and arteries and chambers, its towers, its ladders and lofts, its updrafts and downforce, its ever-ringing silent bloody bell, that I cannot separate it from my sense of who I am. It *is* who I am, only better-sounding and more reliable. It is the version of me that does not lie or change itself or fail or succumb to narcissism or under- or overreach or jump the lights or sit on the sofa for too long or worry about the wrong things or not worry enough about the right things. It's the version of me I always like.

It's the version of me I'd like other people to know.

I look at all that music I can't hear any more, latent and inaccessible, stacked within its cardboard and plastic sheaves, and I find myself asking:

What on earth was that all about?

2

The first record I bought with my own money came from the sort of place my parents shopped. It claimed to be the second oldest music store in England. It certainly looked the part. Miller's long glass frontage wrapped itself voluptuously round the corner into the next street, a facade sufficient in its handsome wooden frame to accommodate two sets of doors without looking pushy. But then that was the tenor of the street. As I remember it, Miller's shared a pavement with a jeweller and a posh travel agent, whose window was dressed not with felt-tipped special offers to Malaga but with a velvet curtain, a large model aeroplane and a palm in a pot. It did not occur to me at the time that buying a record in such an environment might reflect badly on me one day.

I'd thought about doing the deed at the market in the city centre, where there was a record stall. The thing would have been 16p cheaper there, for a start, which in 1973 was quite a sum: 16p represented the price of two return bus fares into town, four Mars bars, a quarter of a seven-inch single, a twelfth of another album. But market stalls were a challenge to a thirteen-year-old of my sort. The record racks were high and deep and I could not reach easily to the back of them, where the letter N was. Furthermore, the heavily muscled hippies who lurked in the gloom under the striped market awning were intimidating. As were the rituals of this kind of transaction. Supposing they smirked at my voice or my clothes or my hair? Or, worse, an uncontrolled widening of my eyes revealed that I was ripe for the taking? I felt my lack of sophistication weigh like a placard around my neck. Also – and this was the clincher – I was not confident that the records sold on the stall were entirely proper: the plastic sleeves encasing the LP covers were fogged up and dog-eared. And the covers were compressed tightly together in the racks as if in a vice. This meant that pulling one out resulted in crinkle damage to the spine, and that really wouldn't do. Besides, how could one know where the stock had come from in the first place? It did not look as if it had seen the inside of a distribution depot in months, if ever. And there are no stock-rooms on market stalls.

They also sold bootlegs.

So I went to Miller's, which, under the hygienic blaze of its ceiling lights, sold pianos as well as records. It smelled of furniture polish. It was a proper shop, respectable and respectful. Here, you could be confident that no one would rip you off or, worse, laugh at you. In token of that, the racks were stocked loosely with record covers clad in the better kind of plastic sleeve – the stiff, shiny sort which did not lose transparency on contact with air. Their pinch-welded structural integrity was immensely reassuring.

And at Miller's you had the option of listening to the music before taking possession. Attached to the wall next to the counter there was a row of head-and-shoulders listening booths into which you inserted your person like a pencil into a sharpener. Oddly, given that the object of these emulsioned, hardboard head-boxes was to convince customers that the gift of music is the gift of life itself, the music which drib-drabbed at barely audible volume from the single speaker behind the fascia was monophonic, opaque, leaden, dead, as if the sound had trickled slowly down miles of thickly lagged pipe to get there, accreting stuff as it went: music with added silt. Nevertheless, once you'd heard enough of a track to be confident that within the silt there hummed the harmony of the spheres, you were entitled to stick your head out of the box and ask the assistant behind the counter if he wouldn't mind jumping the needle on to the next track, and so on until your mind was made up.

For several weeks that summer the journey home from school was punctuated by visits to Miller's, where I would absorb the first thirty seconds of a new track on the LP onto which I had fastened my heart and possibly my soul as well. I could never bring myself to ask the assistant to jump the needle. I went one track at a time, one per visit, the intro followed by a verse, sometimes getting as far as a chorus, if the song had a chorus. 'Razamanaz', 'Alcatraz', 'Vigilante Man', 'Woke Up This Morning', 'Night Woman' . . . Afterwards, I would leave by the side door without a word, shoulders up around my ears, nodding affirmatively, conveying a clear message to whoever was behind the counter that it was only a matter of time before I got the £2.15 together that would make Miller's indulgence of me worthwhile. In those days rock 'n' roll was a clandestine business conducted in full view of the unaligned gaze of authority. Its chief by-product was embarrassment.

Still, I got there in the end. I eventually exchanged money for the object that was going to rewrite the co-ordinates of my existence and got home without really noticing the five-mile journey. By the time I was in the living room, the sweat had dried under my school shirt.

The family radiogram stood in the corner, not far from the television in its bookshelf recess. The radiogram was a dark brown lacquered wooden box on ferruled legs with bakelite knobs and a dial on the front which told you in both numbers and words whether you were tuned in to Hilversum or the Light Programme. My dad would sometimes address himself to the Third

Programme. At least he did theoretically. I have no memory of him doing so or of him listening to any of his modest collection of records, which consisted of Bach mostly, Wagner, Warlock, David Munrow, Julian Bream, things which were northern European and pretty old or, in the case of Warlock, modern-sounding but somehow concerned with old things.

My father was a musical man. He ran music groups for both local children and adults. He sang in the church choir. He composed for his domestic music world. He also owned a small collection of unusual instruments: a vintage Boehm clarinet, a reproduction Renaissance viol and a medieval krummhorn, a 'German guitar', a cittern, and a number of tatty recorders of varying lengths and diameters. He'd have been happy to half-master them all if only they'd been in working order. Instead, he sang to himself at the piano when the weekend weather stopped him from doing the garden. Sad English lute songs were his staple. I think he had music going on in his head a lot of the time, which was convenient for him. He certainly never allowed himself to listen to music in the car, because it would distract him and he would find himself stationary at green traffic lights with his mouth open. I have only one memory of him listening to a record on the radiogram.

'Ah, let's see now . . . What have you got there? Ah-hah. Mind if I join you?'

It was, I'm quite sure, in a spirit of simple curiosity that he sat down next to me as the black vinyl disc was removed from its sleeve by fingertip degrees, both of us facing the radiogram at a slight angle at not-quite-touching distance. I don't think he was expecting to be censorious. I'm pretty sure he wasn't alarmed at the prospect of his solemn but not entirely joyless son falling into bad company and taking drugs as a consequence of buying a rock record. He was curious. I think he wanted to get inside my head and see if there was anything in there he might recognise. Music can be helpful like that. So we sat there for the thirty-six minutes it took to play both sides of the LP, my dad in his habitual music-listening attitude, inclined slightly forward in his upright chair, mouth ajar, eyes unfocused; me frozen like a haddock.

'Razamanaz', 'Alcatraz', 'Vigilante Man', 'Woke Up This Morning' and 'Night Woman' came and went, a freight of over-loading amplifiers and squeals, passing through time like a train in the night: invisible but out there. My father sat on in silence. At the end, as the final chorus of the last song faded in the radiogram's thuddy underbelly speaker, he came out of his trance. He smiled kindly. I looked at my hands.

'Yes, well,' he said evenly, 'I quite liked "Vigilante Man". But I have to say it's not really my taste. Remind me again: what are they called, this group?'

'Nazareth. They're Scottish. It's called hard rock, as opposed to glam rock or heavy rock. Or soft rock. It's like blues but harder and much louder, with different chords – a hint of pop but not poppy, obviously. I think their guitarist is really good. You've got to admit he's good.'

'Well, as I say: not really my taste. Thanks for that.'

And he was gone.

*

'Not really my taste.'

I say it all the time. And not only because I am now the age my father was when we engaged in our earnest transaction with Nazareth. I've always said it. I say it when I hear Coldplay or Tchaikovsky or Sonny Rollins or Frank Zappa. I say it when I know something has virtue but don't like it much. In other words, when I don't want to offend or, worse, be wrong. No one will ever convince me that Coldplay have anything to say or that the things Frank Zappa had to say were worth hearing; but I know Tchaikovsky and Sonny Rollins are good – I can hear that they're good. Or at least I used to be able to. They just don't do anything for me.

So taste is partly about good manners. An armature and a way out of trouble. People are always wounded if you show disdain for the things that are important to them. But, actually, we all know that taste amounts to more than that, in the same way that reading amounts to more than the scanning of written information. My dad would have called it 'discernment', which has nothing to do with good manners at all.

'Taste does not come by chance: it is a long and laborious task to acquire it.'

That was Sir Joshua Reynolds, the eighteenth-century painter and academician.

'Hard is his lot, that here by fortune plac'd / Must watch the wild vicissitudes of taste; / With ev'ry meteor of caprice must play, / And chase the new-blown bubbles of the day.'

That was Dr Johnson, the eighteenth-century wit and compiler of one of the first dictionaries of the English Language. Yes, I've been poking around in a *Dictionary of Quotations*. There are more than thirty entries in the old Oxford under the word 'taste', most of them relating to the verb 'to taste'. But it's the noun I'm interested in; the seventeenth-century noun which became in the eighteenth-century a tool of social calibration.

The taste armature, in its most protective application, might insulate the Coldplay fan from my sniffiness and me in turn from his or her indignation. That is taste's nice aspect. But taste can go the other way too. By the time of the eighteenth-century Enlightenment, Taste, with a capital T, had become a way of life, a value so absolute that you might embody it with an ample woman dressed in a wisp of samite prancing around an emas-culate column with her sisters Caprice and Folly. Taste was got, as Sir Joshua suggests, by cultivation, the implication being that there was a moral dimension to aesthetic judgement. 'Understand this,' Reynolds seems to be saying. 'Taste is a remote and forbidding mountain to be climbed and not all of us are endowed with the means – taste not only makes us better men but better men have it!'

Taste as a social trophy. An accomplishment. Dear me. That would not have been my dad's view of it at all. Discernment, in his book, was no trophy to be won but a process to be enjoyed. You did not arrive at it, suddenly, as a token of personal enlightenment, as if breaking through clouds to some summit of achievement. It is a journey, an exploration. It takes hard work and sensibility, and it requires thought, naturally. But it signifies nothing. It is certainly no excuse for snobbery. Taste has no moral value. One should never, ever *believe* in Taste. It is *only* a process. I do not know whether he would agree that there is a linkage between the burningly self-conscious act of 'having taste' and that most febrile of all our mechanisms, self-esteem. But it seems likely. He would never admit as much, my old man, but he knew that the act of liking things is not unconnected to the act of liking yourself. Yet it is a more complicated connection than you might think.

It has only to be observed. When I finally got round to buying Captain Beefheart's *Shiny Beast (Bat Chain Puller)* rather tardily in the early 1980s, the spectre behind the counter at the Record & Tape Exchange rewarded me with a grimace as excruciated as any I'd seen in my short and sheltered life. For about half a second I could see the spectre's teeth and they were grinding. Yet the source of his distress was unclear. His eyes offered pain but no direction. Had I committed a solecism? Did the slackness demonstrated by my purchase of *Shiny Beast* more than two years after its release mean that mine was now a meaningless gesture? In other words, was I *too late*?

'Is everything okay?' I offered. 'You look a bit worried. Or is there something wrong with the LP?' He brought his eyes up to meet mine for even less time than it took to form his grimace.

'Well,' he mumbled, looking away, '*Shiny Beast* is all right, but it's hardly *Trout Mask Replica*, is it?'

There was nothing much I could say to that, except to register inward relief that I hadn't tried to buy *Unconditionally Guaranteed* from Beefheart's 'commercial period'. The spectre had felt a taste pang, but only a pang, and had survived the experience. I, of course, understood where he was coming from. We parted on good terms.

The principal agony of my adolescence, then, other than sex, was the agony of taste. Getting it. And having got some, making sense of it.

As with sex, this entailed a lot of longing and bafflement and stupidity and humiliation and, sometimes, orgasmic release. I did not presume to be 'cool'. Cool, in the modern, commodified sense, did not exist in 1973. It was an abstraction relating chiefly to the attributes of older, longer-haired or blacker people and their modes of personal conduct. It certainly was not a thing you might buy in the shops – and I didn't qualify on any level.

Equally, having taste did not embody some manifest personal destiny: it seemed unlikely to me even then that a thorough grasp of the merits of *Razamanaz* was an early indicator of future greatness of spirit. All I knew was that if you had taste then you were equipped – tooled up, as we might say today. Maybe not equipped to compete for things like prizes and social popularity, but certainly equipped to stand alone. The most important thing about having taste, it seemed to me, was that you were defensible. Impregnable even: you might not be taken; you could *hold out*. I longed for that almost as much as I longed to be talented and to get off with girls.

And as with sex I had no idea how you went about it. Rock

'n' roll taste was not a thing you learned about sitting on high-backed chairs in front of a radiogram in the silent company of your father, any more than sex was. Not in 1973. Not now, I hope. And if it had been, I like to think that I would not have been interested. But having taste made you real. It set you on a path. It told a story, a secret story. It didn't matter in 1973 what the ending might be.

Ending?
　Is this the end?
　Have I run out of road?
　What has finished?
　Nothing has finished. But the advent of the digital media age has had a pretty hefty impact on the way taste works. And, indeed, on whether taste might be said to exist at all any more. Yes, we all have our tastes; but does 'taste' mean the same thing as it did in 1973?
　So much has changed since then. So much slack has been taken up. MTV, deregulated radio, the DIY aesthetic, MP3, downloading, uploading, streaming, YouTube, MySpace, pop in newspaper pages every day and on television around the clock, and inside your phone – an evolution best encapsulated in two bearings from the commercial compass: the rise of 'shuffle' and the decline of 'retail', both of which stand as fluent emblems of the absolute centrality of individual choice in a free market – the solvent in which the authority of critical taste just dissolves.
　For a start, you no longer have to do any work – either long or laborious – to have your desires met. There is no need to worry any more about the hippies in the marketplace. Or even to get on a bus into town. No one knows any better than you do. Everything is available to you domestically, all of the time and more or less instantaneously. Thanks to the magic of digital streaming, you don't even have to own the music of your choice

to listen to it – it's just there for you, any time. No need to put your hand in your pocket, let alone go out into the world.

One immediate upshot of this is that there is much, much less incentive to question your desires. The most challenging aesthetic judgement you have to make is 'do I want it or not?' The question 'what does it mean?' is now either redundant or pretentious, depending on your standpoint.

The upside of that, of course, is there is no need to feel embarrassment over your preferences, so it is much easier to exercise them honestly. For a start, you no longer need expose such judgements as you do make to the scrutiny of shop assistants, friends, enemies, parents: just press 'download' at the privacy of your workstation and the thing is yours, and no one will be any the wiser that you have just spent 79p on a song without discernible rhythmic character about how everything will turn out all right if you just believe in the magic in the stars. Our tastes need never be exposed. The social gauntlet no longer exists. Everything is now permissible; access to everything absolute. Access to everything is the *point*. Popular culture is democracy perfected, or so it is thought.

The question is unavoidable though: how much of a culture is popular culture? Isn't culture something that is, by definition, shared? Isn't 'popular culture' now just another way of saying 'shopping'?

*

I had a little cultural moment not so long ago, shortly before I lost my hearing. It was quite enjoyable. I was standing in front of an American abstract expressionist colour field in the Modernist gallery at my favourite provincial museum, the Fitzwilliam in Cambridge. I'd gone there with a chum to see a special exhibition and we'd drifted in to the sepulchral greyness of the new wing, while waiting for the rain to stop. And there it was. Five feet by three of muted tallow canvas, slashed with jags of heavy colour, like a rich Tudor's doublet. I stared at it and nothing much stirred in the pockets of my soul. So I stared at it some more. Still nothing.

'I don't think I want to look at this picture,' I said without thinking, 'any more than I want to listen to jazz.'

'Eh?' said my chum, Emma, sounding startled. 'But you love jazz.'

'I do love jazz,' I said, suddenly feeling very sad. 'I always will love it. But I don't love it now, right now, in this instant – not in the same way that I've loved it for thirty years . . .'

'Why would you want to listen to jazz now anyway? We're in an art gallery. It wouldn't be very considerate.'

Emma is good this way.

'I think I'm losing my modernism.'

'What on earth do you mean? How can someone lose their modernism?'

'I mean that, given the way things are nowadays, I don't want to look at modernist painting and I don't want to listen to modern jazz, which is equally modernist and has equally little to say about the world of the early twenty-first century – which is anything but modernist, not in the classical sense of Modernism anyway. You can't apply jazz to anything worthwhile any more, unless you count your own cultivated sensibilities. Jazz is no longer in the world as a thing in and of itself – it doesn't have a proper job to do. Its primary role is to signify and that's all. To most people, jazz signifies period 'cool', and the clothes and attitudes that go with it. It is an atmospheric adjunct of sandwich-buying in Pret, a style soundtrack. Its only real use to the world in general – from which I exempt all serious jazz fans, who are all dying or driving black cabs – is as scaffolding to support crap acting in bad films. For heaven's sake, ordinary people in the street, who have never bothered to consider the ways in which Coltrane differs from Rollins, have the confidence to take the piss out of jazz, as if there's nothing Other or challenging or hip or worrying about jazz at all. As if they know better about jazz than people who actually listen to jazz. They didn't used to do that . . .'

Emma is very patient in the face of this kind of speechmaking.

'Give me an example of what you mean,' she said.

'Well, whenever Miles Davis comes up on shuffle on the iPod, I think, "Hooray, it's Miles Davis, I love Miles Davis" – and then I jump straight to the next track, in the hope that it'll be something that does have a role to play in the twenty-first century.'

'Such as?'

'Well, I have a thing for *The Basement Tapes* at the moment. I love it when that comes up – it'll shuffle happily with anything and everything. That record could have been made last week in a clapboard shack in the backwoods somewhere by a bunch of wild-eyed young men who haven't yet learned how to feed themselves properly . . .'

'But in fact *The Basement Tapes* was recorded in the Sixties.' Emma's eyes were not rolling up into her head, but they might just as well have been.

'Well, that's kind of my point really. How come modern jazz from the 1960s sounds "period" and culturally disengaged – the phrase "costume music" springs to mind – but a scratchy unofficial Bob Dylan recording from the same decade sounds as authentically contemporary as something done yesterday in a trailer park?'

'I dunno. You tell me. I don't like jazz anyway. Maybe it's just you. Had that possibility occurred?'

3

Music has changed now that I can't hear it properly any more. You'd think it would be me that would have to change, and maybe I will in due course. But as far as I'm aware I haven't changed a bit – music has. Since my collapse, it is now flat and unrevealing, distorted and partially concealed behind the uproar filling the right-hand hemisphere of my head, as if hiding. But the flatness is the big deal.

What do I hear when I listen to music now?

I don't know how you hear music. I imagine that if you like music at all then it has, in your head, some kind of third dimension to it, a dimension suggesting space as well as surface, depth of field as well as texture. Does this count as synaesthesia? Possibly, but I suspect not really. It's just the mystery of music.

Speaking for myself, I used to hear 'buildings' whenever I listened to music – three-dimensional forms of architectural substance and tension. I did not 'see' these buildings in the classic synaesthetic way so much as sense them. These forms had 'floors', 'walls', 'roofs', 'windows', 'architraves', 'cellars'. They expressed volume. They were constructed out of interlinked surfaces which depended on each other. Music to me has always been a handsome three-dimensional container, a vessel, as real in its way as a Scout hut or a cathedral or a ship, with an inside and an outside and subdivided internal spaces. I'm absolutely certain that this 'architecture' had everything to do with why music has always exerted such an emotional hold over me. I think music was the laboratory in which I learned to contain and then examine emotion.

I've always kept quiet about this architecture business, partly because it sounds pretentious and even slightly self-congratulatory (you hear Amy Winehouse, I hear Apsley House), but also because I'd never been entirely confident that 'architecture' was what I really meant. Maybe 'hearing music architecturally' is just me being inarticulate.

But I am confident now. 'Architecturally' was precisely right. What I hear now when I listen to music is a flat, two-dimensional representation: flat as in literally flat, like a sheet of paper with lines on it. Where I used to get buildings, I now only get architectural drawings. I can interpret what the drawings show, but I don't get the actual structure: I can't enter music and I can't perceive its inner spaces. I don't know about you, but I've never got much of an emotional hit from technical drawings. This is what really hurts: I no longer respond to music emotionally.

The celebrated neuroscientist and author Oliver Sacks recently published a book, *Musicophilia*, all about the relationship between the brain and music. In it he tells the story of a Dr Jorgensen who lost all hearing in one ear following an operation on a nerve and, like me, afterwards found music as flat and unengaging as a line drawing. Dr Jorgensen did not get the tinnitus, however. He did not benefit from the hissing and the clanking and the sticky clouds of noise gas, let alone the monkey, his pipe organ and the drowning choir. He enjoyed blissful silence in his duff ear. Yet music for him remained steadfastly flat.

Jorgensen wrote to Sacks to tell his story and to pass on the interesting information that, counter to all logic, after about six months' dogged music-listening he fancied that his single ear was beginning to offer him a 'pseudostereo effect', giving him 'ample compensation' for the loss of real stereo. He speculated on the possibility of his brain doing a bit of surreptitious rewiring: 'Hearing fibres might have crossed in the corpus callosum to receive input from my functioning left ear . . .'

Sacks is doubtful about the possible extent of such rewiring, but goes on in a chapter entitled 'Why We Have Two Ears' to ruminate on what might be expected of a brain in such circumstances, not least with regard to the brain's capacity to register 'space' in music as an active element in its emotional reach. He talks about the recruitment of different brain areas not normally used for the purpose. He refers the reader to a book, *This is Your Brain on Music*, by another author-neuroscientist and musician Dr Daniel J. Levitin, who runs a special laboratory in California in which he has conducted experiments on, among other things, spatiality in music.

It was while I was trying to understand this stuff that I began to do little experiments on myself. I dared not listen to my favourite music for fear of what I might hear (imagine: *Exile on Main St* as a technical drawing; Miles Davis as a papery squiggle . . . No, don't even think about it), but I kept up a steady drip of new and potentially interesting (quiet) music into my one good ear, just on the off-chance that something might happen. And on 11 November I slithered downstairs to watch the Remembrance Day broadcast from the Cenotaph.

I always watch it. I love the Cenotaph ritual. In particular, I get off on the Guards' stacked 'Nimrod', followed by 'When I Am Laid in Earth' (from Purcell's *Dido and Aeneas*) and the 'Beethoven' Funeral March: grey greatcoats, deep trombones, utter stillness. Gets me every single time. So every year I watch and wait for 'Nimrod's' unfailing impact on my metabolism, fascinated by the serpentine passage of emotion through my body from its bed in the pit of my stomach, slow as a Guardsman's dead march. It's an extraordinary sensation, made all the more so because of its complete and utter predictability.

So I switched on and sat there, bricking it. What if nothing happened? What if nothing happened and then I faked it? What if I faked it from the start, automatically, like some actor getting off on his own personal drama? But as it turned out I didn't have to fake a thing. David Dimbleby had only to intone 'And now, from Elgar's *Enigma Variations . . .*' and I was off. Before a single Guardsman had so much as licked his mouthpiece, I was in a flood of tears. Real tears.

Yes, of course I was in mourning for my lost hearing. But also, more than that, quite clearly my psyche was not going to run the risk of me being unable to feel a thing in the face of music of such unswerving dolour. But that wasn't the interesting thing. What was really interesting was that, as I sat there shuddering and trickling, I began to hear the music better. Melody, metre, a little bit of timbre, the puffiest cloud of harmony. Yes, yes: that's a trombone all right, not just a note. And I began to sense the tiniest swelling of architectural form in my head. You wouldn't have called it the Taj Mahal, but equally, this was no papery squiggle.

When it was over, I stuck the Purcell on the stereo. I thought: if I'm getting that much from the telly, what am I going to get from the wide frequencies and thick textures of a good recording coming out of big speakers?

I got only discomfort and bewilderment. The music was close to unreadable. It was certainly unbearable. I turned it off and let the uproar in my head subside.

Several things were now clear: if I am to hear it, and it is to make any sense at all to my brain, music has to be quiet, sonically compressed and preferably yoked to pictures. And it helps no end if I'm already in an emotionally lambent state. Talk about putting the cart in front of the horse.

Oliver Sacks was in London a week or two later, to talk about his book on the *Today* programme. He agreed to chisel out half an hour to have a cuppa.

I found him in the foyer of his hotel, looking a little hemmed in, tense even. We sat down with a pot of tea and he listened, kindly and attentively, taking notes longhand. At one point he did a small drawing. He referred me again to Daniel Levitin's book and seemed interested by the Cenotaph experience and by my uncooked theory of music as emotional Petri dish. He then told me that he'd recently lost the sight in one eye and that it had broken his heart.

It turns out that Sacks has maintained a lifelong fascination with, and experimental expertise in, the subject of stereoscopy. He has tinkered since the Thirties with the science and the showmanship of seeing with two eyes and has developed an almost metaphysical affection for the way stereoscopy makes the world loveable, as well as liveable in. He pointed a thumb out of the window of the breakfast bar and drew my attention to the thick, shifting foliage on the other side of the glass.

'Beforehand,' he said, 'I would take active pleasure in the movements of tricky jungle surfaces, and the way we perceive depth and distinctness, especially in the most complex visual environments. But now . . .' He hesitated, obviously not wanting to labour the point. 'Everything's rather flat.'

The Monophone and the Monoscope felt each other's pain and agreed to correspond.

A few days later I tottered off to watch a preview of the Led Zeppelin concert film *The Song Remains the Same*, which was coming out on DVD with remastered sound. It's a daft film, but I am fond of it; I certainly know it well. And this seemed like an ideal opportunity to test a couple of things: the significance of familiarity in any emotional response to music, and whether there was anything in the vague feeling carried over from the Cenotaph that seeing the music helped with the process of hearing it. (I know what you're thinking: Led Zeppelin? Emotion? What kind of weirdo are you? But the fact is, I have always got an awful lot of emotional pleasure from Led Zeppelin; a pleasure that is, I suspect, not unlike Sacks's emotional pleasure in the shifting of jungle foliage.)

Crash bang wallop. After three songs I had to leave the cinema clutching my head in a state of hopeless disorientation. The reactive tinnitus took me close to the threshold of actual physical pain – the illusion was that the auditory cortex for that side of my head, located due north of my right ear, had become swollen and hot and was trying to pressurise its way out of my skull. Great swathes of the music were simply unreadable. The pressure felt dangerous. Jimmy Page's guitar, in particular, was an incoherent storm of detuned noise, like a train entering an underground station at speed. Weirdly, the kick-drum appeared to be out of phase with the rest of the music.

I sent an email to Daniel Levitin, the author of *This is Your Brain on Music*, to see what he thought, being himself a bit of a rocker. I explained about the flatness, the lack of warmth and timbre and the way some areas of the tonal range in music are just unreadable, especially in the middle and at the bottom end.

This is what he said: 'That would be consistent with damage to the nerve cells in the inner ear. Remember, they're laid out "tonotopically" – like a piano keyboard – so all the low notes activate hair cells at one end of the basilar membrane; those could be the ones that are shot.

'As to depth of field, warmth, texture and timbre, that is a tough one. We don't know much about those higher order qualities. I know about them as a recording engineer and producer, of course, but not as a scientist. I suspect that something has gone awry in the inner ear and so the cortex isn't getting all the information it's accustomed to. In the case of pitch, the brain can fill in the missing information, but with those higher-order properties not.'

So there it is. I can make analytical 'sense' of music most of the time, because my brain can compensate for the loss of pitch, which is the very first quality which differentiates music from pneumatic drills and bickering children. What my brain can't seem to do is fill in the timbre, warmth, texture and depth stuff – what Dr Levitin calls the 'higher-order' qualities. Does this mean that it's the higher-order qualities which generate the emotional response to music? Or is it just me? Does it merely mean that in order for me to be able to register music's architectural dimension, and therefore have a special place in which to cue up and explore emotion, I need warmth, timbre, texture and the illusion of spatial depth? This might explain why even now, if I listen hard to music and grit my teeth through the discomfort, I feel perfectly capable of making reliable aesthetic judgements, even as I feel nothing much at all at an emotional level.

Levitin had something else to say.

'The tinnitus and other strange sounds are quite "normal" in the statistical sense of the word, meaning that once your ear shut off input to your brain (for reasons that evidently aren't clear) your brain "missed" having the input and so created some of its own. The brain isn't very smart at this, ironically, and so it creates a terrible cacophony. This is very similar to what patients experience after an amputation, a feeling that the limb or fingers or whatever are still there – this is the brain generating input to compensate for the lack of external stimulation.'

A week or two later I received a nice letter from Oliver Sacks, enclosing a copy of a piece he wrote for the *New Yorker* about a woman who had 'acquired stereoscopy after almost half a century of being stereo-blind'. It was, she said, 'a constant source of delight'. The neurological basis of her transformation was by no means clear, but the impact of it was abundantly so. Stereo Sue described to Sacks the effect of being 'inside' a snowfall for the first time, because she was able now to see it shifting and flowing around her in three dimensions, as opposed to 'looking in on it', as she had done all her life. 'I watched the snow fall for several minutes,' she said, 'and, as I watched, I was overcome with a deep sense of joy.' She might have been describing how I used to feel when I listened to John Coltrane or Marvin Gaye or the St Matthew Passion or, for that matter, Led Zeppelin. I used to inhabit all of them, as they inhabited me, in three-dimensional space. Saturated. Now I only look in.

Sacks was particularly engaged by the Cenotaph episode. 'What you say about the power of emotion to restore a sense of depth and spaciousness to music is extremely interesting,' he wrote. 'You must have (and will always have, whether or not there is any recovery of the ear) the memory of such spaciousness, and the power to evoke it in imagination – and "imagination" imagery is neurologically almost equivalent to perception. One might expect that such a power, whilst not available (or less available) voluntarily, could occur spontaneously by association with emotion, a memory. But you have to sort this out for yourself . . .'

He told me that he was currently reading a book entitled *A Singular View – The Art of Seeing with One Eye*.

4

What does memory hold? What does it hold that I can use? What lurks in that murky sump that isn't irretrievably decomposed, fungused over or dried up and useless? If I want to hear music again in anything like the way I used to hear it then, according to Oliver Sacks, I have to summon its richness, depth and saturating power through the use of memory.

So what have I got in the bank? Here's one, just for starters.

It is late December 1992, in that null chip of time separating Christmas from New Year. I am driving in an easterly direction out of the Fens, where I have spent the last family Christmas before my parents retire to the West Country. I feel kind of funny about that. (Do I really? Yes, I do.) I'm driving across the Breckland to Suffolk, where I'm going to visit a girl I've just met in London. I rather like her. Hey, she's East Anglian. She grew up in a churchyard. She likes music and books and clothes and parties.

On the way out of the house I'd picked up a cassette belonging to my dad – he'd been playing it on his new ghetto blaster (how I loved to hear him say the words 'ghetto blaster'; almost as much as I used to love to hear him say 'cassette', with the stress on the 'cass'; or 'stereo', to rhyme with 'cheerio').

What's this, Dad?

'*Dies Natalis*? Don't you know it? I'm surprised. Oh, I think it'd be rather to your taste.'

'Can I borrow it for the journey?'

Of course I can.

Dies Natalis is by the English composer Gerald Finzi, who died in middle age in 1956 following a bout of chickenpox. He had already been suffering for some years with Hodgkin's disease. The piece, written in the 1930s, is a sort of cantata for high voice (either soprano or tenor, but usually tenor) and strings, a setting of some of the seventeenth-century poet Thomas Traherne's mystical texts. *Dies natalis* is Latin for 'day of birth'.

I'm tooling through the last of the Breckland and the landscape is beginning to undulate. It is turning into deep Suffolk. Wilfred Brown's bright tenor is swooping above the English Chamber Orchestra like a swallow. The sky is grey, shading in the rear-view mirror to peach at the westerly rim. There are streamers of birds flying across it. Even though it is afternoon, the trees are already black against the light.

'These little limbs / These eyes and hands which here I find / This panting heart wherewith my life begins / Where have ye been? Behind / What curtain were ye from me hid so long / Where was, in what abyss, my new-made / Tongue?'

Thomas Traherne, a Christian metaphysician with pantheistic tendencies, might have been waiting for Gerald Finzi. Finzi, the agnostic son of a German Jew and an Italian Jew, lost his father when he was seven, then three brothers during his adolescence and his music teacher to the trenches. It was not a jaunty life. He liked poetry and obscure English apples, which he cultivated in his own orchard to save them from extinction. His great theme was the loss of childhood innocence to the corruption of adulthood. *Dies Natalis* makes the long look back at infancy into a votive agony and rapture. It is impossible to travel through a winter afternoon with it and not wish to be small again, or to make new things.

The Suffolk girl wears her chestnut hair in pigtails. The

churchyard is dank. Her mother crashes about her cobwebbed kitchen with square pots and pans made out of melted-down battleship girders. The girl's father, who is blind and truculent, roars at me about Benny Goodman. On the doorstep afterwards, as evening gathers, the girl and I shift laterally from foot to foot and do not kiss.

We are married inside the church across the churchyard three years later. At the service my dad reads Traherne on the subject of love, while waving his arms around like semaphore.

*

Here's another one.

It is Christmas 1977. The night before Christmas Eve, in fact. The Ramones have just completed their set at the Corn Exchange. We have checked our watches. Twenty-nine minutes. The group have fulfilled their promise to get it all over and done with in under half an hour, all seventeen songs.

I am slightly pissed – a pint, a whisky and six fags in the Eagle, plus a Newcy Brown among the fen punks gathered on the Corn Exchange's rotting parquet. I am slightly pissed and now I have been comprehensively rocked. The Ramones are without doubt the best band ever. Like a muscle, a single muscle flexing against a single bone. A reflex not a rock band.

I pitch out of the Corn Exchange. I am on fire. Next door but three is Guilders, a pleasant, slightly scruffy coffee and sandwich bar in which I have enjoyed many minutes on other occasions thinking wistfully about girls. There are lights on. For some reason it is open. I walk in. I survey the occupants. I stand in the middle of the floor among the tables, stretch my arms out in cruciform and nod repeatedly, mouth gaping in a silent scream. Nod nod nod. I nod so hard that the sweat on my face and in my hair flicks all around. I then overturn the two nearest chairs with the toe of my Docs, swivel and stomp out, still nodding. I have not uttered a word. On the way, one of the buckles on my leather jacket snags on the door handle and holds. I am jerked to a sudden stop. There is silence in Guilders. By the time I have disentangled myself from the door handle I have decided to apologise to everyone present for turning over the chairs. It seems like the only thing to do in the circumstances.

*

Or there's this one.

My first ever gig. It isn't Christmas. It's spring 1974. I am either just fourteen or not quite. I am queuing in the rain outside the Corn Exchange with Lorry, who is already an old hand at this. This is his third time. The queue of freaks is rank – the musk of damp Navy greatcoats and Afghans is overwhelming. I press myself into the stonework of Barclay's bank and consider myself to be fortunate indeed to be so wet and smelly and yet so free. We are going to see Man, the Welsh Grateful Dead.

I can hear the soundcheck taking place inside. It has been going on for half an hour. It sounds all right. Eventually, having parted with 90p each at the kiosk, Lorry and I sag through the door and into the cavern within. It is high and dark inside, like the interior of a mountain. Ragged sheets are suspended thirty feet above our heads beneath the roof, which is made of glass. Perhaps the sheets are there to catch the panes of glass when they fall, loosened from their century-old lead moorings by the uproar below. What a spectacle that would be: a death-rain of glazing – hippie salami. Or perhaps the sheets are there as a sonic brake, to deaden the sound and stop it bouncing in an unpleasing way off the glass roof. Yeah, probably. Or maybe both. Lorry buys Newcy Brown. I do not. I don't even have fags. After all, I have just spent 90p and there's the bus fare home to consider.

The DJ is playing 'Echoes' by Pink Floyd. Lorry is pleased. We flop against the giant heat pipes which snake around the filthy walls at waist height. I assume they're heat pipes. They're not actually hot, although we are cold and wet. We attempt the desultory, mumbled exchange of diffident views that is the essence of freak conversation.

'"Echoes" is twenty minutes long, man. Wonder what the DJ does while it's playing?'

'Probably has a wank.'

'Yeah.'

Man come on. The lights come on. But it is not a light show; they are just lights. They can be either blue or red or a mixture of the two. They permutate randomly throughout the set, without apparent system. Red. Blue. Red. Blue and red. Red and blue. Blue, red and blue . . . I suppose I should know why they don't make purple when they're on together, but I don't.

Man are absolutely deafening. I cannot distinguish one note from another, nor hear any tunes; and though the drummer is obviously really good, it's kind of hard to tell what relationship his playing bears to the diffuse, unhinged din made by the two guitars, bass and keyboards. I like the quacking wah-wah bits though.

After half an hour Lorry departs. He just disappears. As I consider what to do next, I dimly recollect him muttering something solemn in the queue outside about another commitment that evening involving an older woman. I suddenly feel exposed, perched on the cold heat pipe on my own. I have three choices: leave, stay put or get down with the hippies on the rotting parquet. This means getting down literally. At Cambridge Corn Exchange in 1974 it is evidently the done thing to lie down on the floor, either completely supine or supine but propped up on your elbows with your ankles crossed. Presumably the point is to feign cool interest, while staying plausibly relaxed in the tumult.

I decide to join in. I get down off the pipe and join the fringes of the heap. I lower myself down on to my backside and sit there for a while nonchalantly, legs crossed, forearms draped over knees, and then slide into the approved position, propped up on my elbows. Man thunder on. In due course I let go altogether and go fully supine. I find myself staring straight up at the roof. I can just see between the stained and ragged yards of sheeting a few square feet of glass. I am sure I can see it moving.

*

I don't imagine these are the kinds of memories Oliver Sacks had in mind for me, for all their visual and auditory richness. These are the memories music stores up anecdotally, not neurally. They are to do with music's narrative power, not its power to saturate the nervous system. Whenever I hear *Dies Natalis* I see Jane in her pigtails, and always will do: I don't feel the music because of the memory; I feel the music and then the memory comes. Likewise, the Ramones are forever snared with my jacket buckle on the doorhandle of the coffee bar. The very thought of Man – to whom I have listened perhaps three times since 1974 – brings the scent of wet hippie to my nostrils along with the fear of death in a glass rain. These are psychological not neurological recollections.

Even those memories in which actual physical shock plays a part – you know: ouch, now *that's* going to leave a scar! – are not quite the thing. For that reason I will spare you an account of the birth, to music, of my first child (to the elemental strains of John Coltrane, naturally) and of the occasion a hippie fell out of a tree on to my head at the Knebworth Festival in 1976, although it is hard to decide now which was more shocking at Knebworth: the hippie on my head or the Stones, who were simply dreadful.

5

In 1971, the year in which I turned eleven, the fens of East Anglia were an empty place. They still are relatively empty, but only relatively. They were really empty then. Then, you could lie in bed and hear for miles. The emptiness could be felt almost as sound can be heard. It had a presence, a slightly obtrusive one. There was a level crossing half a mile down the road from our house and whenever a small fen train went over it, it was possible to hear the moan of every nut, bolt and bearing in its trundling bogeys. There have never been whippoorwills in East Anglia but you did get trains – little ones going to Peterborough – and they made the silence come alive. Otherwise, the quiet was sprung only by the tooting of wood pigeons against the rustle of chestnut trees, and by church bells, cockerels and the whine, skitter and thwack of teenagers crashing their Hondas into ditches.

I think and talk mauvely like this about my fen childhood as if its very fenniness confers a kind of special identity on me. But even that half-baked fantasy is compromised. My fen life was a shallow one. I was born in a home county for a start, to Londoner parents. I was four years old before the family moved to the Cambridgeshire village where I grew up. I do have an ancestor who tenant-farmed Grunty Fen outside Ely in the nineteenth-century, but that's it as far as depth goes.

Just as compromisingly, the village where we lived constituted the southernmost tip of the Cambridgeshire fens. The absolute extremity. Cape Horn. Look in a northerly direction from our house, past the old people's home, the psychiatric hospital and the hospital's dormitory estate, and yes, the fields would open out then fade into the distance like so much brown-grey coastal seawater in a flat calm, broken by skimpy stands of trees under a simply huge sky. But stand at the back of our house and turn your gaze south and you looked *up hill*. It wasn't much of a gradient, but it was enough to allow small naked boys to lose control of their tricycles on the slope and plunge headfirst into the rose bush which grew up the back of the house like a claw. These were the junior slopes of the Gogmagog Hills, the chalk escarpment which hems Cambridge to the south; the same chalk escarpment which ensured that only marrow would prosper in my dad's shallow-draft vegetable garden (plunge a fork into the ash-grey soil and you hit solid white about five inches down) and which completely screwed up radio signals from the BBC.

This was perhaps the reason why my dad listened to the Third Programme only theoretically. J.S. Bach never sounds as good when he reaches you in a thunderhead of hiss jagged with forked lightning. Believe me, I know. My mum got a half-decent Radio Four signal in the kitchen on her modern tranny, but only half-decent. Meanwhile, upstairs I was going nowhere on the strange chipboard and sticky-backed plastic contraption my gran had presented to me with some ceremony, when she replaced it with the most up-to-the-minute radio the family had ever seen. It was red, my radio, the plastic was peeling off the chipboard, and the dial on the front enjoyed only nominal acquaintance with the transistor inside. Nevertheless, it did reach shakily out into the void and in favourable climatic conditions it would fasten on to certain signals and then hang on, like a man clinging to a ceiling cornice with his fingernails. Usually, it would let go after a few minutes and flump into miserable silence.

The only station it would get reliably was Radio Two. Radio One, on medium wave, was a jungle of static and weird flanging sounds. Radio Luxembourg was an exotic fruit which would swing out of reach as the breeze shifted. Then there was Radio One's antecedent, Radio Caroline . . . Actually, the signal from Radio Caroline wasn't bad. But by the Seventies Caroline was not the energetic, whooping thing it had been in 1964. It was now run by a bunch of offshore hippies with a secular religion to evangelise (they were, I believe, in favour of Loving Awareness and against Defensive Awareness). They had a small record collection sliding back and forth on the shelf in their heaving studio cabin – Santana, Keith Christmas, Barclay James Harvest mostly – and an apparently unshakeable aversion to getting up in the morning, or even in the evening.

So I listened to Radio Two as I pretended to do my homework; as I did when I got up in the morning and when I went to bed. Occasionally, I would hear a good record and that made it worthwhile. Before I had taste, I had Radio Two.

This is important. Well, it's important to me. It was great not having taste, not knowing about it, just allowing stuff to reach me haphazardly, as if by accident. Also, in a perverse, deferred-gratificatory way, it was compelling to know that I'd have to slog through hours of drivel to hear one song that would make my girlish curls straighten. The ratio of jovial pap to hair-straightener was, at a belligerent estimate, about twenty to one. But it was worth the effort. T. Rex, David Bowie, the Animals, The Kinks, the Hollies, the Beatles, the Stones, Elvis – every now and then Radio Two would play them, presumably on the basis that if the record wasn't already a golden oldie, then any minute now it was going to be. And, thrillingly, at the age of eleven, I began to re-open the channels I'd shut down at the age of four, when I first beheld the Rolling Stones on the *Arthur Haynes Show* on television.

My first cataclysm.

I'd watched the awfulness unfold from the relative safety of my grandma's lap while a thunderstorm lashed the living-room windows. Dead-eyed youths with doorstep mouths, not shaking but slouching. The spectacle had shaken me to my rubber soles. It had filled me with the knowledge that there were some things going on out there that were not encompassed by the justice of the Lone Ranger. Zombie insolence does not begin to tell the story. The Stones in the Storm has hardened to become my official earliest memory. I am still paralysed by thunder.

What I am trying to describe here is the Edenic state which existed before the desire to have taste began to make life difficult. It was a time of real innocence; of a world only nominally mediated, in which one's response to external stimuli went unfiltered by sophistication, knowledge, understanding, informed guesses, experience or smarts of any kind whatsoever.

The wait for 'Space Oddity' or 'Satisfaction' or 'House of the Rising Sun' was an indivisible part of the pleasure of hearing them. The sex analogy is unavoidable again – the longer the wait, the greater the buzz at the moment of consummation. Apart from anything else, the contrast was thrilling. Hour would follow upon hour of disc-jockey burble and Engelbert Humperdinck. Sometimes whole listening days would go by without a sniff of a loud guitar or a displaced beat and then, like a god out of the machine, Marc Bolan would descend on pillows of distortion to rock me in my bedroom casing like a baby in his arms.

And so the process of weeding-out became the point of the exercise, while the rewards generated were proportionate to the exerted effort of will, patience and near-erotic self-sacrifice. The germ of taste was sown deep.

*

I do not pretend that there was anything unique about this. On the contrary, my experience was merely a variant on what was then an absolutely standard one, up and down the provinces of a country that was still in the throes of post-war acclimatisation.

What was it acclimatising itself to? How much time do you want to spend on the subject? Other books have been written about the spasm of economic and social modulation which bridged the gap between the end of Austerity and the accession of Austerity's daughter, Margaret Thatcher. Dozens of them. This isn't one of those; not really. But be assured that, in the early 1970s, even for non-aspirational middle-middle-class juveniles of my type, the promise of excitement to come was thickly but foggily manifest. It had something to do with America, but not everything.

If you were born in 1960, as I was, then the relationship with America as it existed in 1971 was not special; certainly not as governing to a kid of my generation as it had been to the previous one – say Keith Richards' – or as it would be to my children's. We were on friendly terms with America, but we didn't go to bed together.

For an eleven-year-old, the dualities of life in England furnished by a solidly liberal Anglican upbringing were comfortably stable. There was no politics as such. But there was right and wrong, good and bad, happy and unhappy, holy and unholy, war and peace, starving and fed, white and black, clever and stupid, dull and exciting . . . At the age of eleven I knew that South Africa was the bad place the orange juice you didn't drink came from and that Biafra was a terrible place, whatever its principal export. I knew that massive violence was consuming distant Vietnam and that Northern Ireland was too close for comfort. I knew that if Ramsey hadn't substituted Bobby Charlton against West Germany in the quarters, then England might have won a second, consecutive World Cup. I knew that Boycott and Edrich made a stodgy but effective pair at the top of England's batting order and that Blücher rescued Wellington at Waterloo. I knew that Bach was better than Handel, but not as warming. I knew when Whitsun was, which is more than I know now, and I knew more or less how to fix a puncture on a bike (which is also more than I know now). I knew that every year the ditches of the Fens would claim another boy as a matter of course. But that was nature. The horizon was wide and my view of it uncluttered.

Full media penetration did not exist in 1971. I can't imagine what it must be like to be eleven now and to be penetrated all the time, fingered by info-tech digits, nudged by the fist of commerce; to know that a bead has been drawn on you; that the horizon is expressed in binary code; that *you* might as well be expressed in binary code. In this sense, at least, my childhood was closer to my father's than it is to my son's. My dad didn't have the Rolling Stones to be both scared of and turned on by; on the other hand, he had Hitler. My dad didn't have to animate the void beyond the chestnut trees by picturing himself on the train to Peterborough; but then again, he did have the Woolwich ferry. By the age of eleven, the age at which I was beginning to think that Radio Two might have something to say about how the void might be filled, my dad had been evacuated out of London and was living an estranged life in a peculiar woman's house in Tunbridge Wells under the flight path of Heinkels. His heightened sense of discernment was, I suspect, founded in the need to recover home. Mine was to get away.

6

I can remember the first seven records I bought, and then detailed memories of that kind of thing stop. I think the reason for this is that the first seven were acquired without the exercise of taste. After that first seven, some time in the middle of 1974, I suppose I began to rationalise the expenditure of what little cash I had in a far more self-conscious way. Suddenly it became important to consider what buying a record might mean and, even more crucially, how it might look. But not to begin with. The serendipitous spirit of Radio Two invested me still.

The First Seven remain accessible to me on a multitude of levels, and in minute contextual detail. I can call up the desire and the sensation of meeting those desires more readily than I can call up memories of first sex. I have access to just about every note. I know who played what instrument on them, and which record company put them out. I can remember the weight of their sleeves in my hand and on my lap, the texture of the cardboard, the dazzle of the artwork, the sound the inner sleeves made as they slid out of the gatefold, the name of the printing firm which printed the sleeves. I can recall how the music made my bedroom change. Here they are, in order:

1. Nazareth: *Razamanaz* (on the Mooncrest label)
2. Lou Reed: *Transformer* (RCA)
3. Genesis: *Nursery Cryme* (Charisma)

4. Yes: *The Yes Album* (Atlantic)
5. Derek and the Dominoes: *Layla (And Other Assorted Love Songs)* (Polydor)
6. Gong: *Camembert Electrique* (Virgin)
7. Rolling Stones: *Goat's Head Soup* (Rolling Stones)

If you know your stuff, you'll see that I was no Mod, and therefore in no sense cool in pop-historical terms. The Mod is English pop culture's most idiomatic stylistic gift to the world. But Mods did not exist in East Anglia in the early 1970s. Soul boys and freaks did (or, in the local demotic, Smoothies and Wallies). Skinheads might be found in certain dark regions, and Rockers were everywhere in their devolved Biker estate, forerunners of the Fen Grebo I would later learn to worry about slightly. But Mods? Nah. East Anglians did not go to such lengths.

English pop history has sentimentalised the Mod. You might even say it has idealised him. Certainly no tribal figure in pop anthropology has been endowed with quite so much retrospective sophistication and glamour. I know men now in their fifties and sixties who shiver with pride at the thought that they once wore the Crombie and button-down livery of Modhood – not as a costumed revivalist at the start of the Eighties, but as the kind of authentic sharpie who troubled old ladies and transport caffs in the Sixties with a sheaf of soul 45s in his pannier and a robust attitude towards the hippie armpit. Your Mod was a working-class hero of the first order (especially if the individual wearing the Mod gear had enjoyed a middle-class upbringing). He was a trailblazer. A modernist, clean as a piston. He was all selfhood – unlike the ego-denouncing hippie or the id-ridden rocker – and his values were marked visibly upon his person, in his tailoring, his coiffure, and in the seething attributes of his musical taste. Mods deployed taste as an offensive weapon in the class war.

Not in the mean ditches of the Fens though. We didn't do Mod. No one did in the early Seventies, unless you count the devolved Modishness of the Smoothies, and I don't. My great friend Lorry, a self-styled working-class anti-hero, would bunk off whole days from school by merging with the cow parsley in the ditch at the edge of his estate. You couldn't do that in a tonic suit. My other great friend Andy . . . Well, his elder sister Linda – one of four sisters – she went out with the lead singer of the local prog group Hamilton Gray (Hamilton Gray was the group's name, Howie was the singer's). She was terrifyingly good-looking. I'd see her at the bus stop outside our house in her afghan coat, kohl-eyed, absently pouting at the sky, a beautiful hippie Bardot standing on one leg, the other foot braced against our fence, smoking menthols, radiating. What use are a tonic suit and panniers in the face of that? She'd laugh her famous throaty laugh, garnish the clouds with her lambent gaze and you'd be done with. Better to merge with the cow parsley. So we did, Andy, Lorry and I, and we took the soundtrack to that activity from such fragments as we could snatch of life beyond the rim of the ditch. These fragments were, on the face of it, arbitrary. But actually they weren't – not quite.

History tells us that in 1973 Nazareth were an entertaining Scottish hard-rock band with a working-man's-glam edge, and that *Razamanaz* was their finest thirty-six minutes. Its second side bore two hit singles, the sanctified pop shuffle-cum-stomp 'Broken Down Angel' and the wild, ball-bursting rave, 'Bad Bad Boy'. History also tells us that groups like Nazareth belonged to their time and to their provincial place. Theirs was not music for the ages but for the moment. The group might – in those passages of solemnity which all men go through from time to time – aspire to seriousness (what do you think my dad detected in their vivid processing of Woody Guthrie's 'Vigilante Man' if not a heartfelt clutching at seriousness?). But really Nazareth were Edvard Munch's *The Scream* with the artiness taken out. Lust and angst barely mediated – shrieking, edgy, oppressive. Almost gory. In 1973 they burst through the surface of the day as would, six years later, the baby alien from John Hurt's chest. They were literally sensational.

I liked Lou Reed's *Transformer* because I was turned on by the deadpan ambiguities of 'Walk on the Wild Side' and 'Satellite of Love', its two singles, also overheard on my red radio. I understood nothing of the Velvet Underground and Andy Warhol in 1973; I knew even less about ambiguity. I could hear it, though. I was very pleased, too, by the way I could see ambiguity on the back of the sleeve, where the hero/ine of 'Walk on the Wild Side' ('And he was a sheesh') cocked a nyloned shank and pouted at a stevedore with a belaying pin down his trousers, who pouted right back. The guitars in 'Vicious' were sufficient on their own sometimes to stir my own belaying pin. David Bowie produced *Transformer*. History suggests that it was his attempt to make urban decadence work as a suburban style. History is probably right.

Nursery Cryme was a fallback position. Deploying my new stevedore's swagger, I'd bravely gone to buy Genesis's latest album, *Foxtrot*, at the stall on the market in town only to find that they'd sold out. Miller's were out of it, too. Not one of the three other, lesser, record shops had it either. Consternation. Andy had been quoting passages of *Foxtrot*'s side-long epic 'Supper's Ready' at me for days and I had a hunch that its surreal yet baroque outlandishness would fit me like a glove. Given that Andy's sister Linda was also known to be a Genesis fan – Hamilton Gray owed quite a lot to the fine-boned Charterhouse boys – it might have given Linda and me something to talk about at the bus stop, should such a frightening yet wholly desired event ever transpire. In the circumstances, therefore, it just had to be

Genesis. And so, in the absence of *Foxtrot*, the group's previous record would have to do. It was cheap too: £1.69.

I still have the thing and still love it, even though I can now only hear it properly in my head, and even then not very clearly. I hope that my own children will love it in due course, too. History says that Peter Gabriel-era Genesis were a slightly unnecessary *folie amusante* arising from rock's need in the late Sixties to expand its formal horizons in a way that matched its artistic ambitions and enlarged social scope. History also sneers at Genesis for being posh; for not being even slightly Mod. Well, history can do what it likes. The middle-class boy writing these words was wholly transfixed at the age of thirteen by the defiant remnants of the shut-down old man who voices 'The Musical Box' and, now that he is partially shut down himself, the boy sees no reason to pretend that pastoral English prog rock didn't have its moments of outlandish emotional clarity.

There are none of those on *The Yes Album*. But there were at the time – there just had to be. The group posed on the front cover in aqueous green light with an empty chair and the head of a showroom dummy. I had seen this enigma pass before my eyes in a school corridor under the arm of a sixth-former and decided that, given the recent success of *Nursery Cryme* in my bedroom, an artefact as explicitly strange as *The Yes Album* might actually expand my horizons still further. You know: make my bedroom go aqueous green, perhaps, and in the extra-mural context even inspire Linda Peacock to think that I was a person worth talking to. My God, the cover was thick, too, as thick and heavy as the language it contained. Whereas Nazareth were provincial and belonged to their time, Yes were cosmic and belonged to infinite space. This would not be the last occasion on which I bought a record by a group I'd never heard.

History says that *Layla (And Other Assorted Love Songs)* may be the best thing Eric Clapton ever did. It says that this tingly summit meeting between the English guitar god and his putative American legatee Duane Allman stands as one of several high-water marks in the pick-up-your-guitar-and-jam school of turn-of-the-Sixties rock, in which golden prodigies with luxuriant moustaches sparked off one another's technical chops, and artistry flowed in a river. It's not an area of music I'm very fond of. Jamming is good in jazz, because jazz *is* jamming. But rock is essentially a music of form and structure. Just look at the tools of its trade, which serve to create mighty building blocks of sound; blocks of real, almost tangible heft and density (and if you're not convinced by me, just ask Little Richard: he'll be happy to straighten you out). Rock actually enjoys being hammered into shape by the strictures of song form. You can hear that this is true on records like *Layla*.

Layla does have songs on it; quite a lot of pleasant ones, too, in the broken-hearted, sozzled-hippie romantic mode. It is by no means all jamming. But the spirit of the jam infects the album to such a degree that the songs are required to act like gooseberries on a date, as if their primary creative duty were to chaperone the guys with moustaches to make sure they don't get too jiggy with each other's chops. In the end, the atmosphere of gallant restraint which pervades the thing is actually rather charming and one can easily afford to have sentimental feelings about it, historically speaking, feelings that I dare say might be felt universally. And viewed in that light, I am quietly amazed that I have only ever met one child of the early Seventies endowed with the name Layla – and very happy she is too with it. But, come on, there must be thousands of you out there. Or did you all change your name by deed poll to Sophie?

Not that I cared at the time. All I cared about was that *Layla* was a double album and I really wanted a double album. Size matters to fourteen-year-olds. In fact, I really wanted anything I could get my hands on. *Camembert Electrique* was 49p, so I got that too. Didn't listen to it much, though. And history hasn't had that much to say about it either, except that it was 49p. That's the price you pay for being cheap.

Meanwhile, at the other end of the cheap-expensive scale, *Goat's Head Soup* lurked in its fat gas-yellow gatefold. *Goat's Head Soup* is another enigma, only instead of it being wrapped inside a mystery, it came cloaked in a fog of ennui and musicianly torpor. History has it pegged as the first record by the mature Rolling Stones not to measure up – not since 1967 and *Their Satanic Majesties Request* had they contrived such an unfocused, listless piece of work. It didn't measure up because, history says, the group had begun to sink in the quagmire of their own celebrity, to succumb rather than to thrill to decadence. It is exactly how a record made on a Caribbean island by a bunch of knackered tax exiles with unlimited access to drugs ought to sound. Stoned. A bit depressed. Uncertain. I bought it partly because of 'Angie', which Jagger mimed on *Top of the Pops* in a ridiculous hat, as if to his mother. And partly simply because it was new and it existed. What it revealed to me was that The Time Had Come.

The Time?

How can I express this in clichés of three syllables or less . . . ? The way I saw it, it was time to lay the ghosts of my tortured, directionless pre-teen past and to face up squarely to my future as a heavy-duty music head. To, in other words, start wearing long flared trousers. Following the *Camembert Electrique* debacle, I decided that I was not going to participate any more in the inane passing rituals of consumerism. I was going to take music seriously; I was going to be *into it*. *Goat's Head Soup* was the decider for the very reason that it was a qualifiable disappointment: because it lacked the energy of 'Satisfaction', 'Brown Sugar' and 'Honky Tonk Women' and spoke in woolly, cheerless language of things beyond the scope of my experience; because it was now clear to me that the art of making rock 'n' roll records was a contingent art and therefore an infinitely explorable one – just like life, but more fun. That's how I rationalise it now. At the time I just thought I was being interesting, maybe even sexy. I still love *Goat's Head Soup*.

So there it is. I offer these reflections on the First Seven not because I imagine that you need to know what they sounded like, or want to hear what I think they had to say, or because you yearn for insight into the sociology of fen adolescents in the early 1970s. I offer them simply because there is a tide in the affairs of schoolboys which cuts across the currents of history. History might give us the matured view, but schoolchildren occupy the moment. They give it its charge. It is important not to forget that.

I also want to make the point that even before you have taste, taste has you. It is drawing you in, snaring you in its coils, drenching you in its digestive juices. There you are in your recently acquired long flared trousers, innocently rejoicing in your sense of absolute freedom from history's tidal tug – for such is the glory of the post-war consumer society – and all the while and without knowing it you're being spooned on to a plate. In 1973 I would have no more cared about what *Razamanaz* and *Nursery Cryme* might come to mean than I would give thought to the future economic well-being of Durham miners. Yet within a year I was fully engaged in the solemn process of judgement. This was a social process, as well as a private one, and never less than self-serving in the sense that, ultimately, selfhood was the thing at stake.

*

It began at the bus stop, as important things often do.

Without really knowing what we were doing, or why, Lorry,

Andy and I hauled our burning adolescent bodies on to the bus to our respective schools in town and into position to engage in the great taste-making struggle over life and death. But mostly, it has to be said, over life.

The debate concerned what was better and what was worse, and why. We were not particularly bothered by what being better or worse (and why) might mean, not to start with. And not being Mods and not having any money to speak of, the debate was conducted slowly and in disorderly fashion over time, without a clear agenda, without intellectual discipline and without a great array of evidence to call upon other than those paltry things we could afford to buy. But there was a lot of passion involved. We simply went to the market stall when we had the money, purchased what we fancied on a basis broadly exemplified by the story of the First Seven, and then sat in Lorry's bedroom and listened to them. And argued.

Andy and I would smoke the occasional Number Six and sip small draughts of Dry Blackthorn, although it was quietly acknowledged that drinking was really Lorry's preserve, he being the largest and most experienced in the world and all. Lorry would also decide what order the records were to be played in, because it was his bedroom and his stereo. His album first, then, and in full; although words would be had – sharp words – if he came home with a double. He would also set the terms for the debate by announcing that his latest acquisition was superior in every way to whatever pathetic items Andy and I might have brought along. As social scenarios go, it was a distant precursor of the modern book group, but with less gracious manners and a lot more sulking.

We were unstoppable. We certainly would not stop for each other. The debate would revert back on to the bus, to and from school and in due course to and from gigs at the Corn Exchange in town. We never agreed about anything. And although we fought, we only fought verbally, often to a standstill. Lorry would always get crossest and I would always get sneeriest. Andy was simply too sunny to get sucked into that kind of posturing and would laugh at both of us.

Yet sometimes a strange form of collective enlightenment would descend upon us, like a dove, and we would agree that there really was no correct answer to be had by anyone, not as things stood in the moment, and that we would leave it to history to decide.

Indeed, it was after dark one autumn evening on the top deck of the 114 going through Teversham that Lorry drew his zippy boots up on to the seat-back in front and sighed deeply. It must have been at that moment that the dove landed on the roof of the bus, because Lorry then made an announcement.

'Most freaks would have "Stairway to Heaven" as the National Anthem,' he said portentously, staring out into the weather. 'Not me though. I mean, "Stairway" is great, but it lacks something. Or maybe it's got too much of something. I dunno . . .' He fell silent for a moment, scratched the mossy stump of his chin and then did something he had never done before. He asked what Andy and I thought.

'What do *we* think?'

Predictably, consensus was as hard to find as ever, despite the proximity of the dove. The debate raged all down the Teversham Road and, by the time we'd reached Lorry's stop, we still hadn't managed to agree on a nine-minute, multi-section prog suite that would properly dignify state rituals. Faced with such an impasse, and with Lorry halfway down the stairs to the platform, it was accepted that it was most freaks who were in error, rather than the three of us.

Being right – or at least staking out a position and then defending it bloodthirstily – became for a while the point of listening to music. And at some juncture in early 1974, as our tripartite relationship matured into a round-the-clock bickering contest, I found myself ramping up my modest interest in Yes on the basis that doing so was good for a bicker. This bickering took flame to become what Lorry would fondly recall in later years as 'The Prog Wars'.

Yes, Genesis and Pink Floyd were the Big Three of English progressive rock during prog's commercial high summer between 1973 and 1975. There were others, of course, and the term 'progressive' could and would be applied with a taxonomical diversity which touched the borders of jazz, folk, classical and, in particular, early music (anyone for Gryphon?). But the three big bands ruled the high middle ground. They defined the idiom.

The least conventionally proggy of the three, the sonorous, spacey, socially dolorous Pink Floyd had *Dark Side of the Moon* in the charts at the time, as they would do for years to come, casting a fenny gloom everywhere. All of a sudden that year the Floyd had become big-hitters, even if their home run had only arrived after several years of swinging and missing and falling over. Moreover, they were a local band, an authentic Cambridge band – they were ours in a way that no other band could be. The group's fallen *primum mobile*, Syd Barrett, lived a couple of miles up the road with his mum on the outskirts of town, and Syd-spotting was a local sport among junior elements of the freak community, who would excitedly report Syd sightings to each other with wide eyes and much empathetic shaking of heads: Syd on his bike wearing a Yogi Bear suit or Syd coming out of the off-licence on Cherry Hinton Road dressed only in his pants. We all staked a claim to the Floyd at the narrative level. But really the Floyd were Lorry's.

Genesis were also by now entering the top ten with every LP release, and had even troubled the lower reaches of the pop charts with a catchy, English-surrealist single. They were already Andy's.

Yes were . . . well, they were strange, elaborate, aqueous, unremittingly cosmic and 'pretentious' in ways that brought fresh nuances to the expression. What they were pretending to was largely immaterial: what was important was the nakedness of their pretension and the way the group were unashamed of that nakedness – in this slender sense at least, they were the Swedish naturists of rock. And it was quite clear then that – with Genesis and the Floyd already spoken for – Yes had to be my prog group, the free-floating cosmic hillock on which I would make my stand. And so I started working through the Yes catalogue, album by album, piece by suite, strong in my belief in the ultimate value of aqueousness, but never entirely confident that the moments of joy I would get out of the experience – most often on the spasmodically lovely *Close to the Edge* – amounted to much more than an inelegant straining after something far-fetched, something so elusive and recondite that no creature of flesh and blood might find it reachable, let alone the soul who made solitary study in my bedroom of Dalí's *The Great Masturbator*. I'd actually much rather listen to the Stones, Zeppelin, Skynyrd and Bowie. Even Genesis and the Floyd, if truth be told.

Nevertheless, it was a position to be defended and so I did defend it, as steadfastly as a Saxon housecarl at the shield-wall. I learned the opening stanza of *Tales from Topographic Oceans* off by heart (I can still recite it today, you will be enchanted to know). I surveyed vistas of rapturous twiddling for examples of transcendent musicianship (this was money for old rope: if nowhere else, Yes kicked Floyd and Genesis butt in the technique department). I studied the artwork of Roger Dean for . . . for . . . I'm still not quite sure what. I attempted to make the case, both to myself and to the boys, that because Yes were so incomprehensibly, overweeningly, baroquely far out they stood a much better chance of taking you somewhere you'd never been before. And this, in short, was the very coin of true art.

I'd then listen to Zeppelin's 'Whole Lotta Love' alone in my bedroom and get a hard-on.

7

The coin of true art, eh?

It seems funny, now, that it was once important to all sorts of young men that rock 'n' roll might count as art. Or not, depending on their individual needs of both art and rock. But it was important once to have the argument.

That rock is art is the only thing Lorry and I have ever agreed on. Although it's probably truer to say that we agree only that rock *may aspire* to the condition of art – it isn't an absolute requirement that it get there. After all, where would we be without the simple pleasures of a good time?

But then British rockers have always worried about art and about whether what they do is *real* or just something clipped together on a whim out of bought-in components – you know, as a sort of hobby. It's because our rock 'n' roll didn't grow in cotton fields and freight yards. We imported it along with a lot of other gear in the immediate post-war period, and then we learned how to copy it; even, in due course, to improve on it in some rare instances. The upshot of that was that we British have always been self-consciously aware of rock's status as a commodity, even as we treasure its peculiar artistic reach.

It hasn't always been an easy fit. Art into commodity; commodity into art – how does that work then? It was certainly uneasy in 1973, following the no-show of the hippie revolution and then the corporatisation of its imagery by – among other early adopters – Coca-Cola. Even Mods worried about art a bit, although not as much as hippies did, nor in the same way. Mods fretted about the metaphysics of style (Pete Townshend: 'The Who were an installation!'), while hippies read Gurdjieff, threw the I-Ching, gazed at Surrealist paintings and meditated upon the implications of rock's innate theatricality.

At art schools – the seat of British rock's early learning – students of rocky inclination spent their nights finding ways to ensure that rocking was contiguous with coursework. Art schools became schools of rock. If you discount the valuable contribution made over the years by the provisions of the welfare state (specifically, Social Security and Unemployment Benefit), art school was the closest rock 'n' roll ever got to government sponsorship. Well, until the 1990s it was.

But more than that, British rock has always wanted to embrace the idea of art not because art was interested in rock (with the notable exception of Peter Blake's Pop Art generation, it generally wasn't), but because intrinsically 'inauthentic' British rockers had so much of their jam invested in visual language and the ironies of camp contrivance, in *identifying* themselves correctly. It is one of the dearer myths of rock 'n' roll that it is intrinsically classless. Actually, rock is as riddled with class anxiety as Jane Austen and situation comedy. Indeed it shares quite a lot of features with both.

Even at its most rarefied and musically challenging, British rock always had to have a look – that is, it had to comport itself with some overt demonstration of style. Style, after all, was a reliable way of either identifying or transcending class, depending on what you wanted to do. Moreover, we British, feeling so compelled to be socially observant, were never in a position wholly to adopt the heroic authenticity of American style, with all the classless unself-consciousness that such transparency implied. And so, for us, the rock 'n' roll experience has always been something of a fancy-dress party.

We wore costumes. We attended social events – noisy, dark ones – in which the wearing of costumes was in itself a form of communication, a creative act. It is only a quirk of history that, for my generation of provincial schoolboys, the dressed-up look was a spangled cape and wizard hat. Mostly, unless you were a Smoothie, it was the fashion then to dress down. The idea was to look like shit; downwardly mobile, as if nothing more than the decomposing afterthought of a revolutionary moment that had belonged to someone else. My generation was the tidemark left behind by the 1960s.

Not that we knew as much or cared. All that mattered was *now*; now and what happens next. What counted were the things which belonged to us alone, regardless of their heraldic position on the wallchart of history: Genesis, Yes and Pink Floyd, then, with a supporting cast composed of Free, Lynyrd Skynyrd (the American Free), Can, King Crimson, Hawkwind, The Faces, Van der Graaf Generator, Jethro Tull, ELP, PFM, Man, Focus, Greenslade, Barclay James Harvest, Isotope, Hatfield and the North, Caravan, Soft Machine, Kevin Ayers, Rory Gallagher, Deep Purple, Uriah Heep, the Rolling Stones, The Who and Led Zeppelin. And Andy rather liked Früup.

But of even greater importance to thirteen- and fourteen-year-olds than the stuff they do like, is the stuff they don't. None of us liked Bob Dylan. Why would we? Why would we be bothered? He was of no relevance. To us, Dylan was a tired and intractably bonded figure, tangled up in the moribund values of literary minstrelism, of remote American superstardom and the general unravelledness of the American hippie vibe. He was 'Establishment' somehow, an approved purveyor of wordy songs to those who require rock music to be *worthy*. This group would include parents, teachers, social workers, vicars, government mandarins and, probably, policemen.

I felt that way about the Beatles, too, to Lorry's abiding disgust.

I didn't hate them, of course. No one could hate the Beatles. But I did feel that the Beatles stood for something behind which I could not, in all conscience, stand.

Even now, when the Beatles' manifold virtues are as palpable to me as the useless ear on the side of my head, there is a part of me that rejects the Fab Four's sound on contact, as a reflex. The reflex takes the form of an admonitory wagging finger and a hard, cold voice which says, 'Not here, son; there's nothing for you here.' You see, even though the Beatles are obviously great in every way – what tunes! what musicality! what talent! – what I get first in my head when I hear them is the sound of ingratiation. The sound of wanting to please. The sound of boyish charm. The sound of the end of the pier, of Saturday night television, of music hall – I hear it even when the Beatles are being grumpy or soulful or revolutionary. It's in the sound of their cherry-cheeked voices and the cheery, four-square, swingless thump of Ringo's drums; it's in the self-conscious skilfulness of their songwriting and studiocraft; it's in the mannered counterpoint of McCartney's sentimentalism and Lennon's studied rage. Later on in their career, it's in the mandarin authority of their discourse.

It's in the fact that whenever I hear the Beatles I feel once more the clamminess of the tea towel I used to do the wiping up with when I was a kid. My mum and dad didn't like the Beatles, not as such. They didn't *like* any pop music. But, crucially, they didn't *mind* the Beatles. They didn't mind them to the extent that they bought a Beatles tea towel in the hope that it might encourage the children to participate in the most undesirable of all domestic chores. The tea towel was adorned with badly executed images of Beatle faces and Beatle guitars and drums and, worst of all, incorrectly written musical notation – quavers with their tails on backwards – all of it spread over a greying weave in a patternless sprawl. In due course, the tea towel wore thin with wiping. It rotted away on the rail on the back door. One Sunday night I put my thumb through George's face.

What chance did the Beatles ever stand with me, then? They stood for the washing-up, as well as the expediencies of show-business, mass culture and, most hideous of all, commodification.

At thirteen I was above showbusiness, mass culture, commodi-fication, anything at all that smacked of ingratiation: the will to be universally popular: *self*-commodification. I could not have articulated such a premise at the time, let alone teased out of it a clever rhetorical position with which to baffle the straights at school, but I felt it all right. Anyone who offered themselves – their talent, their appearance, their nature, their selfhood – as a package of desirable goods for widespread consumption was of no interest to me whatsoever, except as an object of derision. People like that were beneath contempt. I thought that they were narcissistic fatheads who had no idea of what was good for themselves or for the rest of us. I felt that they were the kind of people who would be displaced in the end by people like me. I was quite as sure of the rightness of that as I was sure of the wrongness of unearned privilege. But the worst of it is that as an adult I still struggle with the same reflex – it remains auto-matic in me to presume that there is no value where my delicate sensibilities perceive arrant self-commodification. I suppose I just don't like people who suck up.

This reflex is grounded in something fundamentally old-fashioned, austere, religiose, anti-materialist, something at least as old as Bob Dylan and his stock suspicion of all things 'phoney'. Such feeling has no comfortable place in the twenty-first century, any more than my parents' rooted, post-Victorian liberalism had a fun time of it amid the kaleidoscopic circumrotations of the 1960s. It's the kind of knee jerk that stops me from enjoying the easy, uninnocent pleasures of *The X Factor* and which finds almost nothing to be entertained by in today's alt.showbiz pop world. Mind you, back then it was priggish high-mindedness on my part; now it's high-mindedness plus old age. Please feel free to sneer. After all, the part of me that turned a blind eye to wizard hats in 1973 also found it necessary in 1977 to wear a biker jacket and brothel creepers, and in 1983 a zoot suit; yet it really will not stand to see the youth of the twenty-first century offering themselves up – their matey clothes, their hedghog hair, their wounded sense of entitlement – as grist to the celebrity grinder.

I am not pleased that this reflex still exists in me, even in residual form. This is because I despise priggishness almost as much as I loathe snobbery. But I cannot, in conscience, pretend now that I didn't have a need back then to feel that I was trying to be *better* – better than the early Seventies equivalents of our twenty-first-century hedgehog wannabes: the squares, the straights, the Smoothies, the swots, the rugby team, the cadet force, the lickspittles, the phoneys, the boys and girls who recognised that life has in it some of the qualities of a competitive game, and then played it as if winning the game were the point of life. The people who were on-message. I was definitely on a better track than them and I could prove it. For I had an attribute that none of them possessed. It was an attribute born of sensibility and taste. For want of a funkier expression, we had better call it artisticness.

'Art' meant something very particular to me and my chums in 1973. Well, to me and to Lorry. Andy wasn't fussed about art – he just liked Genesis in the same way that he liked horse racing and football: they represented a stimulating way to pass the time while lying on the sofa. But to Lorry and me, the Prog Warriors who actually bothered to go to war, art was the magic ingredient – the mysterious chemical in life which made change happen.

Lorry was (and still is) a year older than me (he and the even more august Andy were friends long before I joined them on the bus into town). As a fourteen-year-old he blotted out the sun. He was a very big fellow in a very big straw hat rammed down hard on very long straight black hair and black beetling brows. He wore zip-up cardigans and zip-up plastic boots. He walked slowly on his heels with his toes pointing outwards like the hands of a clock at ten-to-two. He spoke with a Norwich accent. He nearly always looked cross. He was never, ever seen in public without an album under his arm. His extra year of life counted for a lot; that and the fact that, like Andy, and unlike me (who had two younger ones), Lorry had an elder sister.

Julie was twenty or thereabouts and lived elsewhere with her equally young husband. Whereas Andy's sister Linda was remote in her beauty, Julie was just remote. I never saw her or knew what she looked like or sounded like or anything. However I was very much aware of the things she liked: the Beatles, the Moodies, the Floyd, the Strawbs, the Stones . . . She was not a heavy-duty music head but a typical serious-minded chick of the period, who took music to be an expression of the really important things in life – not an ancillary soundtrack to her lifestyle but a continuation of those really important things by other means. Lorry attributed his superior sophistication and maturity in freak matters to time spent with her. They used to listen to music a lot together when he 'was a kid', Julie nurturing, maybe even steering his enthusiasms in an elder-sisterly way. Her authority was unchallengeable. 'Oh yeah,' Lorry might announce, as he manoeuvred *Caravanserai* on to his purple turntable, 'Julie's really into Santana,' and that would be that, the very last word on the Mexican Sustain King. Music was what they did together, although Julie liked to dance. Lorry has never danced.

So Lorry came equipped to tackle adolescence with special knowledge. In particular, he came armed with the certainty that the world was an irredeemably corrupt place populated by liars, bullshitters, phoneys, arseholes, wankers, over-vigilant publicans and politicians, all of them in thrall to a system that was organised to benefit the elite by keeping the ordinary man, woman and child under the yoke. This was not a system driven by political expediency and folly so much as by man's innately corrupt nature, and by the engine of material privilege itself. Politics was no solution, any more than religion or obliviousness were. The only force that could save humankind from the corruption to be found everywhere was art. And the only art equipped to do the job, apart from the imagery of René Magritte, Salvador Dalí and Tony Benyon in the *NME*, was rock.

You can see why I was impressed.

You may have got the impression that my outlook on life in 1973 was not the same as Lorry's. Let me refer you back to the 'dualities of life furnished by a solidly liberal Anglican background' and their 'comforting stability'. You are right. It was not the same outlook at all.

Let me take you in a little closer.

There is no surer way to the inner child than through his bedroom. Mine was still essentially a child's room. The fetor of hormones and underwear had long since overpowered the scent of Airfix glue and Humbrol paint, but my bedroom was still the domain of a solemn kid, decorated with the arrangements of books and pictures and models and artefacts that stood in miniature for the ordered world I expected to enter.

Lorry's bedroom was different. His room was a model of havoc; of the world he *knew* was coming. Every inch of wall space was covered with dog-eared cuttings from the *NME* and *Melody Maker*, posters, scraps, trophies, booty, emblems of the havocking events he required himself to identify with. There was the obligatory stolen traffic cone and flashing roadworks lamp, which you switched on and off with a matchstick poked into a hole in its yellow casing. There were piles of magazines, music papers and reference books (but no novels). Along one side of the bed was Lorry's record collection, eighteen inches long at least – massive then for a kid of fourteen – and next to and above it, contained in some hacked-together box arrangement, the exotically powerful stereo he'd inherited from some elder freak: a purple-painted turntable, a great big amplifier with thunking switchgear and the special box which allowed the sound to be wired to not two but four mighty speakers. The speakers were acned all over like the walls with stickers and cuttings. They so dominated the room, one in each corner fore and aft, that everything else in it apart from Lorry was forced to the edge, as if by centrifugal force.

Lorry himself would sit on the bed in the middle, the undisputed captain on his bridge, while Andy and I would perch on the windowsill like particles thrown to the rim of the universe by the mighty *woomph*. And there we would stay, perched on one bum cheek, one leg dangling, rewarded by the theoretical proximity of fresh air and with a good angle to see into Jackie Copsey's bedroom over the road. Besides, any prospect of movement around the room was deterred by Lorry's artistic creations. These hung on wires from the ceiling, in some cases right down to knee level: toothbrushes fused with light bulbs fused with melted vinyl 45s fused with ashtrays fused with electrical parts fused with things unnameable. I felt that everywhere here were clues as to what might fill the void.

This, to my mind, was what art was for: void-filling and going places you hadn't been before, metaphorically speaking, to negate the effects of the void. This was not pure escapism, by any means. No way. One's destination had to be meaningful. It was no good going to the artistic equivalent of Benidorm, where everyone and everything was basically the same only hotter. That would not be artistic; it would be tourism. In fact, deep cogitation on the matter of art revealed that having a destination, real and/or metaphorical, was rather less important than the travelling one did to get to wherever it was. Being transported was the true object of art – being transported so that you were no longer in the same place.

Lorry's art ideas were rather less flouncy. He took the view that it was the job of art to press your face up against the shit. Reality was all that counted. Not the reality which the system fobbed you off with, but the real one, the one described by the Floyd and Zappa and Lennon and Can and Crimson and Kevin Coyne. The one you only experienced if you truly opened your eyes. It was important in that case to not read novels ('fiction is all lies, man – by definition') and to avoid bullshit wherever you encountered it, on telly, at school, on the bus, in the street and, naturally, given that it was the seat of all bullshit, in church. This included avoiding drugs and fags, though not, interestingly, Dry Blackthorn cider. Sometimes Andy and I on the windowsill with our Number Sixes didn't know where to put ourselves.

Nevertheless, despite the fundamental differences in our sensibilities, Lorry and I did find ourselves standing on the same spot sometimes.

In December 1973 the Sensational Alex Harvey Band appeared on the BBC's rock show for grown-ups, *The Old Grey Whistle Test*. *Whistle Test* studio performances were not known for their excitement. Standard practice required the artist or group to roll up and wedge themselves in to whatever space was available in the schedule, on a minuscule sound stage in a junk room somewhere behind the walls curtaining the BBC's Shepherd's Bush keep. Performers performed to cameramen all of three feet away. Cameramen responded by pointing their cameras at the performers. The alchemy of live performance seldom ensued.

But Alex Harvey was sensational in actuality, as well as in name. He performed Jacques Brel's bleak *chanson* of ripped innocence 'Next' right into the camera's mouth, as if trying to bite out its tongue. He hugged a Telecaster to his chest and showed all his teeth while executing a perfectly baleful Gorbals *Sprechgesang*. Behind him, three violinists in mutant masks sawed for all they were worth, while SAHB's clown-faced guitarist made the fingering of barré-chords look like vivisection. Lorry, Andy, everyone of my age I've met since who saw it at the time, thought it was the best thing they'd ever seen on telly. I thought so, too. I certainly didn't breathe for several minutes after it was over, and since it was past my official bedtime, I didn't like to draw attention to myself by letting air out in the long, exultant, orgasmic shudder that would surely loosen mortar in walls for miles in every direction. Christ Christ Christ. I can remember thanking God Almighty that my mum and dad were in another room so that they wouldn't see me like this.

True, the effectiveness of the performance was partly achieved through the oath sworn crisply 'on the wet head of my first taste of the kiss of gonorrhea'. There is no hiding place in the psyche from lines like that, not when they reach you through so many regular yet strangely tiny teeth. Also, 'One day I'll cut my legs off, burn myself alive / I'll do anything to get out of life, to survive / Not ever to be next. *Ne-e-e-ext!* . . .' It's good material for a boy to conjure with. Alienation, sex, dismemberment. But Christ, was this art or was it art? Not only did it take you to a place you'd never been before, but it pressed your face right up against the shit. It was art all right, any way you sliced it. It was also a polka.

That same December, Lorry's sister Julie turned twenty. Four months later, on the last day of April, she took her own life. It was her husband Spencer's birthday. He had been killed in a car crash in February the year before. Julie had been five months pregnant at the time. Following Spencer's death, she gave birth prematurely and then lost the child.

'I bought a copy of the Floyd's *A Nice Pair* twofer on the market stall on the Thursday of that week, May the second,' said Lorry, many years later. 'I was thinking it would impress her. It was just after I got home with it that the police came round – I remember going upstairs later that evening and playing the *Saucerful of Secrets* half of the album and thinking how different it was from *Dark Side*, which Julie had turned me on to.'

Lorry did not tell me about Julie's death for five and a half years, even though we continued throughout that period to listen to music together and to disagree about everything. I still don't know what Julie looked like, but I can imagine her as keenly now as I did then. She hasn't changed at all.

8

I opened my eyes, then closed them again.

Everything was too bright – the ceiling, the walls, the light coming through the windows, the light reflected in the edges of the white-painted bookshelves which line the loft in which we sleep. It was evidently an overcast day in the world beyond the half-open blinds. The clouds sagged like weary gussets towards the treetops of north London. Yet the grey diffuseness of the light in the bedroom felt aggressive. The edges of my vision were unstable; something – I'm not sure what – was moving there. I dragged myself together and felt every nerve in my body shape itself as full consciousness returned. This was the first morning of my new life. I was out of hospital, back in my bed at home, barely mobile, deaf, deafened, nauseous and dazzled by dirty clouds.

I braced myself to turn on to my side and contrive the series of lunging yet smooth movements I'd have to make to get to the bathroom. When every little movement you make ends with a struggle not to throw up, you not only limit movement but you predetermine it. You look at the space you have to traverse and you make plans. You think: okay, from here to the corner of the bookshelves you can do in one longish stride; but getting up from the bed and into that stride is going to be awkward, because it will entail twisting and travelling in two directions within the same movement – so break up the movement: make the twist into one motion and the launch into a second, then give yourself a second or two to stabilise body, head and vision before lunging for the bookshelf, then keep the movement going smoothly, because if you pause for too long it will allow time for the nausea to get a grip and you want to be well on your way to the bathroom before that happens, so that if the worst does occur you can evacuate into the handbasin, while the other end makes use of the toilet bowl, plus you can support your head in your hands with both elbows on the rim of the basin while everything lets go. Thank God Jane insisted on the en-suite bathroom when we got the loft extension done.

And so on.

That was the morning routine for a number of weeks. That and the ingestion of medication and the relentless flipping of my right earlobe with a fingertip. I did the flipping more or less continuously in the hope that I wouldn't miss the first faint crunchings of renewed auditory life – so that I'd be there, so to speak, when it happened. But nothing ever happened, even when I was convinced there were stirrings. On more than one occasion Jane would be woken during the night by excited yelps: 'Yes, YES! I heard a crunch! I'm sure of it. Well, I'm pretty sure. Ssshhh – don't move. Let me try it again . . . Keep the duvet still. I'm sure I heard something. Sure of it . . .'

'Fucking hell.'

But on that first day back at home none of these routines had been established. Everything was new and everything was frightening. I sat aslant the toilet seat with my temple resting on the cool rim of the washbasin and listened to the havoc engendered inside my brain by the splash of my own urine. My private Presleyad. The compass of my vision was now widescreen and slotty, its outer edges a blur. Nausea no longer came in waves, but hung in me like fog. The sensation of pressure in the front-right quadrant of my head felt hydraulic. I would surely feel better soon.

I didn't though. Not unless you count the slide into oblivion every night, ushered in the soft hands of Temazepam, or the terrific, hungry euphoria which followed digestion of the morning's steroid dose; the euphoria was short-lived, of course, and swiftly followed by a sudden slump into inanition. Instead, as day followed day, the overbright world darkened quickly and I sank like a stone, faster than I thought it was possible to go. With neither diagnosis nor prognosis to act as a line to drag me into the future and with no sense of improvement to buoy me from within, I plunged into depression; not any old depression but a kind I did not recognise from past experience.

I no longer wanted to be awake; not ever, not even for a minute. Being awake just rubbed it in. Yet every night without fail I would emerge from sedation in the small hours. *Ping.* Oh no. And I'd lie there like a carcass till dawn, unable to move or think, unable to register anything other than the disfigurement of my inner world. I felt I had no life and no prospect of life; that I now constituted nothing more than a resonating chamber – empty, inanimate, unstable, LOUD – the sole function of which was to transmute every sound in creation into pain. Every night between one and four I'd awaken to the pitch-black vision that I was sealed up in the hold of a ship and the ship was going down.

One night Jane woke up too, disturbed by my 'weird breathing'. That's what she said anyway.

'I can't stand this,' I whispered.

'I know, darling, I know.'

'No, I mean it. I can't stand it. I can't *do* this. I think I may have to ask for your help.'

'You don't have to ask – you can have whatever help you need.'

'That's not the kind of help I'm talking about.'

Silence.

'I mean it, Jane. I can't do this. I cannot bear being alive like this. It is unbearable. It's not life. I can't do it. I really would rather be . . .'

'Don't you DARE talk to me like that.'

On the fourth morning back at home, the thirteenth since my collapse, when Jane had gone to work and her mother – who'd come down from Suffolk to hold the fort and get the children from school – was out at the shops, I took my longest trip out of bed yet. It involved some planning, but the execution was perfect.

I scythed out from under the duvet and was at the top of the stairs in an instant, shoulders pressed into the flank of the airing cupboard, as fluidly gymnastic in my flight as any free-running urban athlete in big trainers zooming around the rooftops of Paris. Maybe more so. I don't suppose those guys have to swallow their own vomit every time they leap from pediment to fire escape, plus they can see where they're going, so I rate my achievement in reaching the airing cupboard in a bound-and-a-half as of an altogether higher order.

That was the easy bit. Next I had to get down the loft stairs, which are steep, narrow and double back on themselves. This would take some time, because I'd have to slide down the wall, making sure that the side of my head maintained full contact with the plaster at all times, which, in turn, made it difficult to see where I was putting my feet. I could not look down. I might as well have been doing it in total darkness. But I did it anyway (we urban athletes have to maintain aggressive positivity of attitude at all times) and finally got down to the landing in reasonable shape. There I took a breather to make a tactical assessment of how I might traverse the length of the first-floor landing to the back bedroom where the computer is before Granny came back and my courage ran out. Yes, why not? Go for it! Once again the athlete's instinct took over and within a matter of several minutes I was at my desk, breathing heavily, listening through gritted teeth to the fuzzy *pnnnng* of the computer's switch-on note.

You may not be aware of this, but you move your head all the time. You are doing it now. You are. Well, you are if you're not lying down or you're not supporting your head with a pillow or a wall or a stick. You move your head all the time because it is in the nature of the balancing game to do so – adjustment is continuous and unconscious, and so tiny in scope that you can't actually feel the movement you're making, even if you think about it. The balancing game is ruled by your brain, supported by your eyes and by your joints (especially your knees), with the hair cells in your inner ear acting as the brain's conductors and gatekeepers in the series of linked vestibules that go to make up your auditory system. Do without all or part of these cilia and all those minuscule adjustments are no longer possible – not without inducing the nausea and whirliness that you will probably only know from being completely sloshed.

The difference between sloshed vertigo and the sort I was now experiencing is one of degree, context and quality of whirl. Past experience of the drunken whirlies tells me that they are at their emetic worst when you are lying down with your eyes shut, trying, for Jesus and Mary Mother of God's sake, to go to sleep. Not at all pleasant. My new, cilia-free whirlies were different. They only got a good hold when I had my eyes open and when my head was not supported back and sides in the soft grip of pillows. In other words, most of the time that I was not stupefied.

There are degrees, of course. Forward motion on your own two feet is pretty bad, but not as bad as standing still, presumably because the act of moving forward brings the eyes and knees into play. Standing upright and motionless is virtually impossible.

This must be, I imagine, because standing motionless negates the usefulness of eye-adjustment in relation to a moving visual field, and there's only so much knee-flexing you can do with straight legs. But the least comfortable of all the many positions a human body can be in – and I tried them all – is sitting upright on an office chair at a desk in front of an inanimate visual field, your knees a dynamic irrelevancy. It's in this position that you're solely reliant for micro-balance on the hairy friends buried in the middle of your skull; and when you've lost half of them, the half on the other side get confused – the signals they send are conflicted, so they give up on the job of helping you make all those imperceptible adjustments we make with the neck muscles supporting our great big heavy heads. Sit down at a desk in front of a computer in my condition and the whirlies go into overdrive. Within seconds you are chewing on the leading edge of your own vomit. Your neck feels as if it will snap.

I Googled 'assisted suicide'.

I don't know what I expected to find, but I knew what I wanted. I had it in mind that I'd discover a to-do list of subtly worded ways and means. Coded stuff. Abstruse discourse on the most painless method of first getting to Switzerland and then getting the juice into your veins. I imagined there would be a profusion of what American screenwriters like to call 'schematics': blueprints which show you the technical layout of what lies ahead, enabling you to silence the guards and tiptoe through the security network without tripping the lasers, to pull off the heist efficiently, maybe even with style. Above all, I expected to find thoughtfully worded documents taking you on a circuit of the maze of your moral responsi-bilities. How do you minimise the distress of those you're leaving behind? How do you ensure that they do not fall foul of the law? How do you *make good*? I wanted practical advice. Tips. That sort of thing. Information that would make the prospect of leaving life seem easier than the prospect of continuing with it.

Nevertheless, I was slightly anxious because I have never been any good with manuals or handbooks and I was concerned that detailed instructions in the antisocial craft of killing yourself might make my head spin even more than it was already doing. What I discovered was even more troublesome than that.

Look up 'assisted suicide' on the Net and what you get is not practical advice but moral debate. Miles and miles of it. Euthanasia.com, dyingwell.org, carenotkilling.org, endoflife. northwestern.edu . . . The alternatives are endless, the rhetoric profound, the positions taken painstaking in their arguments for and against. I read and read and read and felt my eyes harden in my head and my neck muscles scream. No blueprints, no tips. After five minutes or so I got down on my knees to rest my chin on the edge of the desk for support. I read for the sixth time how statistics show that nine out of ten people who consider suicide are actually making a desperate plea for someone else to *feel* their desperation; for someone else to push through the isolating membrane of suffering and join you, through the power of empathy, there on the inside in the sanctum of your pain; that what nine out of ten people who consider suicide want is not to die but to co-habit.

I knew that I was one of the nine.

I knew that I was not like Julie.

I didn't burst into tears. I swore and went back down the landing and up the stairs on all fours. I crawled into bed and rang a friend who used to be a rehab nurse and also happens to be the cleverest person I know. She came round the next day and held my hand while I cried. I'm not entirely sure what she said to me, but by the time she'd finished there had been a measurable rise in the levels of my enthusiasm for life.

Soon after she'd gone, Granny set off the smoke alarm in the house for the third time. *WEEEER-uh! WEEEER-uh! WEEEER-uh! WEEEER-uh!* The alarm was attached to the ceiling three flights down and Granny was unable to reach to turn it off.

9

Art was helpful at school. No, not helpful: absolutely critical to my survival.

I was not at the right school. By some unexpected twist I'd done very well in the Eleven-plus and been rewarded with a scholarship to the direct grant independent school in town for well-off and/or clever boys. My family was not well off and I was not clever, but a scholarship was a scholarship and so I went. Lorry and Andy were already at the two local grammars, one or the other of which was where I should have gone.

I envied them. I was not built for the strictures of private secondary education: not for the conformity, nor the hierarchy, nor the privileges, nor the competitiveness, nor the money and certainly not for the show. All of it was embodied in the school heraldry, which was purple and required to be on display at all times when pupils were at large in the public domain. Punishment for failing to abide by this rule was weirdly exaggerated and always exacted. The school cap was roundelled in purple and black, like some Victorian elite sporting club titfer, with thin white stripes dividing the main colours to make them really yell. (I Zingari? I Privileged Tosser, more like.) To say that I cringed every morning over the last half mile of the journey to school – the distance at which the risks arising from not wearing the cap just about outweighed the risks entailed in keeping it on – is to say that I only walked on two feet because crawling on all fours would have invited even more trouble. In the effort to be invisible, I ate myself alive every morning, and then again on the journey home every afternoon, especially over the last bit, walking down the hill through the estate where Nicky Wise and his brothers lurked (although I always removed the cap from my head once on the bus out of town, and was therefore beyond the reach of the cap police, Nicky and his brothers had a way of finding it stashed about my person, filling it with soil or leaves or snow and lobbing it up a tree – and the consequences of not being in a position to wear the thing through the school gates the next morning did not bear thinking about).

In between, all day at school, I devoured myself, too. Or I would have done if I hadn't snacked on the small fruit spilling from the cornucopian grail that was art. Art it was that stopped me dying the spiritual death that has shrivelled tougher souls than mine. I did not mind that the very word – 'art' – sounded a slightly foolish, unworldly note in this new ultra-masculine environment devoted to pragmatic achievement. On the contrary, I liked it a lot. Art itself – both art the curricular subject and art the stuff of life – was not a priority at the school. The school's priority was the preparation of its pupils for Oxbridge entry (Cambridge always a clear preference) and then for eminence in whatever field was fortunate enough to receive such alumni, in government, science, industry, the colonies, the cultural establishment, business and the City. Conformity was the basis of everything. Non-conformity was held to be a form of stupidity. Boys from the school did not, as a rule, go on to art college, although some of them did become rock stars. The school's most famous products were the literary academic F. R. Leavis, the theatre director Peter Hall, David Tang (the Hong Kong entrepreneur beloved, I think, of Baroness Thatcher, whom I remember as a highly polished prefect directing post-assembly traffic in a tailored suit) and David Gilmour of Pink Floyd.

Roger Waters and Syd Barrett had gone to the High School, where Andy went.

Things for me were never any good at 'that school', as my dad called it, something like disgust riding in his voice. On the very first day of the very first term I was hauled over the coals by the headmaster in front of the whole assembly for reading during prayers. 'YOU, BOY!' he roared, stabbing a pudgy digit from an Olympian height on the stage in the hall, an unexpected aftershock to the collectively grunted 'Freveranever'aahmen' at the end of the Lord's Prayer. 'You were READING! See me AFTER ASSEMBLY!' I trembled and tried not to weep. His finger somehow ruffled the outer tissue of my soul in a way that left permanent ruching. I can feel it now, all rucked up and tender. What was I reading so impiously? I was reading a copy of the school rules, which I had been issued with that morning and told to ingest as if my life depended upon it. Nevertheless, and despite my snivelling protestations of moral innocence, from that day on the headmaster had my number and he prosecuted it with a porcine enthusiasm which bordered on the truffly, never missing an opportunity to delve in the bole of my freaky tree. He seldom came up with much. I was not a particularly bad boy, just the wrong sort of boy for that kind of place. I responded by becoming more and more long-haired and arty with every passing day. I found relief where I could.

There was at the school an art room and inside it an art master, a leisurely individual called Roland Waring. He had a pudding-basin haircut, a sharp nose and buggy eyes, which he liked to strain for dramatic effect. The effect was André Previn with a groin injury. Waring was caustic, flamboyant and freckly. He liked to shoot favoured boys with a large staple gun. I liked him a lot. He used to call me Colefreak, with an extra roll on the r in 'frrrreak' when he was displeased with my idleness. Either that or Freakville. He'd tell my parents on parents' evenings that their son had an 'artistic temperament'. This was as popular as I ever got to be at the school.

Freakery did not endow you with eminent status there, as it would in some institutions, where it could make you a legend. At this school it endowed you with undecorated outsiderhood. You were simply null. This was fine by me. I knew I lacked both the will and the necessary charisma to make something of myself with the exercise of sheer unusualness. Furthermore, I could see there was a smattering of other outsider-freak ghosts floating around the school corridors, silently, behind curtains of hair. They went all the way up to the top of the sixth form and hung together in small, detached, greasy clouds. I admired them silently and wished to be considered one of their number.

How to join though?

If the school taught me one thing it was that one had to take one's opportunities ruthlessly, as they presented themselves. And so it was during my first year at the school – my memory of the weather says it was autumn 1971 or spring 1972 – that I found myself perched on the bench at the bus stop outside the gates next to a prominent fifth-form freak who happened to be nursing a lilac-coloured album on his lap. He was engaged in earnest conversation about it with a henchman. He had a terrible cold.

'Yeah,' he said to the henchman, 'it's the latest Ned Zeppelin.'

Their talk drifted opaquely over matters of which I had no understanding, such as 'heaviness' and 'vibes'. I canted my head to one side and managed to steal a look at Ned, who was pictured on the album cover with a bundle of sticks lashed to his stooping back. A country man. A man of the earth. A woodsman. A charcoal-burner. I imagined the vibes emitted by a heavy charcoal burner; conceived that Ned must be the last of his kind, recorded in his forest hovel by some enterprising anthropologist (although I was not confident of the meaning of the word 'anthropologist',

I assumed that there must be people who did stuff like anthropology for a living – this was Cambridge after all, where there was a museum of it). I imagined Ned playing a zither and croaking songs lost to modern memory, maybe accompanied by a group of young musicians with a feel for the woods. Either that or it wasn't Ned himself on the cover, but a projection of how the real, comparatively juvenile Ned would like to be seen. I conjured the image of someone not unlike Bob Dylan, whom I'd heard of and seen on the bedroom walls of my friends' elder siblings. Unkempt, twiggy. But I much prefered the idea of the ancient charcoal-burner.

The next day I scored 'Ned Zeppelin' into the leather of my satchel with the point of a pair of compasses and filled in the etching with Quink.

My foot was in the door.

*

My favourite book about the doing of music was written by the twiggy one.

Bob Dylan's *Chronicles Volume One* is both hilarious and serious. It isn't an autobiography exactly, although it is highly autobiographical. It is a selective tour of his sense of being, in particular of his selfhood in relation to creativity. Throughout the book he watches himself coolly and listens carefully; we get a lucid picture of what he thinks goes on inside himself. It's a warty self-portrait in the spirit of Rembrandt's self-portraiture. Unrelenting. Episodic, too. Lots of interior. No attempt to disguise brushstrokes. The Rembrandts, which were painted at intervals throughout a relatively long seventeenth-century life, actually constitute an extended meditation on the very idea of self-scrutiny and reveal not only the cool passion of the painter's vision but also the heat of his questioning. The pictures take your breath away, even as you feel Rembrandt's, full in your face.

The Dylan book is obviously shot through with essential truths and half-truths and maybe even big fat whoppers, but it is also heartily honest in its contemplation of its main theme, which is the theme of subjectivity. You can see his brushstrokes. He wants you to see them. He asks, What do I see and feel? And what is the consequence of me seeing and feeling those things? What then happens? What is it about objective reality that colludes with me in the invention of this other weird thing, subjectivity? What in the name of Beelzebub *is* this shit?

My favourite passage comes when the author hogs out of New Orleans on his Harley and fetches up on the stoop of a tourist-tat shack in some swampy boondock – yep, another one – with no one for company but an unnamed wife, who waits in the long grass outside while Dylan attends to the rambling of the proprietor, a man named Sun Pie. Bob is in fugitive mode just for a change. Things are not going well in town, where he is stuck fast in the recording of his *Oh Mercy* album with the producer Daniel Lanois. Sun Pie is all conjecture. He loosens up Bob's sense of himself. 'He was the right guy to run into at the right time,' says Bob, 'a guy who grooved on his own head.' A master of subjectivity, in other words. A man happy to take his own conjectures as the basis of a serviceable truth in the world.

Sun Pie predicts that the Chinese will soon reclaim America for their own – it was originally theirs, you see, before they, the Chinese, turned into Cherokee, Sioux and Narragansett. You feel Bob nodding along, mouth slightly ajar. Sun Pie trucks on about fate and the impossibility of equality even within the races. He likes Bruce Lee a lot. Is convinced that Elvis was a woman, the last of the race of Amazons. 'I think all the good in the world might have already been done,' he concludes, varnishing a chair.

Bob is in heaven. He is released into himself in a flood and, swollen, he hops back on the Harley with his missus and races back into town like the tide.

The album turns out well.

Sometimes it is not only more creative but also more useful to conjecture than it is to assimilate facts. Bob Dylan knows this. Lorry knew this (even though it went against his First Law, which was only ever to deal in facts, the enemy of bullshit). My eleven-year-old son knows this. Whether or not I knew it sitting on the bus stop bench outside school considering all the possible lives of Ned Zeppelin, I do know it now.

It is certainly true to say that the freedom to speculate offered by Ned enabled me less than twelve months later to see Stevie Wonder clearly in my mind's eye for what he was (in my mind's eye): a badly drawn cartoon yob-superhero, with layered shoulder-length bottle-blond hair and stubbled chalky skin, clad from collarbone to knee in skintight sky-blue spandex, a purple W emblazoned on his chest, a portable keyboard slung around his neck, his heavily muscled legs ferruled by the least sensible pair of stack-heel boots yet seen in England.

How did I know this? I knew it because I'd heard 'Superstition' on the radio and it was clear to me that that was what Stevie Wonder looked like. I can back this up. There is a moment in the song when that remarkable *boing-y* clavinet riff arrives at a cadence and detonates with all the vindictiveness of a tea trolley crashing into a china cabinet. It goes *crash-tinkle-smash*. Beneath the sound of the impact there is the screeching of castors on lino. You can hear it if you really listen. I still have an absolutely indelible picture wired into my memory of the pose struck by the pasty-faced yob in the moment that the trolley cadence hit – so indelible I always see it whenever I hear the record thirty-five years later. Stevie is rearing back on one leg (he's a cartoon superhero, for heaven's sake: they do that) one hand crashing down on the keyboard, the other held aloft to support a single, quivering digit pointed straight at the heavens. His head is back in a scream of ecstasy. The peroxide hair is everywhere.

It is a part of nature that eleven-year-olds believe in things that they don't understand – apart from anything else, it's the stuff that makes them fall in love. And they don't appear to suffer too much; they certainly don't deserve to be punished for it.

*

There is another way of looking at this, though, which is to observe that the sound of music is not a reliable narrator. It does not tell lies – not often anyway – but it is always possible to be misled by it, or confused, or left wondering. Music can be saying one thing with great truthfulness, while we hear something else altogether, also with great truthfulness.

This very unreliability is, of course, one of the miracles of art – it's what makes art beautiful and contingent – but it is especially true of music, where there is no materiality, nothing of any substance you can grasp in your hand and hold up to the light. You can do that with books and films and pictures and actors and installations. But music has no heft. It will not hold still. Its meaning is not demonstrable. You can take a movie out of time by freeze-framing it – you may not have the whole movie in that frozen image, but you do have something to study, to hold and take away with you, to interpret and to fetishise. And you can repeat the exercise. Paper your walls with it, if you choose. Try doing that with music and all you're left with is silence, or a meaningless sliver of noise. Because as soon as you try to trap music, it abandons its form. It becomes nothing. Yes, it is always possible to listen harder, of course, but that will only give you more of what you and music do together. It won't result in more objectivity. Besides, before you know it, time has passed on its merry way and the notes you were poring over so assiduously have gone, leaving only ripples. Music is as slippery as eels.

To eleven-year-old ears, it is even slipperier than that. An eleven-year-old has very little to grip eels with. He is pretty much naked in the world; he is certainly not wearing ribbed rubber gloves. He will hear things for what they are within his own compass of the world, such as it is, whether or not it agrees with what is actually out there. What is out there is of consequence, no doubt, but of no real substance. The void is a void because there is nothing in it. An eleven-year-old is discrete, alone, like a little god on the edge of nothingness.

By the time I was thirteen, however – two years on, riding the crest of the year of the Sensational Alex Harvey – I no longer felt quite so discrete or alone. It seemed important to make contact with something real, something which perhaps contradicts or even confounds godlike innocence. I was certainly keen that I should see Stevie Wonder as he really is. I had already discovered the true identity of Ned. I wanted to be real in the world, as you do when you are no longer a little god.

*

Any event of measurable worth in school life took place in the art room, or so it seems to me now. These were not great events, either: they were tiny moments that passed virtually unnoticed at the time. Atoms of time. Particles of no weight yet great eminence. In the precise moment that I am now trying to summon to memory, I may or may not have just been shot by Waring's staple gun; I may or may not have failed to do my art homework again; the playing fields may or may not have been billowing with coloured smoke and resounding to shouts and bangs as the school cadet force exercised its right to lie down on wet grass. Possibly, some boy was at that moment staring unseeingly at the walls of a toilet cubicle, fighting tears, as he wonders what the word 'cunt' really means. Possibly, another boy was explaining to a junior that objective hierachies do indeed exist in social relations and that it is quite possible for one person to be better than another – as was being demonstrated by this very conversation. QED. Almost certainly someone was wishing his cock would not harden involuntarily whenever some other part of his anatomy made contact with male skin.

In this most pregnant of moments I discovered that there were two other boys who liked science fiction, prog-rock and skiving. Cuthbert would have been designing a wholly practicable real-world space ferry – portholes, portholes, portholes, portholes, thrusters. Thompson would have been pissing around cleverly. I was possibly working on my epic series of pink splats. These were small gouache paintings of pink artefacts falling out of the sky to splat into mountainsides and valleys. Planes, rockets, grand pianos, the feet of gods. They were, to my mind, a rather splendid continuation by enigmatic means of the *Très Riches Heures du Duc de Berry* – for every prayerful day of the year, a new splat. 'Pink Icarus' was their collective title. They were a bit Monty Python too, if I'm honest, which I wasn't at the time.

But the moment was pregnant, of that I have no doubt. It almost certainly revealed something important. But it has gone now, like the coloured smoke. A now-obsolete usage of the word 'conjecture', incidentally, is to denote 'the interpretation of signs and omens'.

10

Another room I liked to be in, other than Lorry's bedroom and the art room at school, was the Peacocks' living room. Andy's family were the warmest, friendliest people I had ever met. They seemed almost exuberant in their preparedness to relax. They dwelt in a modest 1950s detached house over the road, just around the corner from our house, almost opposite my gran's. I'm not sure how they all fitted into it, but by the time I knew Andy well enough to go round his, the two eldest girls had left home and Linda was on the brink. The front garden was unfenced and barely gardened. There were no gates.

Andy's dad ran a carpentry business, his mum was a direct descendant of the Queen of the Nile. You could hear her coming round corners, the clack of her heels, the tinkle of her hooped earrings, the swoosh of her sleeves, cuffs, collars and piled ringlets always alerting you to her arrival seconds before the person actually materialised. When she did materialise, she came aureoled in perfume and chortles. Pam Peacock was a passionately optimistic woman. I adored her.

She had known her husband virtually all her life. They'd gone to the same school in a village at the other end of the Gogs and, according to family legend, fell in love side by side in their pushchairs. I later learned that while Geoff Peacock was uncut East Anglian as far back as could be traced, Pam was the product of the union between a Cambridge college bedder and an Indian undergraduate. Not a descendant of the Queen of the Nile after all, then. But I thought so; I thought of her as the bountiful fruit of Nefertiti's line (Cambridgeshire branch). According to Andy, Pam's glass was always half-full because of her striking good fortune in being fostered out as a child to the village in which Geoff lived. That's what she said, anyway.

All Peacock family members, and anyone who came into their orbit, were given nicknames. Geoff liked to issue them as signs of approval; at least I hoped it was approval, although I often doubted it. My nickname was Nickelarse, with the stress on the third syllable. Geoff's youngest daughter Miranda was always known as Shinnie (a corruption of 'shingy' – and there we'll leave it: life really is much too short). And much as I was in awe of Linda and sought to bathe in the sunshine of Pam's approval, it was Shinnie who blooded me in the world of women.

I know what you're thinking. No, is the answer.

Shinnie was two years younger than Andy, a year younger than me. But she was fiercer than both of us put together. She was also a Smoothie. She ruled the living room with the exercise of iron will and a gaze as baleful as a wolf's. Her word was not law so much as the basis for a butcher's negotiation in which Shinnie carried the cleaver. 'YOU WHAT?' she'd explode, leaning forward in outrage from her pouch in the black quasi-leather which cushioned the perimeter of the Peacocks' living room. 'You really talk a load of CRAP sometimes, Nickel*arse*!'

I talked crap quite a lot of the time, as it happened, and she would duly tear me to pieces in a way that I found thrilling. She would then make everything all right with unexpected displays of kindness. The record Shinnie liked above all others was *Motown Chartbusters Volume 3*.

Motown Chartbusters Volume 3 is a magnificent artefact. For those readers who go that far back and care, it was the silver one, the one with metallic radials issuing like fans of light from a cosmic vanishing point in the navel of the front cover. It kicked off with Marvin Gaye's 'I Heard It Through the Grapevine', pulsated straight into 'I'm Gonna Make You Love Me' by the Supremes with the Temptations, then Stevie Wonder's 'My Cherie Amour' (so confoundingly different from 'Superstition'); it thundered like a train through 'This Old Heart of Mine' and 'Dancing in the Street', reached a late secondary peak with Edwin Starr's 'SOS' and achieved maximum load, sixteen songs after it began, with the small poetic miracle that is Smokey Robinson's 'Tracks of my Tears'. What a thing.

MCV3 did not belong to Shinnie. It was a hand-me-down from a departed elder sister and was deemed to belong to everyone. It was consequently a little dog-eared at the corners, its silvery lustre a little dimmed. It was not treasured. It was neither a totem of anything nor a fetish, and certainly not an object of any sort of faith; it was a thing to be used in the house when inclination and circumstance demanded, like curling tongs. Nevertheless, it served as Shinnie's main armament, other than her mouth and her stare: her proof if any were needed that Andy and I were imbeciles and that Genesis were imbecilic.

I could not agree with her, of course. But I really didn't mind *Motown Chartbusters Volume 3* being on. I already knew several of the songs from the radio and *Top of the Pops* and I considered 'I Heard It Through the Grapevine' unusual among soul records in that it appeared, even on my red radio, to have mysterious properties. Issuing from the radio's small plastic speaker into my bedroom, these properties were attenuated, brittle, spindly but unmistakable: even in stick form the record radiated mystery. But thickened up in the circuitry of the Peacocks' music centre, and projected through larger plastic speakers into domestic space occupied by *other people*, it became as pervasive and unifying as weather. The song loomed. It invaded the room, dominated it, reconfigured everything, somehow contriving to join up space in a new contiguity, as if all the stuff contained within its walls were being described for the first time. People, things, the spaces in between people and things – they enjoyed new relationships while 'Grapevine' played.

Permit me to invade it back.

Soul – as all Rhythm and Blues-based pop music made by black Americans was called in the early 1970s – was then an established commercial force in the British top twenty, every bit as dynamic in its anthropological implications as the other pop genres. More so, in fact. Soul came loaded with implications, not all of them at odds with the environment those implications modified. What did it imply in the fens of East Anglia in 1973? Depends on who was listening, of course, and for what purpose.

Who listened to it? In one sense everyone did. It was not possible, if you had the slightest interest in pop in 1973, to avoid soul music (although, of course, if you weren't interested in pop music, it was perfectly feasible to avoid the lot of it, if you wanted to – popular music was not as meteorological then as it is now: as in universally unavoidable). Soul came in many forms, although it took a giant effort of will on the part of your average white thirteen-year-old long-hair to bother to distinguish between Philly and Motown and all the lesser variants of the semi-sophisticated, pre-disco urban soul vibe then prevalent in the charts. It was easier to expend that effort on trying to ignore it altogether. Except that you couldn't, not if you liked music. You might as easily ignore your own brothers and sisters. Southern Soul? Wouldn't that be the kind they like in Hampshire? As opposed to the kind they like in Wigan and Stoke – Northern Soul. Cambridgeshire had its own, extremely virile Northern Soul scene, based in and around the fen outpost of St Ives, conveniently located within the golden triangle of East Anglia's American air bases. So why wasn't that Eastern Soul?

Yes, I knew a soul record when I heard one, but I didn't know what *kind* of soul it was. To tell the difference you needed to be a soul boy and wear different clothes, strike different attitudes, be virile, wash your hair more than once a week. Soul boys and girls – always happy to be known as Smoothies – extracted special juice from soul records, something to do with the sense of self in relation to the tribe. Soul committed you to a view of things; perhaps not a world view, but certainly a view of your immediate surroundings. This view differed in just about every conceivable way from the freak perspective.

If I liked a soul record, I liked it. If I didn't, I tried to think about other things until it was over. Soul did not, as a rule, arouse what I liked to think of as my more interesting parts. I liked 'Me and Mrs Jones' by Billy Paul, but it didn't engage my curiosity. I thought it was quite sexy, I suppose, but I did not aspire to penetrate its mysteries any further than was sufficient to get a superficial grip on the story it told, which was the story of an adulterous couple trysting in a café and feeling bad about it. To sing the song, Billy Paul cushioned his adenoidal tenor with strings, while he sloughed his toes through his confessor's penthouse shagpile, cooing softly, obviously slightly upset about this 'Mrs Jones' he was maybe or maybe not humping. But why so lush? Why so draggy? 'Me and Mrs Jones' was *languorous*, and its atmosphere seemed to be at odds with its theme, the theme of anguished, isolated, guilty compulsion: 'Me-ee-ee-ee and Missus, Missus Jones, we got a thiiing going on – we both-a know it's-a wrong. But it's much too strong to let it go now.' Nice tune, but who gives a shit about what goes on between consenting adults in cafés, man? And frankly, what does this have to do with rectifying our perceptions of reality? It was against nature for a freak to give thought to the quotidian, let alone to dig beneath its surface.

Yet soul was everywhere, every day, which meant that soul itself was an issue.

The soul issue was not a race issue. It was a class and culture issue. What disbarred the Temptations from any serious freak interest was not their skin colour but their clobber, plus their footwork, their respectability, their cleanliness and their determination to please. But mostly it was their clobber. All five of them wore identical baby-blue crimplene suits with collars like spaniels' ears. Showbiz or what? No one wore gear like that round our way. Our vision of harsh reality rested on an uncompromising rejection of crimplene. Yes, there were black people in Cambridge – hardly any, but there were some. I knew what they looked like, and sounded like; had a pretty solid grasp on the fact that where there were differentials, they were social differentials. And one thing that was incontrovertibly true about the black people in Cambridge was that they did not go around in baby-blue suits, dropping to their knees, pirouetting in and out of shop doorways going 'woooooo!' The big soul worry was not race but aspiration. We didn't disdain soul because soul singers were black but because the people who were into soul were Smoothies.

Anyone could like soul, but not everyone could be into it. To be into it, you needed to aspire to the good things the world had to offer. Love and sex, obviously. Showbiz success was another one – 'superstardom' was a desirable destination in life even then, if not quite the standard career option that 'celebrity' is today. But material things, too, like cars and jewellery and fine clothes and food and comfortable furniture and the all-encompassing virtues of a 'happy home' – the happy home somehow got more air time in soul records than seemed strictly necessary. Less materialistically, soul seemed to be rather keen on upward social mobility, respect, religion, children, work, the disposal of garbage in the street, the avoidance of drug dealers and gangsters, not being taken for a ride, not being framed, getting a fair deal, not being killed.

By and large, these were not the sort of concerns which

disturbed the sleep of rural white boys, whatever their station in the English class system – and especially not the brotherhood of freaks, to whom all forms of social mobility were anathema (because to admit to the possibility of social mobility is to concede that society's structure is immutable, and that is simply not on). The fervently aspirational crimplene-suit stuff seemed shallow and credulous to me and my chums, even as it was blandly accepted by the Smoothies who turned themselves inside out and upside down at the Black Diamond disco in the village hall. Social control, hanging on in quiet desperation and the evils of money – these were *our* big themes. Much more serious. All in all, soul appeared to have very little to do with our lives and very little to do with art.

'I Heard It Through the Grapevine' had something else in it, though. It's the Marvin Gaye version I mean, of course, not the Gladys Knight one, which is splendid, robust, soulful, passionate but almost completely devoid of the thing which made the Marvin one reach out and zizz resistant freak nervous systems.

The record is all edge. It begins with a perfunctory report. A sort of slap, or is it the sound of a door slamming somewhere else in the house? Actually, it's the sound of a tapped snare drum overlaid with a curt biff on a tambourine. So perfunctory. So unfreighted. As declamatory moments go it does not compete with the famous biff at the start of Bob Dylan's 'Like a Rolling Stone', a detonation which has launched many great thoughts down the decades. This little finger-slap is a sneaky little shot at your cheek while you're looking the other way.

Then, your attention having been secured, the rest of the song issues into the mind like smoke under a door: electric piano, kick-drum, hi-hat, bass, fluttered tambourine, guitar, another chopped guitar fingered high up the neck, strings, horns – they ghost in singly, one after another, each shaping a new emphasis in a rapidly evolving metrical scheme and, in the case of the first guitar, hinting at a different tonal centre to the dark minor key we'd already thought we'd settled for. Before Marvin Gaye has even licked his lips, we know we are into the deeps.

The song barely needs its words. The first one is an utterance: 'Oooooo-ooo'. Beneath that, the lollop of tom-toms which rolls the voice into the song is one of the most exquisitely placed and executed rhythmic figures in all popular music (right up there with the cymbal crash which ushers Miles Davis into 'So What'). It somehow describes both time *and* space in the passage of a second and a half. It also imparts to Gaye's voice instant momentum, as if tipping it out on to a slope with a caressing shove: Marvin, just *go*.

Listen to the thing. But don't, for once, listen to it from the top down. Listen only to what's going on underneath the voice, the instrumental accompaniment. I am willing to bet you have never heard anything that so cogently expresses the ideas contained in the words 'economy' and 'restraint', 'austere' and 'spooky'.

These are not Motown words. Not usually anyway. It might be glib to suggest that Berry Gordy's most far-reaching achievement was to take the church out of black pop, thereby making it easier for whites to buy it. But it's also not far short of a workable thesis: as a rule, you don't get much gospel to your Motown pound. 'I Heard It Through the Grapevine' goes the other way, though. It may well be construed as the label's all-time greatest hit, yet there is no churchier record in the entire Sixties Motown canon. Not if churchy means what I think it means.

But it's not churchiness on its own that makes 'Grapevine' singular: it's the combination of churchiness with something you're not supposed to find in church: anxiety. 'Grapevine' is also the most neurotic record Motown put out in the Sixties, the one most fraught with worry. And you could go further, I suppose, as some have done. So pent up is its arc of emotion, you might say that the record is an expression of high paranoia. After all, its subject is the pain inflicted by adverse events – or at least the perception of adverse events – shaped by forces beyond the individual's control. The song is partly about impotence. 'Grapevine' emerged scowling into a frightening year, 1968, when paranoia was in the very air that you breathed, especially the air breathed by African Americans of draftable age.

But I think you'd be wrong. It's not a paranoid record, it's an anxious one. Anxious as in fretful, as in twitchy, as in self-absorbed, as in self-dramatising. Let's go back to the music and to Marvin's singing.

The first thing you notice when you listen hard to it – the right way up – is how hard Gaye sings; hard both tonally and in the way he presses against the pulse of the music. One of the loveliest aspects of the rhythm track is the tension between the plunging off-beat stress and the float of the strings, piano and percussion on top – especially the congas, which pitter-pat continuously, evenly, round and round, appearing to pull the edge of the rhythm to its outer limit, as if stretching a sheet. It's not unlike reggae in this respect, and not only because the biggest metrical shove falls on the third beat in the bar.

But it's quite unlike reggae in several other respects, chief among them being the singer's relationship with time. In 'Grapevine' Marvin sings close to the ragged edge. He is neither floating with the strings, piano and congas, nor plunging and bobbing evenly like everything else. He is driving forward. This is not normal Motown behaviour either. The Motown school placed great emphasis on its singers maintaining a comfortable, even elegant relationship with the pulse of time. Motown singers were certainly permitted to go off at the deep end in terms of frequency and amplitude (think of the Four Tops and the Isleys just for starters – a bunch of berserkers in shiny shoes), but Motown voices in the 1960s were not supposed to fray with unmanly screwiness as they did so, to the point where individual pathology threatens to run amok. It would be as easy to pass Diana Ross through the eye of a needle as it is to imagine her self-loathing driving a performance, while even the abundantly urgent Levi Stubbs (of the Four Tops) never sounded as disturbed as Gaye does here. Stubbs's great gift was to make the articulation of volcanic passion sound like heroism. 'Grapevine' doesn't do that. It is anything but heroic; and it has barely a mote of elegance in it, apart from the feigned kind, which was always Marvin's cover for everything.

One of the reasons for this inelegance is that for the entirety of the performance, Gaye sings on the cusp of his two primary registers, on the torn edges of his throat voice and his head voice, right there on that awkward, inhospitable fault line separating angry rasp from sepulchral whoop. Perhaps Motown's Norman Whitfield, who both co-wrote and produced 'Grapevine', should take creative credit for this, and for never letting either the singer or the listener off the hook. Marvin begins in relative comfort, flicking from tessitura to tessitura with urgency but handsome control. But as the iniquity of the singer's situation is revealed and more air is required to push out the heaviness of his feelings ('Losing YOOOOO might end my life, you see'), the envelope begins to stretch. Listen to the way he sings the word 'surprise' in the line 'It took me by sur*pri-i-ise*, I must say': this isn't moral indignation and its portal to the high ground; it's the door to what Muhammad Ali, in a different context, used to refer to as 'the Near Room' – the place you go to when you are no longer wholly inside yourself.

All of that got through to me, all of it, at some unplumbable level.

I'd sit in this happy place, in Peacock sunshine, softly gripped in black quasi-leather, breathing Pam's air-freshener, the racing on the telly with the sound down, Shinnie giving me what for,

Pam giving me another cup of Nescafé with enough sugar in it to stand the spoon up, Linda out with Howie but due back later, maybe, Andy shushing Shinnie as his nag came in, Geoff taking the mick out of every life form within his compass, including his eldest daughter Marnie's husband Pogle, who seldom uttered a word – and I would shudder. This was not a sexual shudder like the Sensational Alex Harvey one. It was the shudder of one who recognises the viability of a contradiction. To me it seemed suddenly that even if it were preposterous – pretentious even – to argue that ecstasy is the handmaiden of despair, and vice versa, then it is demonstrably true that at least they might lounge around simultaneously on the same furniture. As might Shinnie and I, for all our differences.

Furthermore, soul music did not have to be all about tribal aspiration, slick moves and alpha clothing. It could be all about soul.

11

I am standing almost alone in near darkness. The gloom is punctured only by the light of two candles guttering in long brass portable candlesticks. Their flames are sheltered from the draught by the hands of my two seraphic accomplices. Their hands are small and orange-pink.

It is dark because the lights in the church have been switched off. I am almost alone because the three hundred people occupying the church are invisible to me beyond the circle of light; and because my accomplices do not have bodies, only hands; and because Turkey, the crucifer, with his brass Cross on a pole, is out of sight behind me. He is at the front of the choir, which snakes back behind him into the vestry, if a choir of nine can be said to snake anywhere. The vestry is in a transept, slightly off to one side of the main body of the church, behind a white-washed pillar. I can't actually see anyone at all. Just the candles and the orange-pink hands protecting the flames and the faintly glowing curvature of the pillar. I might as well be alone. It is the Sunday before Christmas 1970. I am ten. It is my turn this year to open the carol service by singing the first verse of 'Once in Royal David's City' solo and unaccompanied in front of the entire village.

Out there in the blackness I know my mum, her mother and my youngest sister, Deb, are standing in their pew in the thick of the spluttering throng. I know my mum is attempting to reconcile opposing impulses: one is to swell with pride, the other to constrict with anxiety. I imagine her left hand, with its rings, gripping the back of the pew in front, white at the knuckles. My dad and the elder of my two younger sisters, Becca, are togged up in their cassocks and surplices in the choral snake behind me.

I know the time has come because a lot of solemn hand-signalling has passed between the choirmaster, the rector and the sidesman at the back of the church to indicate that the lights should be switched off. The lights have just gone out all over St Vigor's with a gravely reverberant *thunk*.

It is so dark out there.

The organ sounds a note. It is my note. I now have to open my mouth and let it be. And in that fraction of a beat of time I feel a familiar hot, tingling sensation bubble up inside, just below the buckle on the belt holding up my trousers. This can mean only one thing. If I don't start singing I will wet myself.

And so I do. I sing. I would hope in these circumstances to be singing to the greater glory of God. And, in one sense, I am – God's prestige would not be greatly enhanced by me weeing down my leg and leaving a puddle to steam on the vestry step after the choir has gone. But, in fact, the glory of God is not at the forefront of my mind in this moment. Getting into the music is; getting in as far as I can go, so that no part of my mind is left behind to dwell on, and thereby further stimulate, the coming urological apocalypse.

'*Once in Roy-al Daaa-vid's city [breath] stood a loooowly ca-a-ttle she-e-ed . . .*'

I am a decent boy treble. I have a 'nice' voice, an unaffected, unwarbly, mid-range sort of pipe, which makes up in accuracy and reliability for what it lacks in oomph and tone. I am not one of your golden wonders, gifted by Apollo with the power to move grannies to fluttery hand gestures and choirmasters to ungodly ambition. I am more the sort of choirboy you'd want next to you in the trenches. So I am well enough equipped to survive the crisis developing south of my belt buckle – just by concentrating like billy-o and breathing in the right places and pinging (not swooping up to) those top notes. And. By. Not. Rushing.

'MAR-y was that moth-er mild, JEEE-sus Christ her li-i-itle chiiild.'

Touch down.

The beauty of that moment is not describable. My shoulders drop. The task is complete. I didn't muck up. But no time to bask because something else is beginning.

There is a beat's pause. The choirmaster has insinuated himself into the circle of candlelight and is now visible not only to me, but to the choir and much of the congregation. He lifts his arms and his surplice sleeves open like wings. It is an upbeat. The downbeat falls and the entire church opens its lungs. The sound that comes out is warm, rounded, buoyant, thick; loud in the building but soft in the transepts of the mind. Amazingly, the nerves that afflicted my bladder had driven my intonation only fractionally sharp during the first verse, so there is no great jarring when all three hundred voices plus the organ settle into their way, like a great ship launching.

'He came down to earth from heaven . . .'

There is more flapping and Turkey emerges from behind me with his Cross. The choir processes slowly through the darkness to its stalls, singing as it goes, borne on the ship of voices. It is not necessary to put one foot in front of the other. We float on the sound. The candles float with us. Shadows climb the vaults in flickering runnels to pool in the recesses of the roof.

' . . . And he leads his children on, to the place where he is gone.'

There is a dark tail of organ chording left behind after the voices have stopped. Then silence.

The lights come on again, but this time there is no thunk.

The silence is broken only by coughing. I wonder if my mum has relaxed her grip on the pew in front. I can certainly no longer feel the tingling in my bladder, only a different kind of tingling all over my body, like a rash on the inside of my skin.

*

Although I always knew I liked music, it was church that first saturated me with it. It's possible that it was church which created in me the feeling that, once inside the mind, music takes on architectural form. This whole process began when I was quite a small child and I have never been able to enter a church since without being visited by a sense of warm anticipation: the feeling that any minute now I might hear something that will stop my feet in their tracks and make my jaw go slack. For many reasons, I am a sadder man for the fact that I seldom go into churches at all now.

My family was and is religious in varying degrees. But it's very hard to say precisely what those degrees are. This is because it is canon law in our family that religious belief is a private business, neither to be shared with nor imposed upon anyone else – even within the family. Affairs of the spirit are far too complex to be kicked around on common ground in the half-deflated football that is language. Furthermore, the evangelistic impulse is to be resisted at all costs. Evangelical behaviour is the Great Wickedness: there is surely no more ignorant conviction than the one which tells you that you have the right to convert other people. (Saint Paul? Nutter.) That doesn't mean that religion can never be the subject of amusing allusion – heavens, no – but it does mean that the subtleties of individual faith, or its lack, are always reserved *in camera*. Always.

For this reason it is very difficult indeed for me to describe what went on and what continues to go on in our family in the name of religious belief. What can be revealed – hold on to your hat now – is that those family members who do subscribe are Protestants, loosely grouped around the liberal, pro-intellectual, middle-ish theological strata of the Church of England, with, in my dad's case, a streak of latent Quakerism in him so antsy that I often used to wonder why he didn't just say to himself, 'Oh, what the hell . . . Where's the tricorn hat department?' But then my dad's greatest fear in life was always shopping.

I spent a lot of my childhood in church. I spent a lot of it playing football, too, but I have far more vivid recall of enuretic near-things on the vestry steps than I have of diving saves in fen mud. I would like to be able to say that this was because of overriding spiritual conviction, allied to uselessness at football, but it is, in fact, because of music; music and a nervy bladder.

Which is not to say that I didn't believe in God. I certainly did. He was a given in my cognitive landscape, in the same way that the Internet is a given in my children's – a source of universal wisdom and benevolence, but with a beard. He had long hair, too – naturally, this being the Sixties; and, for a period, full Anglo-Saxon harness, God being the model on which Alfred the Great based his look. Alfred was my hero when I was a small boy, despite the incident with the cakes: a fugitive, law-giving, bookish warrior king who invented the navy, fought the Vikings to an honourable draw, was a proto-parliamentarian (which is to say that he enjoyed an amicable relationship with the Witan, the Anglo-Saxon equivalent of the House of Lords) and who reigned for a very long time, despite Anglo-Saxon plumbing. All through the Sixties God/Alfred looked down benignly and involved Himself in my interests without partiality, as befitted an Anglican deity. He was not a wrathful God. In fact, the chances of His having read the Old Testament were slim.

The landscape upon which He bent his eye was as immutable as He was. It rose and fell in concentric agrarian ripples from its centre in our village. Beyond the fen and the chalk there were hedgerows and fields, hills and woodlands, rivers and streams; features across which man sailed and ploughed and sowed and reaped and plucked, as he does in the *Très Riches Heures du Duc de Berry*. And every now and then the flux of countryside was broken by a city. There, people busied themselves glamorously at the very edge of God's peripheral vision. For one thing was as sure then as it still is: if you are to escape God's gaze, then the city is the place to do it. God is a gardener. His chief concern is to be left alone to potter. His great interest is the integrity of the fields, hedgerows and streams, to which preoccupation a little moral stiffening is brought by a concern for the starving of the world. He has no eye for streets, buses and skyscrapers. That is chlorophyl you see between His toes. Mine was not a complex theology (although I do like to think of myself, with hindsight, as a kind of juvenile forerunner of the modern Green religionist).

God was into music, too. Must have been. Otherwise why would we always be singing to Him? Imagine God not caring for music! Inconceivable. Must be torture for Him anyway; worse than the Queen's problem with the national anthem. She might have to endure that dirge every day, but at least she is only obliged to sit through single performances of it, one at a time. God has His music playing everywhere, all the time: Handel's *Messiah* going off simultaneously with 'Onward Christian Soldiers' and Gregorian plainchant and the *Nunc Dimittis* and 'The Old Rugged Cross' and 'Jesus Wants Me for a Sunbeam' or whatever crap it is the happy-clappers are into now . . . An unimaginable din.

So what happens if God decides that what He really wants today is to hear the choirboy singing 'Once in Royal David's City' solo on the vestry steps for the first time, and nothing else? Well, in that case ordinary mortals would have a problem, because all the other choirs and congregations and organists and solo choristers going at it hammer and tongs would be jamming the signal. But not God. That's one of the benefits of being Him. If you're God, you can tune in. You can edit, live. Indeed God has many natural advantages, rather as you'd hope. His great musical advantage over the Queen – apart from His editing capabilities – is that He has a far wider range of music to choose from, virtually all of which is better than the Queen's. He can exercise a sense of taste. God has the best tunes. Everyone knows that.

He has a lot of duffers, too. 'Onward Christian Soldiers' is a notably duff one, as are all muscular Anglican calls to arms – a good two-thirds of *The English Hymnal*, then: so four-square, so muscle-bound, so attritional. Similarly, all strummy, modern 'Lord of the Dance'-type music, which suffers from the multiple (crypto-evangelistic) deficiencies of being ingratiating, trendy, whiningly metaphorical and cheerful. I used to imagine God rummaging frantically in drawers for earplugs. 'I am not the bloody Lord of the Dance!' Puff, pant, scrabble, rummage. 'I am the Lord thy God and I HAVE NEVER DANCED!'

But the good tunes are simply unbeatable.

The organist at St Vigor's throughout most of the twentieth century was Mrs Beeton, a farmer's wife from over the road. She was not a very good organist. Under her fists, chords would put themselves together like a rabble, in their own good time. And her pedal work was at best vague. From my position in the choir stalls, I'd sometimes watch her ankles criss-cross on tricky cadences with frantic indecision, swinging first one way, then the other, her feet hovering, tangling, hovering, then plunging like laden buckets on to the wrong pedal, sending dissonant shudders through the foundations of the building. Most of the time she didn't bother with the pedals at all.

But Mrs Beeton had soul. There were certain pieces she

played with real confidence and feeling, no doubt born of endless repetition allied to a deep affinity with the emotional charge of the music. Judging by the way she played it, her favourite hymn was 'The Day Thou Gavest, Lord, is Ended', which she rolled out with a steady, melancholic passion I found utterly compelling. She made it into my favourite hymn, too.

Because they are written in a set of standard metres and are therefore vulnerable to misrepresentation by tone-deaf vicars, Anglican hymn tunes frequently acquire familiar names, just for the purposes of no-nonsense identification. The melody of 'The Day Thou Gavest' is usually called 'St Clement', presumably on account of the fact that it was written by a man called Clement Scholefield in 1870, a man I imagine to have had a tall head and hard, sad eyes, the sort that are filled with longing yet masked with piety. 'St Clement' is high Victoriana, as romantic and sentimental as it is solidly engineered. The melody is an epic roller – its up-and-down motion brings to mind the swells of the open sea. Its harmony, in the best Anglican tradition, supports the tune with plain chordal ironwork, hinting at the intricacies of counterpoint from time to time, but never actually delivering anything inessential to the efficient functioning of the machinery, apart from the occasional glancing harmonic suspension. These tiny passing moments, like glints, serve only to heighten the tone of golden solemnity so warranted by John Ellerton's beautiful words.

The day Thou gavest, Lord, is ended,
The darkness falls at Thy behest;
To Thee our morning hymns ascended,
Thy praise shall sanctify our rest.

This is not great poetry, but it is great hymning. It is wonderful to sing. Following the pitch and yaw of Mrs Beeton's introduction, that opening verse would get the pictures going in my head as I sang the words, as vivid as cinema, and I'd try to sing further into them as the hymn went on. This seemed to be the point of doing it – singing into the pictures. Reading the words of 'The Day Thou Gavest' now, I can still call up the exact same scroll of images in my mind, of darkness settling like feathers across a weary world as it lays its burdens down, village by village, country by country, continent by continent; and I can feel the tightening of my chest in the drive for the line, the hymn's destination, as if singing it were a means of going somewhere.

The last verse is not as beautiful as the first one but its scope is truly epic. By now we have circumnavigated the globe on a tide of fading light.

So be it, Lord; Thy throne shall never,
Like earth's proud empires, pass away:
Thy kingdom stands, and grows forever,
Till all Thy creatures own Thy sway.

Mrs Beeton would always pull out a couple of stops to give the last verse some welly. She'd toe the right pedals, too. And afterwards the thing would linger in the air for what seemed like minutes, like a taste in the mind. An atmosphere. The sacred as a form of weather.

*

But Christmas was the time.

My dad had a thing about Christmas and we all got infected to some degree. In him, Christmas was a well of emotion without bottom, to which certain rituals were fixed like rungs on a deep-reaching ladder, all of them involving music.

In fact, the very idea of Christmas seemed to drop my pa into a different space, a column of clear, streaming air in which he breathed deeply of some special oxygen suffusing him with both energy and pleasure. I suppose the rituals of the season enabled him to decompress from the year-long stresses of fatherhood and his job at the University Press, but there was more to it than that; more than recreation, more than symbolism, certainly more than self-indulgence. In my dad's view, the value of Christmas has nothing to do with the relief a good time brings, everything to do with revelation. Christmas has to be done properly – its emotional meaning revealed – because the natal feast is all about the fundamentals of being alive. It has to do with childhood. Not the usual, recollectable sort of childhood we have stored in our memories, but the passage of infancy which goes before memory: the mystery of nativity and its immediate consequences, when the entire world is made different, even new.

Around the beginning of Advent you'd hear the first repetitious plunking of the piano downstairs, and, later on, as we became teenagers, the scraping of the viol. In due course a new arrangement of a medieval carol for krummhorn, bassoon, viol and voices would be forthcoming. We'd all show up and play it amicably enough. My dad was not visibly moved by this process. He would just inhabit it more fully than he did most of the other activities we pursued as a family.

That kind of earnest, Victorian domestic music-making did not get me off, though, much as I was perfectly happy to join in. This was not an aversion so much as a failure to connect. What got me off were the numinous aspects of choral singing in church, with the echo and the darkness and the empty vaulted spaces in which both sounds and imagination could run and play. There were girls in the choir, too, other than my sisters. And candles.

There are Christmas carols and there are Christmas carols. Oddly enough, the largest yet most inscrutable category is the category of blockbuster carols, the ones everyone beyond a certain age knows and can sing without thinking and which may only be fairly judged according to the deviations of your personal sentimentalism. In some respects the blockbuster category transcends taste, because blockbuster carols are all good and all bad. Their impact is contingent not on their musical content but on the context in which you hear or sing them. I don't actually rate 'Hark! The Herald Angels Sing' much, either for its words or as a piece of music, but, by heaven, there is no more heartfelt sound at the end of a midnight mass than a battalion of pissed yeomen and -women giving it some stick in preparation for the chilly slither home to bed (especially when you have enough sopranos in the congregation with the swank to have a go at the most sock-it-to-me of all carol descants). Equally, 'Away in a Manger' is a puppy on paper and a stillborn puppy in the school hall. But hear it coolly sung by competent voices capable of negotiating one of the better four-part arrangements and it is utterly disarming. Or perhaps I am just my father's son.

Then there is the category of 'show' carols. These are carols which are not familiar to everyone. They are not for joining in with but for marvelling at. Yeomen beware. Only accomplished choirs can sing them; only accomplished people would wish to. It is for the rest of us to take what we can from the experience, dependent on our capacity for enjoyment of Latin or medieval English allied to complex chord voicings and metre. A full-strength show carol is always about other people.

And then there's the Hardcore Private Choker category.

Everyone has a hardcore private choker carol, don't they? In the same way that everyone has a hardcore private choker soul ballad. Surely. Having one is a prequalification for continued membership of the human race for those under retirement age – always bearing in mind that the choker carol is, by its very nature, a different beast to the choker soul ballad, because it presses different buttons using different equipment and with slightly different objectives in mind (although not nearly as different as you might think).

Mine is the Harold Darke setting of 'In the Bleak Midwinter'. Harold Darke was a composer and organist who gave lunchtime recitals on Mondays in a church in the City of London for more than half of the last century; a bald, scholarly, kindly-looking man of the sort I wouldn't mind becoming one day (but won't, being neither scholarly nor having the right-shaped head). He also stood in for Boris Ord as organist at King's College Chapel in Cambridge during the Second World War. He died in my home town when I was sixteen, although I didn't know it at the time. If I had, I'd have broken off from whatever self-regarding activity I was currently engaged in and sought out the funeral. I'd have dressed smartly and hung discreetly at the back, hoping they'd got a choir in. I'd have made myself respectable as a mark of respect.

The words to 'In the Bleak Midwinter' were written by Christina Rossetti in a Christmas poem first published after her death and most famously set to music by Gustav Holst. That's the version you sang in school – a nice enough tune if a bit four-square and folksy. It is, at least, easy to sing. The Darke version is easy to sing too, but is anything but four-square and folksy. You've certainly heard it if you've ever tuned in to the *Nine Lessons and Carols* broadcast every Christmas Eve from King's. My mum always had it on in the kitchen while doing her Christmas Eve catering. Always. The holiest of all days in the calendar would be properly consummated at midnight, but the *Nine Lessons and Carols* at four o'clock in the afternoon was the leg-up, the boost which shoved you into the heart of Christmas. I would always make it into the kitchen in time for that, although I'd sometimes be chased out again.

The Decca record company owns the definitive recorded version of the *Nine Lessons*, in the same way that it owns the definitive version of '(I Can't Get No) Satisfaction'. It was committed to tape in 1962 when King's choir rejoiced under the direction of David Willcocks, another kindly organ scholar who became synonymous with the King's sound in the way that Keith Richards is synonymous with the sound of the Rolling Stones.

Willcocks' recording of 'In the Bleak Midwinter' is far from technically perfect. Consonants pop right, left and centre in a way that would not be countenanced by a producer of popular music, then or now, and microphone placement in the chapel was such that the performance reaches the ear as if across a mountain range through a cloud, which is certainly not how it reaches the ear in the chapel. The sound is toppy, underpowered at the bottom and vague, even puffy, in the midrange. There's even a hint of tape hiss, suggesting that recording levels were set too low. And so I reject, utterly, the value of perfection.

Perfection is an irrelevance, anyway. The Darke/Willcocks 'Bleak Midwinter' is a distillation of tenderness. Not the tenderness of close familiarity but of another kind: the transcendent tenderness associated with the toils and exhaustion of new birth, as meditated upon by Thomas Traherne, longed for by Gerald Finzi, imagined by Christina Rossetti.

The poem locates the reader/listener/singer not in the stable, nor in adjacent fields, and certainly not in some advantageous theatrical position, watching events unfold from the front stalls, but in his own space in the here and now, looking back in his mind. This is explicitly an *imagined* bleak, snowbound midwinter of the distant past, an imagined stable, an imagined frosty wind stirring the hinges of an inadequate stable door; and angels and archangels 'may have gathered there'. On the other hand they may not. Because, for Rossetti, the beauty in this conjured event is that it is all 'enough for Him': the breast full of milk, the manger full of hay, the ox and ass and camel, which adore. The entire scenario is a projection of the wonder and sufficiency of childbirth, and there is no real attempt made to differentiate between this birth and any other birth which has taken place over the past two millennia. On the contrary, this birth is the universal one. It is only incidental that cherubim and seraphim may have thronged the air.

The effect of this is twofold. Firstly it fixes the act of imagination, not the events taking place in the imagined scene, as the sacramental act; secondly, it seals the psychological integrity of the poem. You may inhabit it with absolute confidence, because what the poem describes is not figurative but real and universal. The poem describes the act of thinking, and having authentic feelings, about something; something which on this occasion just happens to have been a divine event as well as a biological one. It articulates feelings as if they are real and being experienced here, now, and only in this way. And we can all, as Curtis Mayfield once observed, get behind that. That is the essence of soul.

And the music?

The Darke/Willcocks setting establishes itself with a fragile intensity Rossetti would have doubtless found agreeable. You'd expect an organist to make a big deal out of the organ accompaniment, but Darke doesn't do that. The organ – high, tip-toeing notes – comes in like a creeping chill. To listen is to watch frost form; the phrase is tiny, cold, brittle. Then, after six seconds, *ping*! A solo boy's voice. Or is it three or six of them (the score says 'trebles')? He, or they, are singing one of the great cradling melodies by an English composer, singing in unison in the disciplined Willcocksian style, without affect, winged with fifteenth-century reverb, modulating dolefully through 'snow on snow' as if the cold is starting to bite, then following a methodical scale step by step up the syllables of the title phrase to a sustained plateau for the final cadence of the first verse: 'Lo-o-o-ong ago.'

The echo decays.

Then the ship launches. It is the most beautiful launch in all English music, the whole choir surging under full canvas: 'Our God, heaven cannot hold Him, nor earth sustain . . .' The joy of it is like wind in the face. Yet it isn't even the best bit. That comes after the interrupted cadence at the end of the third verse, which has been sung by tenors and basses and apparently closed off by the organ.

'What can I give him, poor as I am?'

The re-entry of the boys at this point is so stunning in its guttering delicacy that I am not sure I can find a way to write about it. Perhaps it would be easier simply to wonder whether art has ever possessed the power and subtlety to express the idea of tenderness in a way that corresponds with the experience of the emotion. If it has, then I haven't felt it. For me, this is as close as it has ever got. There is no Nativity painted by a Renaissance master which will give you such quiet, and no poem which can, with words alone, describe the sufficiency of such a feeling. It is as if, at the end of the carol, it is time for the words to run out.

'Yet what I can I give him: give my heart.'

12

Six weeks.

They said I would get my hearing back in six weeks or not at all.

After five weeks I was back in hospital. Not Bart's this time but the Royal London in Whitechapel, its twin, where cables hang from holes in the ceilings of corridors decorated with empty-eyed sitters, and every space that isn't a corridor is a partitioned void.

I sat at an angle in one such space with my head cocked against the partitioning, looking at the doctor diagonally. The doctor looked at his computer, at the space on the floor in between us, at my wife. He looked in my ear. He made me stand up as straight as I could manage with my eyes closed and caught me when I began to fall.

'We just can't say,' he said, with an effort at kindness. 'It is literally impossible to say. All that can be said is that it was either viral or vascular, the cause; and that we have to wait and see what happens. As regards the return of your hearing, I wouldn't hold your breath once we go beyond the six weeks . . .'

I hadn't been holding my breath, just flipping my ear. We had grown accustomed to no news, no views, no diagnosis, no prognosis, no attempt to address how I might be feeling, no way of knowing anything or having anything to hang on to. We were inhabiting another kind of void. Jane was really angry by now.

She drove home as smoothly as she could, taking the big roads to avoid speed bumps, while I kept my head wedged and my eyes fixed on as distant a point as can be found at dusk in Bethnal Green. I did not throw up. I went straight back to bed and slept.

I was woken by Jane clutching the phone. 'It's the doctor at the hospital . . .'

'Look,' the doctor said, 'there's one more thing we can try. I've spoken to the consultant and he thinks it may be worth a go. It's an American treatment. It's ideally carried out right at the start of the problem and it's been, what? . . . five weeks? Hmm. Well, you have nothing to lose really, and I'd like you to feel as if everything has been tried that could be tried. Can you come in the day after tomorrow?'

Two days later I found myself flat on a hospital gurney, listening to my mother's voice. She was up in London reinvesting her role as a mum and doing it with panache – cooking, cleaning, coralling children, making decisions, making me do the crossword with her. (I had been complaining that I couldn't think properly any more, let alone read books.) She had even worked out the local Turkish grocers and had already struck up a relationship with one of them. But now she was making bracing conversation with the doctor, as a mother would whose son is prostrate before her, rigid with fear.

'Well, it will hurt a bit,' the doctor was saying to us both. 'But not as much as you probably think it's going to.' Then just to me: 'The important thing is that you keep absolutely still.'

Okay.

'Tip your head slightly. That's it. Right. I'm going in now. Keep still. You'll feel two pricks. One is to let the air out of your eardrum, the other is to get the steroid in through the drum to your inner ear. Don't worry, the holes should heal quickly, without too much soreness, and with only a small chance of infection. But you'll have to grit your teeth a bit – it takes about twenty seconds to get it all in. And it'll feel cold . . .'

The chances are that you will not be familiar with the sensation of having a quantity of steroids injected directly into your inner ear through the membrane of your eardrum. It is singular. Never mind the pain – he was right: the thought of the needle going through the eardrum was more excruciating than the experience of it. But the steroids going in was not nice. The human head is a sacred chamber and it is a sacrilege for it to be turned into Baked Alaska. Nevertheless, as my innermost cavity filled with chilly curls of whipped steroid, and terror and revulsion combined to generate heat prickles all over my scalp, a fatuous pudding was what I became. I lay there as if on a rack fresh out of the oven.

My mother's silence was eloquent. She didn't move from her position somewhere to my right. What is to be done in such circumstances? What can be said? I was instructed to stay absolutely immobile for thirty minutes and then the ice-cream man withdrew without further comment. I kept my head exactly where it was, face up, reluctant to disturb its new filling even slightly.

'Well done,' my mum said quietly after a while. 'Luckily, I couldn't see what he was doing. But I could tell from your feet what you were feeling.'

Mothers are like that.

*

Six weeks came and went. The ice cream in my head achieved nothing, as I knew it would. I don't know how I knew, but I knew. Perhaps it was the hullabaloo in my brain, which was getting louder and more insistent, more confident, like the bully who sees that resistance is dwindling and takes larger and larger handfuls of what he can get, because he can. Furthermore, the eel music underneath the hullabaloo was fading. In fact, now I came to think about it, it had disappeared. When did it go? I certainly didn't notice it go. How come? Why? Did I say it could go?

Whose head is this anyway?

A kind friend had brought me the audiobook of *Moby-Dick*. I love the idea of *Moby-Dick* and Melville's prose is, to say the least, oceanic, but over the years I'd tried and failed to hook myself into the thing three times. How come? It's an amazing novel – everything you could want in a story about a man pursuing a whale-sized obsession. A monster. An unassailable monster. What is it with whale-sized books? Does it always follow that as body mass increases so pace slows unbearably? Something to do with resistance. Or was the book simply too heavy for my wrists? Perhaps if I listened to the words of *Moby-Dick* intoned by a sonorous American actor with a beard then I'd be able to gear my internal machinery to the tempo of the narrative. After all, I'd be lying down, not moving, eyes shut if I wanted, nothing heavy to hold up in front of my face, nothing else to do or think about. So I lay in bed and pointed my good ear at it, with the volume set as low as it would go while remaining audible.

Ten or so minutes later, the sonorous beard had become a victim of the bullying too. Gradually his vowels and his carefully enunciated actor's consonants had been assailed by waves of distorting noise, then swallowed up. It was as if the tide had come in. I could still hear his voice muttering away beneath the surface, but the effort required to decipher the words diminished my ability to interpret them. I switched the machine off, re-wedged my head and attempted to float away.

That night I dreamed that I was walking along a clifftop with my son Tom. We were burbling away happily about nothing much. And then I realised that he wasn't with me any more. He'd disappeared. All I could see were sky, sea and the grass running up to the edge of the cliff. I ran, choking, to the edge and looked over, and there he was, four feet down and climbing purposefully towards the beach; perfectly safe in his own mind. Quite happy.

I bawled him out at the top of my voice. '*TO-O-OM!*' I yelled. I yelled so loudly in the dream that I woke up. I sat up, certain that my bellowing must have woken the whole street. Yet Jane was sleeping quietly and all was as calm as a pond. I obviously hadn't made the slightest noise outside the pathways of my own brain. No sound had entered my good ear. But in my head the dreamed scream had brought tube trains crashing, and they were continuing to crash.

Even dreams were no longer safe.

*

It was after that that my mind began to change. I don't know precisely what state it was changing from or what state it was moving towards, or what the process of the change entailed. But I do think that whatever was imposing the change had a lot to do with a part of me that seldom gets a look-in, let alone a run-out.

I consider my 'warrior instinct' to be something of a theoretical construct. Generally speaking, I am not very inclined to believe in it. But if it does exist in some small way, it is certainly not to be confused with that rabid part of my personality which cadences into action when my sense of injustice is aroused. That is the berserker bit. I'm familiar with that. The berserker is the part of myself that I have learned to suppress and laugh at, except on the occasions when it has been required to Do Good. And I don't remember any of those. On the vast majority of occasions that the ginger beard worn by my inner Viking has got all foam-flecked, the results have been unhelpful and mildly shaming. I'm talking about road rage here. Local Education Authority Rage and Hackney Council Rage, which is always justified in the moment but regretted afterwards.

The warrior instinct, if it exists at all, is different to the berserker one. It is much more calculated, colder, calmer, more occlusively single-minded. Ruthless. It is never rabid. Nor does it occupy a very large or conspicuous area of my psyche. I am about as attuned to the nature of my secret warrior as I am to the inner lives of sheep I have never met.

But there is some evidence that the warrior may exist. I remember him – or what I assume to be him – emerging darkly from the fog of nerves when I used to play cricket to a reasonable standard, long ago. And I did have to go into battle once in a supermarket, when an extremely disturbed person needed sorting out. The warrior emerged unbidden then and did what needed doing.

And now, after two months' bed-bound misery, I had had enough of this shit.

I decided that I would do what any rational Saxon housecarl would do when he is no longer in a position to stand up straight or sit unsupported, walk fluently, see clearly, hear properly or countenance any sound louder than the intimate scrape of a turning page. I decided to go to the football.

Jane has since rationalised this decision as the neurotic reflex of a tightwad: I simply couldn't bear the waste of my Arsenal season ticket. And it's true. I was missing game after game after game. Other people were using my ticket, to sit on my seat at the Emirates among my friends. Unbearable. But there was more to it than that: something quite weird and atavistic in the impulse. It was an arousing feeling. There was a cold rush in the very thought of it.

Fuck. Yes. Football. That would hurt.

Let's do it.

The arrangement was that Jane would drop me as close to the

ground as she could get in the car, and that I would ring at the first sign of trouble and she would then come and pick me up. If I was outside the ground when trouble presented itself, then all well and good and I'd be fine to make the call on my own. If I was inside the ground, however, I'd have to get one of my chums to do it, because there wasn't a butterball's chance in hell of me distinguishing words bellowed in my ear by my immediate neighbour, let alone a tiny voice inside a Nokia, not in the middle of all that uproar. We decided that at all events I would leave the ground at half-time, call home and she'd come and pick me up from the police cordon in Drayton Park and I would probably regret it for the rest of my days, but what the hell.

So I donned earplugs, headphones and a thick woolly hat that covered the lot, heaved myself out of the car on Highbury Hill and shuffled with two sticks towards the stadium, bent like a tiny cripple in a strange hat in a crowd in a painting by Bruegel.

There is something emotionally ravaging about not being able to stand up straight, or at least as straight as you normally would (I have a slight stoop at the best of times). It is wounding to the point of humiliation. Not for nothing do we straighten our backs when we are beset. We straighten them and we face down whatever it is that's coming. Our pride is in our straightened backs. It is literally there, in the electricity between the vertebrae. But if you absolutely can't straighten your back, not without falling over, and you need to curl your body forward so that your centre of cranial gravity is located for optimum steadiness and balance at a point directly above the quadrilateral space created by two legs and two sticks, then your pride has to go the long way round. You are that tiny cripple in a mad hat.

I shuffled and shuffled. Squinted. Sucked in the burger stench. I adopted the language the warrior would understand. I used it out loud to myself, quietly, as a warrior would.

'Come on, you cunt. Come on. This is fucking *easy*.' And as I approached the stadium a new thought formed.

Oh no. They search bags. You can't take stuff into the ground, least of all weapons or things that might be used as a weapon, like gnarly old walking sticks. They'll have my sticks off me. I'll have to go straight home. Jesus, after all this . . .

At which point a familiar burly figure in a luminous steward's jacket disengaged himself from the thicket around turnstile D and approached at a saunter.

'Yes, all right, sir?' he said.

Oh well. Here we go. Wonder if he'll bother to be polite? Wonder what he's been trained to say? How will I convince him that I am not going to use my sticks to belabour fellow Gooners? Will the fact that I am bent at an angle of fifty degrees convince him that I am not a danger to other fans? Wonder if any of my friends are in the queue? If so, maybe the stewards would hang on to the sticks while I get walked into the ground in the manly grip of Matt or Paul or Kevin? I could pick the sticks up again when I come out at half-time. Yes, that would make sense . . .

'All right, sir, here we go.' And I felt a hand on my shoulder. 'Easy now. Would you like some more help?'

Oh. Right. No, I'm fine, thanks. Just a bit slower than usual. Um, so you're not going to take the sticks off me then?

'*Wha*'? 'Course not. Okay, here we go . . .'

And the steward, one arm out in front clearing a path, the other resting protectively on my shoulder, gently shoved me through the throng to the turnstile, where he offered to put my ticket through the reader, then reached over my head to push the metal bars of the turnstile to keep the momentum going and ensure my ingress was as smooth as a greased baby's.

Once inside, tears came suddenly like a sneeze. They came because of the steward's gentleness and kindness; and because this is what it is to be handicapped. There was a kind of reeling self-pity in the tears.

I waited for them to dry in the gents, facing the wall, as warriors do, then made my way to my seat where football convention required that no verbal fuss was made. Instead I was patted a lot and given plenty of elbow room. It felt churlish to point out that elbow room was the last thing I needed. What was actually desirable was a jovial cramming together, so that I'd be clamped in an upright position. But what can you do?

The hubbub in the stadium before kick-off was grotesque. It took me straight back to the corrugated iron and chickenwire in Bart's car park, a lashing, metallic turbulence seething around the interior of my dome in waves. While I wobbled and grinned and nodded as if I had a clue what they were saying, Matt, Paul and Kev filled me in on everything I'd missed in the season so far, against the background chat of 60,000 other souls.

Splash crash lash. Nod. Grin.

Football hubbub, by its nature, is fervent and slightly edgy. But it is still hubbub. It is the incoherent sound of many voices having their say, rising and falling, weaving and counter-weaving, plaiting and unplaiting, according to the moment-by-moment expediencies of making yourself understood in a busy social environment. It is a chaotic sound and the auditory signal is complex: jagged, spidery, unpredictable, broken, many-layered. A drawing of the sound would not be coolly architectural but a child's angry scribble. And that is what causes me grief. It is not the amplitude of the noise that does my head in but the complex irregularity of the signal. Six voices rabbiting over supper is worse than any pneumatic drill; a scrunched crisp packet hurts more than a car alarm. And 60,000 football voices hubbubing is not significantly different to dinner-table chat or the kind of low-level rhubarb you get in art galleries, except in the details of tone and volume. To my brain all three are equally excruciating. My brain does not do tone any more, and it doesn't do headcounts. It does volume only when it has to.

At kick-off, however, football hubbub is transformed. It undergoes a radical change in nature and we enter a completely different auditory environment, as if crossing a threshold into a new room and closing the door behind us. This room is no longer defined by the random, chaotic complexity that the word 'hubbub' implies, but by the laws of chorus.

Football crowds don't sing continuously as one voice, or chant like RADA-trained Bacchae. Nothing so neat, or organised, or coherent. And thank heavens for that. But they do share a nervous system. They do respond as one to the exact same stimulus, instantly, without thought and with great passion. A tackle goes in, a player collapses, the referee awards a free kick to Wigan, the crowd goes ape. *Crash!* Just like that.

The sound the crowd makes is diffuse in detail, of course. Every imprecation you can think of is poured into the sunshine within nanoseconds of the official making his decision. But the sound is one sound. *Crash!* It is the sound of a single nervous system reacting reflexively. It is what makes being in a football crowd better than watching football matches on television: being hooked up, being wired into the system.

And, oddly enough, peculiar as it may seem and overwhelming as the reality of it was, once the match started and the volume level in the stadium increased to operational norms, I felt less pain: the noise in my head appeared to be less obtrusive, less belligerent, more companionable. It was still there, of course, and growing exponentially with every roar. But there was a focused rhythm to the communal bellyaching that was almost soothing. I seemed to *notice* the discomfort less, even as it crashed through my head like a train. For now there was a general neural connection. We were joined. Every time anything of any consequence happened on the pitch, the connection would be made and my nervous system would either fire or spasm in chorus with everyone else's, spreading load, obliterating self-consciousness, dissipating pain. It is not hard to see why crowds act like crowds, rather than as agglomerations of individuals: our nervous systems are soothed by unanimity. It is, in large part, in our individual interests to submit to the general sensibility. It feels good because, neurally, it *is* good.

Then half-time came and we returned to the agonies of hubbub. I tottered off towards the exit and to thank the steward again, were I to see him, for his help. Once safely wedged into a whitewashed elbow in the Emirates concourse I thumbed Jane's number. I intended to tell her I'd be at the police cordon in ten minutes and I'd see her there – and that, well, it had been excruciating but definitely worth the effort. Hooray for life and so on.

Instead, I told her that I was going to stay for the second half.

*

Boxers talk about how a really good punch will set off an explosion inside your head. And then the lights go out. It is as if the delivery of the punch and the receipt of the punch are two events and the explosion is a third one. It is not a pain that you feel on the point of your chin, but a discrete event that takes place inside your skull as a consequence of the punch, disconnected in feeling from the point of impact. *Boof!* Afterwards, you do not remember the punch landing.

Similarly, after labouring prettily for nine tenths of the match against a resolute Wigan defence, Arsenal scored, their captain William Gallas burying a header. I know this because that is what I was told, but I can't actually remember the ball hitting the net. What I remember is the explosion in my head as the crowd reacted. The neural jolt. And I remember the lights flickering, and I remember being caught by Matt, who thought he was giving me a hug.

Afterwards, he walked me up the flank of Highbury Hill to where Jane waited in the car. I was high as a kite. Deaf as a post, squinty, unsteady as a pig on a frozen mere. But high as a kite. It was as high as I have ever been legally. I went straight to bed and stayed there for four days.

13

One evening in 1963 I awoke in an awful state. I could not breathe. I could not see very well either – the room was dark and I was delirious. I was not sure what was going on. I certainly dared not move.

There was a dog that lived under my bed, a nasty little one with devilish facial fur. It had the dimensions of a Scottie, but the instincts of an alligator. The fur radiated from its snout in curved and tapering metallic blades which cut skin on contact, like butter; I would sometimes hear the points of the blades tapping on the bed springs when the creature stirred during the night. Inside the dog's mouth were rows of needle-sharp yet weirdly tiny teeth. I knew that if I ever tried to get out of bed within snapping range of the dog then I was done for. The secret to survival was to leap well clear. A good two feet. Because the one sure thing about the dog was that it would never venture so far out from under the bed as to expose its rear end. I did not know why it had this vulnerability.

But on this occasion I lacked the strength to make the leap. It was simply impossible because I was consumed by the whooping cough. I ached all over; movement of any kind was out of the question. I was trapped. So I called for my mother. Over and over again I bleated, whined, choked, coughed and spluttered, as I struggled to get air in and out without succumbing to the whoops, which were racking and pinning my body down like a giant's heavy hand. For long minutes the bleating was fruitless. My blood cooked. But I did not give up. Children of three do not imagine what death is like because they are preoccupied with an even greater fear, which is that they will not be heard.

My mother did hear – in the end. She came up and laid a damp flannel on my head, calmed me down, stroked my hair and then leaned over to kiss me good night again. And as she did so her black mohair cardigan flopped down towards my face, its large buttons heavy like plates. I breathed in the mohair, or seemed to. The fibres stuck in my windpipe. I choked once more and the giant's hand pressed me down and down until I thought I might be pushed all the way through the mattress and springs of the bed into the cavity below where the dog waited for me in darkness, panting.

I have been terrified of cardigans ever since. Can't be in the same room as them.

I was not properly ill again for eleven years, discounting bouts of boy-flu and the occasional pox. And then, when I was fourteen, I went down with a kidney infection and was sent to bed for ten days.

Yawnsville.

Well, I say that, but actually there is only one place a fourteen-year-old boy would rather be than lying in his bed, and that's lying in a bed belonging to a girl. Well, I say *that*, but things are never quite so straightforward, are they? At least being ill in your own bed isn't challenging or frightening. You know what you're doing when you're ill in bed, and where you are, and the chances of making a fool of yourself are small. Also, it gives a fellow time to think, explore himself, listen to records.

So I did. I became expansive in my inertia. I decided that I would make the utmost of my situation by listening deeply and systematically to everything I had in my small but growing record collection, and by calling in as much music as I could from my friends. I would penetrate music to new depths. I would become more accomplished. This was an opportunity not to be missed.

'Well, you can borrow *Burn* again,' said Lorry balefully. Borrowing records from Lorry was like punching yourself in the face. It was both painful and virtually impossible to do, and ultimately fatuous. 'No way, man,' he'd say if you had the naked front to ask. His man-of-the-world chuckle would then shade into a menacing scowl: 'I need to keep everything to hand at all times. And besides, if you think I'm going to let you play my albums on that piece of shit you call a stereo, you're out of your mind. That thing *destroys* vinyl.'

It was true that my record player was not as impressive as his. In fact, it was terrible. But still, I found his attitude mystifying, even wounding, especially given that he was always prepared to loan out *Burn*, the most recent album by Deep Purple. Lorry liked Deep Purple rather more than I did and so the logic of the loan was obscure. Perhaps he figured that he stood to lose less if he could be confident that my enjoyment of the thing would be limited. Or maybe he just despised the new singer in Deep Purple, who we all agreed was a tit.

So I borrowed *Burn* again, plus a small handful of albums from Andy that wouldn't cause him undue pain to be parted from for a week or so. I couldn't raise anything from Cuthbert and Thompson at school because, well, they were at school and I was at home. *Burn* it was, plus Barclay James Harvest, Früup and Yes's new LP, *Relayer*, which I had not yet raised the funds to get for myself. Andy had been given it for Christmas by Linda and I'd listened to it round at his house already. I'd been impressed by its uncompromising nature and its muted grey Roger Dean artwork, which hinted at paths out from confined spaces. Musically, it was spiky right from the off. In fact, before the singer, Jon Anderson, got to sing so much as a snatch of melody, the rest of the ensemble had already modulated through half a dozen key changes, at least as many time changes, and seeded a crop of modal scales which thrust upwards from their roots like knives.

Excellent.

The opening song of the three-track *Relayer* was 'The Gates of Delirium'. It occupied the entire first side of the record: not really a song at all; more a piece, twenty-two minutes of it. Better and better. I had all the time in the world. I hauled myself out of bed to impale the disc reverently on my clunky Marconiphone, flumped back under the duvet and assumed the posture.

It was my habit in those days to lie down to listen to music, even when not ill. This was partly because a year of going to gigs at the Corn Exchange had taught me that supine was the approved listening posture for freaks. It made sense, too. The imagination will gape wider if the body is neutralised. Plus it's comfy. Also, I found that lying down made it easier to concentrate on the buildings in my head; and then, having conducted the statutory room-by-room search, to flit into my other favoured listening mode, that of participant.

I was an accomplished recumbent air guitarist. I could never bring myself to do it standing up – that would be silly – but on my back and with my eyes closed tightly to abrogate the dull familiarity of my bedroom, I was a master of the pinch harmonic and hammer-on: an expressive artist not a masturbator. I liked best to stand in for Mick Taylor of the Rolling Stones, both in the studio and in front of stunned crowds – me and Keith rocking impassively together like brothers, my lyric-poet sensibilities bringing a certain romanticism to bear on his gutty swagger.

Yet I could find no way into Yes's guitarist. None whatsoever. I lay there with my features contorted in a rictus of creative pain, the guitar strapped high across my chest like his, but found that the substitution would not take. Steve Howe is a technician of outstanding severity, an ascetic, a virtuoso capable of many things, nearly all of them difficult-sounding. I could not be him even with practice, not in a million years. In 'The Gates of Delirium' he rips impossible-sounding squalls of notes from his fat Gibson just like a heavy jazz guy, but not jazzily. No warming blue notes in here, please, thank you. Or swing. Just edge. Edge after edge after edge, of which Howe's edges are merely the frontal ones – the ones you encounter first. Beyond him, the density of the music suggests a deep forest of moving parts, teeming and growing pitilessly, with no way out for the enclosed wanderer, no end in sight, no horizon, a forest expanding ahead of you like the universe, inexhaustibly.

So it comes as a balm when, after something like fifteen minutes of this, the teeming is relieved by a sudden drop away into no-time and an attenuated series of swooshy keyboard chords, out of which Howe rises again like a wiry spirit on his lap steel. At last, some *tune*. Then the voice reappears and glides off the steel with choirboy lightness and words about the inevitable coming of spiritual enlightenment – 'soon, oh soon' – just ahead at the rim of the trees. In fact, we are now standing facing outwards on the edge of the forest, breathing deeply in the cool vapour of cosmic time, gulping, sucking in . . . until a key-change brings in an organising backbeat for a few bars and the sudden arrival of a final upward-resolving cadence.

And that's it.

'The Gates of Delirium' is extraordinary. It is elaborate beyond necessity, complex beyond desire. That four young Englishmen and a Swiss should want to do something like that with the prime of their youth says almost as much as you could want to know about what northern-European rock culture thought was important in the middle of 1974: twenty-two minutes of unbroken, highly finished, ultra-complex *effort*, enshrining how many hours, days, weeks of work and fight and optimism? Bitterness, competition and hatred, too, I shouldn't wonder. There is something noble in its overreach, as well as indulgent; something almost farcical in its determination to open and close doors. I care not that its haughty agitation of the listening ear reveals its origins to be middle-class and educated, as well as almost parodically fin de siècle (for these were the very 'progressive' brambles which sealed off rock's first historical cycle). I care not at all. For all that the surface of 'Delirium' seethes with fantastic stuff, as a creation it makes no provision whatsoever for common sentiment. It is music without interior. It isn't even empty. To be empty, you need first to have some capacity.

Rucked up in my sweaty bed wrestling with brambles, I wondered about the ache which now permeated every thought and fibre of my body. I wondered if this is what loneliness feels like and tried to soothe the ache away by turning off the music and listening instead to the chestnut branches outside. But it didn't work.

*

Later that spring I was delighted to be invited by a village elder to 'spin some discs' at the village fete.

The fete took place every year on the recreation ground, in aid of the church fabric. The rec was unattractive and the fete was always dull, a festival of diffident meandering and poking. There were coconut shies and games which involved small children chucking huge lumps of agricultural pig iron over minute distances; pet dogs were encouraged to participate in a behaviour contest, and, more often than not, a pony would be deployed in a ring of hay bales by a member of the local gentry so that, in return for a few pence, the tinies might circle on its back for five minutes, quaking, mouths turned down at the corners. The sky was always grey and the coconuts could not be dislodged from their wire cups even with a direct hit.

But I was chuffed to be asked to DJ. This amounted to the first public recognition ever of my status as the parish's foremost music head. How can they have known?

'Throw something new in, Nick,' the elder said, winking. 'You'll have the box of the usual records, of course, and what you play should come from there mostly, because that's what people like – let's not forget that this is a public event in aid of the church roof restoration fund. But I don't mind if you include the occasional record of your own, if you think it's appropriate. And fun. You know what I mean, don't you? Of course you do. You're an intelligent lad.'

So on Saturday morning, in traditional grey light, I installed myself at the DJ console in my navy greatcoat, collar up, head down. The console consisted of a single 1950s turntable mounted in a wooden crate. To put a record on you had to approach from above and reach down into the crate to the turntable, which sat on top of its amplifier some nine or so inches below the rim. This meant barking your elbows on the splintered edge as you twisted your forearms and bent your wrists at painful angles to operate the mechanism. The tone-arm was as heavy as a cucumber. A double helix of brown flex emerged from the base of the crate and coiled up a metal pole above the DJ's head to enter, eight feet up, the back of a single PA speaker in the form of a loud-hailer. The loudhailer was welded to the top of the pole.

This rig had been put together in a shed by a local tinkerer a dozen years before out of parts which were even then grievously obsolescent. The entire contraption looked like a man-eating flower in a sci-fi B-movie (I have no doubt that, hunched at its foot, I resembled the remains of the teen freak the man-eating flower had been unable to digest). So there I sat in the lee of the men's toilets, like something that has been spat out, positioned so that the mains wire might pass from the base of the amplifier through the open window of the toilet to plug in to a socket on an inside wall of the sports pavilion. It seemed somehow inevitable that the turntable only worked at 78 and 45 rpm.

This was awkward because, naturally, I had brought along a bag of LPs with which to enlighten the meandering throng – you know, to really get everyone off for once, to shake them out of their diffidence; maybe even to make girls come over to my console. Nothing too radical of course. Even then I was a sensitive soul and knew that 'The Gates of Delirium' was not for people buying cakes. But I did think that 'Bad Bad Boy', 'Walk on the Wild Side', 'Whole Lotta Love', 'The Jean Genie' and some of the more jauntily pastoral bits of Genesis might help to move things along a little. And, of course, there was 'Layla'. Everyone loves 'Layla' – or at least, they do once they've heard it a couple of times.

But I possessed those songs in long-playing form only and the machine only worked at 45 and 78. Which, with two exceptions, left me with the box of 45s provided by the fete organisers, and there was absolutely no way I was going to play 'Chirpy Chirpy Cheep Cheep', 'Mouldy Old Dough' and 'Tie a Yellow Ribbon'. No way. So after I'd played both sides of the first of the only two 45s I had brought along in my bag – Ace's admirable if unexciting 'How Long' – I had to resort to 'It's Only Rock 'n' Roll (But I Like It)' by the Rolling Stones. Only moments before, the church bell had struck ten to signal the grand opening by the retired Dean of a leading Cambridge college, who lived in the village.

It's a factoid seldom acknowledged, and apparently only foggily recalled by those who were there at the time, that 'It's Only Rock 'n' Roll (But I Like It)' only has two serving Rolling Stones on it: Mick and Keith. The bits that aren't Mick and Keith – which amounts to quite a lot of it – were put together in Ron Wood's basement in Richmond by some other people. At least, that's how one version of the story goes.

Wood was still a member of The Faces at the time, but he had been busily chiselling out a home-made solo album with a bunch of mates, as you did in those days. 'It's Only Rock 'n' Roll' arose from a slovenly two-chord acoustic guitar riff devised by Ron and filled out by Faces drummer Kenney Jones and the American session bassist Willie Weeks into something resembling an archetypal Stones groove. The details of precisely how this skeleton of an idea evolved from casual weekend knock-off to full-blown Rolling Stones hit is naturally lost to ravaged memory, but it would seem, in this account, that during the course of Mick and Keith's participation in the solo project round at Ron's, Keith and/or Mick took a shine to the basic track and took possession, as you're permitted to do when you're Keith and/or Mick. The somewhat lo-fi home-recorded Wood/Weeks/Jones rhythm was duly smeared with claggy layers of additional guitar, Jagger hacked out some disjointed, sarcy lyrics addressing the relationship that barely exists between a rock and roller and his critics, and lo, a Rolling Stones record lurched half-dressed and unsteady on its feet out into the middle of Richmond Road.

In some ways it's a frightful piece of work. But in other ways it is a work of genius. The finished record is murky, harmonically vague, slow and squished – there are so many layers of bounced-down instrumentation on the thing the music sounds as if it has been a victim of geological time: still wriggling just about, but close to succumbing to the pressure of all the weight piled on top of it. The melody, such as it is, is a modal plank balanced on the chords of E major and A, relieved with the odd passing reference to G and D (the easiest four chords for a guitarist to play when he's pissed and stoned); the singing is one long emetic groan with a bellowed chorus and yelps in both voice and guitar parts to suggest that, really, everyone is having a tremendous time in here – how about you? 'It's Only Rock 'n' Roll' passes through the listener's mind like a cortège of drunks. It is a record I love so much I would like it played at my funeral.

And by 10.15 that spring morning, immediately following the Dean's short speech, I had played it three times in succession over the PA and was beginning to warm to this DJ-ing lark.

'Said, aaaah know-wuh . . . 'sonly rock 'n' roll-uh, buh ah laik-i', laik-i', yessaaah *dooo!*'

It was soon after the start of the fourth iteration of this first chorus that the village elder approached, smiling. 'Well, Nick. I was wondering whether you might get around to playing any of the other records – the ones in the box . . .'

'Um, yes. I mean no. I mean yes. Um. But they're not very good, you know. I'm not sure that anyone wants to hear "Mouldy Old Dough" any more. And I've never heard of Frank Ifield . . .'

'Well, I can't say any of it's up my street, either. But well, you know, it is a bit *shouty*, this record you're playing, and it is getting a little repetitious, hearing it over and over again. Especially at this volume. We have other people to consider, you know –'

I must have looked as stricken as I felt. I felt trapped. My features prickled all over, as if I had pins and needles in my face. How do I get out of this one? There was a principle at stake, after all. I could not possibly, in all conscience, play 'Mouldy Old Dough' and 'Chirpy Chirpy Cheep Cheep'; and yet neither could I desert my post nor offer a viable alternative other than forty consecutive plays of 'It's Only Rock 'n' Roll' – which would have been fine by me but, well, there were other people to consider, many of them quite elderly.

'Well, I did see "Needles and Pins" by the Searchers in the box,' I blustered, 'and I've a feeling that that may be all right – I think I've heard it before. I'll play that. But, but . . .'

'Look, tell you what, Nick,' the elder said through his smile, which had ossified into a sort of facial exoskeleton, 'if you're troubled by all this, why don't I see if someone would like to take over from you. I know it's all a bit square, the fete, and pretty boring, and I'm sure I've never heard of Frank Ifield either. So why don't you leave it with me and I'll see what I can do? In the meantime,' he added on the half-turn, 'do you think you might see your way to changing the record now? I mean *right* now?'

By the time 'Needles and Pins' had come to an end my place by the toilet had been taken by the traditional fete DJ, who had to pass the care of his pig iron-chucking stall on to another family member and looked about as pleased about it as a man can when his brand new vision has been ruined by the weakness and narcissism of others.

14

Cambridge in the 1960s and 1970s admitted the modern world grudgingly. It is less grudging in the twenty-first century, but I suspect that that is partly because what serious damage can be done to it by modernity – if damage is what it is – has all been done already. The city is a living, breathing, choking experiment in radical traffic management. New housing estates have spread like metastasising cancers outwards into the fen. The ring of satellite villages, which for centuries were divided from the city by open fields, is being drawn into the main body as the green belt is sold off for development.

My old village is no longer separate. It has become a suburb. The psychiatric hospital has been subsumed, the majority of its buildings now forming the hub of a vast business park and housing estate conjoining village and city. The hospital's strange central tower, which once stood as proud of the surrounding fields as a grain silo on an American prairie, is now just one perpendicular among many. New roads snake all around.

Lorry's dad was a nurse at the institution adjoining the hospital, the one which bled the hospital campus into the village: a sprawling residence for mentally handicapped juveniles. His mum and sister Julie worked there too for a while. It has been closed for a couple of decades. The handicapped people now occupy what was once the hospital's dormitory estate with the nursing staff who look after them in cohabitative attendance, and that includes the house where Lorry grew up. New eyes stare out from Lorry's bedroom window into what used to be Jackie Copsey's boudoir.

These are the margins of Cambridge life, the frayed edges. It is probable that the edges are no more nor less frayed in the twenty-first century than they were forty years ago, when strays from the hospital would occasionally attempt to batter our back door down in a haze of terror and alienation, looking for home, no doubt. I'm certainly willing to bet that the essential character of central Cambridge life – the life lived at the heart of the city, where the fabric is strong and as stain-resistant as it ever was – has not changed at all. Cambridge really does have much to preserve, after all. As well as lovely buildings and ancient streets, it has an ethos, a way of life, a purpose, a purview, a tradition which serves to neuter the effects of passing time. Cambridge has only got rid of the bits which are not profitable.

You have to go back a bit to witness the start of it. For instance, the half-timbered medieval warren which gave excitingly on to the semi-popular shopping street next to Boots, called Petty Cury, was pulled down in the early Seventies and replaced by a multi-storey car park and shopping mall. A classic of the carbuncle genre if ever there was one, it is as ugly and contaminating now as it was in 1971. Nevertheless, that car park, in all its brutalist novelty, serves as the setting for a jointly held but independently experienced memory of almost immeasurable import to me and to one of my friends.

We weren't friends at the time; we didn't even know of each other's existence. Nevertheless, I vividly recall, as does Rob, being on the upper floors of the car park at Christmas 1972, me sliding into the family car in a pubescent funk after being taken to the pantomime at the Arts Theatre. At the same moment and in the same place Rob was up there 'hanging around with David Joyce', for reasons that escape him now. The higher levels of the car park gave a direct view over cold concrete bastions straight down through the windows on to the stage of the Corn Exchange over the road. Both Rob and I have transfixing memories of the muffled roar that billowed through the glass and out into the night air over Corn Exchange Street, and of the partially visible – in fact, headless – shape of a spotlit checked shirt and electric guitar bobbing on the stage forty feet below. I can hear the boom now, edgeless as fog but as exciting as a storm. I can still see Rory Gallagher's Stratocaster and shirt. And so can Rob, who has enshrined the memory in the same way that I have. That would have been four or five years before he and I actually met. For each of us, it was our first encounter with live rock 'n' roll.

Another exploitable part of the city was the run-down kite-shaped area of scruffy housing to the east of the centre, which was known to everyone, funnily enough, as the Kite. By the time I was venturing into town on my own in 1974, the Kite had evolved into a maze of sub-Bohemian squats, bookshops and hippie eateries mingled with a few remnant renters and roofless shells. A significant number of the houses were occupied by people who had been born in them but did not own them.

Back then I used to skirt the area out of sheer uncertainty. What happens in the Kite? Was I welcome there? If not, what might happen to a skinny boy intruder who doesn't know what he's doing? Does Cambridge have a *dark* side? Nevertheless, the rush of confidence which came with turning sixteen allowed me to succumb to the allure of cheap foreign food and scraggy people with too much to say for themselves, their music, their scented candles, their hive lighting schemes created by carefully deployed ethnic scarves, and by the obvious proximity of their drugs. And so I scratched the Kite's surface for a couple of years as one does an insignificant itch, just for the pleasure of it.

It was a brief exaltation. Following a couple of decades' struggle, the city council and Jesus College finally got their way and flattened the area to make way for another mall, every bit as hideous as the Lion Yard one, maybe more so. And that was it as far as major city-centre redevelopment went, until only recently and the wonder of the new John Lewis Xanadu. Central Cambridge's real-estate options are guarded jealously and effectively. This is because the city does not own itself. The colleges do.

There is nowhere else in the country quite like Cambridge. But then no other city in the country is owned in the way Cambridge is owned, by the yoked yet private interests of the institutions which, combined, give the city its irreducible identity. Cambridge only exists because of the university. It has no proper industry of its own (and no, I don't count the hi-tech bricolage which goes on in the name of science in 'Silicon Fen'; and I don't count the brickworks, lovely as Cambridge bricks are). The city is where it is, hiding in its low-lying spot behind a barely there chalk escarpment, only because a huffy bunch of fugitive clerics in the thirteenth century settled there, miles from civilisation, detached from the vulgar realities of high feudalism, in the avowed hope that their pursuit of knowledge might not be disturbed by, well, you know, *all that crap*. The city was conceived as a bolt-hole.

And as the colleges grew up over the medieval period and acquired royal accreditation to go with the money and influence which found their way to this obscure fen outpost, what was conceived as a bolt-hole developed into a city, with all that that word implies in the way of people, property, crime, transport, services, trade and all the other manifest unsightlinesses of urbanised society.

In the face of all that it was only to be expected that the colleges would evolve their own discrete micro-society with its own anthropology, its own hierarchies and its own way of managing money. They also owned the land; nearly all of it.

And the great thing about holding all the cards – by which I mean the land – is that you can influence to a profound degree who and what goes where and on what terms. Especially the unsightlies. You know: scurvy knaves can go and live in a housing estate over there, behind a big hedge. Mental defectives can be parked on a village somewhere else. And yonder, the best part of a mile out of town, that's where we'll build the railway station, because it would not do to make it easy for the young gentlemen to get to Newmarket.

Meanwhile, the centre of the city can be reserved for the beautiful buildings which house our beautiful thoughts.

Tidy.

And it is. Cambridge *is* a beautiful place. I can't help but love it and part of me yearns to return there, even though I left it thirty years ago vowing never to go back. But I also shudder when I remember the social organisation of the place; in particular, the strange relationship that exists between 'town' and 'gown' – the ugliest part of my socialisation, the bit I know is weird and disproportionate and somehow not *real*, not in the way most people think of reality, but which nevertheless corresponds with the sort of artificial bilateralism that Protestants and Catholics grow up with in other less privileged but equally divided environments. I am riddled with prejudice in this respect. I love Cambridge, but find it hard to like.

My parents were university employees, not members. My father graduated from Clare with an MA in Law, but he emerged from that experience firstly determined never to practise law and secondly not to spend a minute longer in his university town than was strictly necessary. Somehow, though, only a decade or so after taking his leave, he found himself back there with a middle-management job at the University Press. He'd had enough of his London commute; he evidently felt that the medieval bolt-hole he'd bolted from soon after graduation might make a good environment in which to bring up a family, and in lots of ways he was right. In due course, to thicken things up a little, my mother became assistant librarian at Magdalene College, with an additional gig upstairs looking after the private library of Samuel Pepys.

My parents were outsiders endowed with a selection of insider privileges and I don't think they were ever very easy about it. Not my dad, anyway. My mum loved her job, loved the peculiarity of the college world and its irascible denizens, inexplicable rites, extraordinary buildings, unfathomable laws. She loved having somewhere awkward to organise. Nevertheless, I was brought up in an atmosphere of wariness and circumspection regarding 'what goes on' in the world behind the high walls and studded-timber gates of the colleges. The issue was not morality but snobbery. It was not turpitude that made Coleman blood boil, but the hierarchical attitudes which serve to support such deeply rooted, charismatically traditional institutions – the same as the ones you find in royal households the world over, in the Church, the legal profession, the military, government, even in the medical world (possibly the most completely *feudal* voice I've heard in the past two years was the one belonging to the surgeon who boomed over my head in Bart's hospital). For heaven's sake, Oxford and Cambridge universities still have a servant class: these people are identified individually as 'servants' and the servants themselves rejoice in the designation. Nobody minds in the least.

To my Quakerish pa, there really wasn't that much difference between the clerical elitism which so affronted his spiritual sensibilities and the vertical social organisation of the academic world – it was as if one completed an ugly echo of the other. You could sometimes see the unease in his face; sometimes, later on, when he was an older man with a couple of stress-related coronaries to reflect upon, there was nothing at all to be seen in his face.

This was his equivalent of the thousand-yard stare. 'Hel-*lo-oh*,' we children would say perkily over supper, waving the palms of our hands in front of his face. 'Hel-*lo*! Anybody *i-i-in*?' And then he'd close his eyes, open them again and smile slowly. Very occasionally, we wouldn't even get the smile.

As you'd expect, Cambridge is teeming with the offspring of university members and employees. The city now has a population of more than 110,000 souls (perhaps a 20 per cent increase on when I lived there), a significant proportion of that number being the children of academics, researchers, publishers, printers, librarians, lab technicians, school teachers, music teachers and therapists of every discipline. The relative proportions of those groups may have changed a little since the 1960s, but not so as you'd notice. Perhaps there are now more therapists than there used to be. Whatever, the Cambridge middle class is one of the most redoubtable in existence.

They are not the same thing at all as the braying middle classes of Kensington, nor the quietly entitled professionals of Crouch End and Chiswick; they bear no relation to the kind of folk you find congratulating themselves in the Thames Valley and even less to the social adornments of Surrey. As to the elegant creatures who have made Bath into the extremely well-dressed heritage site it is today – well, you'd do well not to confuse a honey-stone Georgian backdrop with the properties of a supra-enlightened mind. Good lord, no. And that's only to list the stereotypes which crop up in your average southern stand-up comedian's class-war routine. It takes no account of Stratford-upon-Avon or Chester or Edinburgh or the nice bits of Yorkshire. Indeed, the only reason you won't have heard many jokes about the weirdos who spin the wheels in the humming engine of growth that is Cambridge is the fact that making jokes about them is fraught with risk: if you know enough about them to make jokes, then you might as well admit that you're one, too. It means you're a bright boy or girl with a Cambridge degree – or the offspring of one. It's one of the peculiarities of such an idiosyncratic and socially inaccessible place that it always takes one to know one. And it takes one to turn a blind eye, too.

Back in my day, the children of the city's elite seethed around its buildings and over its lawns and bridges like flood water. I expect they still do, their confidence as fluid and undammable as ever. I expect they all still attend Holiday Orchestra in the school holidays, too, and fuck each other senseless in their tousled beds while their parents read Flaubert on the other side of the partition wall. Whether the nuances of juvenile society are still the same is moot, though – I'm not particularly inclined to do the necessary research (for fear, in part, of disappointment that it hasn't changed at all, and in part that it has). But I bet they do snooty in exactly the same way. Cambridge snooty is special and it travels extremely well, both through space and time.

That's because it is armour-plated by its own certainties. These guys have *certificates* to prove that they're better than you are. In Cambridge, an individual's worth may always be calibrated: by college, by title, by qualification, by publications, by staircase, by seat at table, by position on shin of bicycle clip.

All right, I made the last one up. The position of your bicycle clip is entirely your own affair in Cambridge; the city is proud of its lack of snobbery in this respect, and justly so. But such is the arcana of status and preferment in the university that it is not inconceivable that once upon a morning by the Mill Pond a junior Fellow may have worn his clip a foolish inch and a half too close to the knee and forever after wondered whether this might not have been the tipping point at which a Chair began to go to ground.

What can always be said about Cambridge society is that it is not materialistic, not in the usual sense of the word anyway. Wealth is less important than academic achievement, beauty ranks lower than brains and conspicuous materialistic display is the one thing you do not do, ever, under any circumstances. Old shoes, old trousers, outdated skirt-suits, leather-capped elbows, bicycle clips – that's the deal, still. Personal elegance is deployed neither as a signifier of economic standing nor as a means of self-projection, but only as a disguise. You don your best clobber in the same spirit that a headsman puts on his hood.

Similarly, your house is a sprawling tip, your car a run-down French *wagon de la gare* and you do not go on expensive foreign beach holidays. There are those in the new Cambridge who have embraced the consumer boom of the past decade with a certain narrow-eyed enthusiasm – where, for instance, did all those vast SUVs with small blonde women at the wheel materialise from? Do they have a precedent? Really, we might as well be living in Chelmsford! – but they are an inevitable by-product of the London-suburban commuter outpress. Money doesn't talk in Cambridge, it mutters darkly.

Which is not to say that Cambridge money is hidden. On the contrary, it is everywhere to be seen. It just manifests differently. It has different priorities. Mostly it is concerned to maintain what is already there in a state of quiet, even sublime stasis. Which is one of the reasons why Cambridge was always in my day a terrifically violent town.

I was once stopped on my bike on Midsummer Common by a large youth of about my age who wanted a light. I matched him and smiled nicely, at which his eyebrows came down like twin guillotines.

'Are you a poof?' he asked.

'You what?' I replied, genuinely surprised. I'd thought we were heading in the direction of firm friendship.

'Are you a poof?' he snarled again, growing into his dismay. 'Or are you a punk?'

I had to admit he had me there – it was 1977 and I was

wearing a leather jacket twinned with a scarlet-and-pink mohair jumper over torn drainpipe jeans. My outfit yodelled ambiguity: hint of poofiness, shade of part-time punk. I made sure that the bike pedal was in launch position before replying.

'Do you know, I'm really not sure today. You choose.'

And away I flew like Hermes borne aloft on wingèd Raleigh. He nearly caught me, too: bruised the small of my back. But I didn't fall off. And in that moment I felt wholly wedded to the gown and not the town. And the gown was *not* my people. It was in that moment that I first hated Cambridge.

Cambridge divides because division is a property of its nature. On the far side of Midsummer Common from Jesus College lie a couple of the estates where the less privileged of the city live their domestic lives, away from the beautiful central area they are there to service and maintain. Back in the Seventies the Common was a highwayman's paradise – the bloody no-man's land which literally divided gilded centre from grotty suburb. And if you were caught in the middle of it after nightfall, with the wrong credentials and no back-up, then you were fair game. Everyone I knew had a story to tell, the best of them belonging to my schoolfriend Thompson, who had fallen into the hands of a marauding pack of highwaymen at dusk, submitted to the ritual kicking and then been pleasantly surprised when, mid-hoof, his principal assailant had suddenly called off the assault and helped Thompson to his feet.

'To what do I owe the honour?' Thompson probably didn't say. His assailant pointed out that he'd just realised that the two of them had been at infant school together and, given that fact, it wouldn't be right to completely rearrange Thompson's internal organs, so they'd leave it at that.

And it was on Midsummer Common, two or three years later, that the Specials played a concert to a marquee full of local neo-Mods and a large body of the group's regular travelling support.

The marquee simply wasn't big enough to get everyone in – a detachment of local skins contrived entry by slitting open the side of the tent – and the violence which ensued resulted in a couple of Specials being charged with incitement to riot and the event making the national news.

It was one ruck among many. 'Too much fighting on the dance floor' indeed. Of the several new things that Cantabrigians learnt to their dismay (or pride) from the post-riot media huffery was the statistic that Cambridge now stood as the third-ranked most violent city in the UK, measured on a per capita basis.

But that didn't stop Holiday Orchestra.

*

Nothing stands in the way of Holiday Orchestra. It still exists, I believe. And so it should, not least because the back row of an orchestra is every bit as stimulating a place for a fourteen-year-old to sit as the back row of a cinema auditorium or football ground. Holiday Orchestra was to the children of Cambridge in the 1970s what the north coast of Cornwall is to today's young Harrys and Annabels of Kensington: a summer playground; a safely familiar social environment away from parental supervision in which to make a firm impression.

I dutifully lugged a trombone to it for two or three years. I was not a very good trombonist and I didn't like the Holiday Orchestra repertoire much either, which tended to comprise the large-orchestral Romantic hits of the nineteenth-century, from Beethoven through to the Russians, plus a bit of Elgar and Holst – high-colour stuff long on tunes and oomph. Not enough badass Stravinsky, in my view, nor Monteverdi, both of which have proper work for trombonists to do. But to be fair, music didn't always seem to be the point of Holiday Orchestra.

As you'd expect, the orchestra accreted around a caucus of

seriously talented young musicians. It was probably dependent on them. These were the gifted ones who had doddled Grade Eight bassoon at the age of twelve and were already eyeing up places at the Royal College for three or four years hence. They were strange, admirable creatures who appeared to move at their own pace in their own space and at their own behest, in a nimbus of glory, as if appearing at Holiday Orchestra as a favour to everyone else. They had about them something of the ghost Elvis at an Elvis convention. Their minds and bodies were there but not there; seen but not seen. They only ever really interacted with their peers and the adult tutorial staff, whom they treated as equals and sometimes as subordinates.

But for the rest of the orchestra it was business as usual in the Cambridge style, which meant unabated hardball jostling for status. I never really got my head round all that, although it was clear that the more successful jostlers had certain attributes that others lacked: a mum and/or dad of prominence at the university, for instance, or – even better – social proximity to a Ghost Elvis. After that you were graded according to the instrument you played. This was a genuinely arcane system governed by a metaphysics which passed all village-boy understanding.

Top of the pile were cellists – don't know why, they just were – followed by first violinists (calibrated by proximity to the leader's desk), followed by the more exotic woodwinds (bassoon, cor anglais, oboe), followed by the obviously noble but suspiciously brass-coloured French horns. The next layer, the orchestral yeomanry, was composed of second violins, violas, flutes, clarinets and double basses, those humble but always well-intentioned operators without whom an orchestra would be merely a bunch of brilliant musicians. The wadding. A trumpeter of exceptional ability might aspire to join that group or even vault beyond them in virtuosic cases but, really, trumpeters ought not to get above their station because, incontrovertibly, trumpets are brass. Oiks.

All brass are oiks, but some are more oiky than others. The tuba/ euphonium is pretty low on the totem pole. Its natural habitat is the brass or military or American marching band, as a hippo- potamus's is African river valleys. But at the very bottom of the heap, next to the beaters of drums and the twanglers of triangles, lurks the trombone.

I can't for the life of me see why. Couldn't then, can't now. The trombone is a beautiful thing, a rich, sonorous, perfectly chromatic tone-cannon endowed with unmatchable weight of shot, handicapped only by a slow rate of fire. Trombones don't do fast and they don't do fiddly, but they are capable of magnifi- cent volleys of ensemble sound that lift audiences right out of their seats. They can also sing, really sing. If you want an instru- ment to suggest in a single lyric line the way a laden human spirit yearns to vault, then get a trombone in. That's what I think.

Mozart thought so, too. Well, he did on one occasion. The trombone is not an obviously Mozartian intrument, not by a long stretch, yet one of the very few great passages of lyric trom- bonery in the classical canon is *Tuba Mirum* in the Requiem: a radiant antiphon to a vocal line.

'*Tuba mirum spargens sonum,*' sings the bass. 'The trumpet, scattering a wondrous sound thoughout the tombs of every land, shall gather all before the throne.' Quite so. It is a call to waken the dead to judgement, so, naturally, Wolfgang got a trombone in.

Unfortunately the Romantic composers of the nineteenth century appeared to have other ideas and generally confined themselves to deploying the trombone as a simple and very occasional painter of tonal colour fields and deliverer of fanfares and other generic parps. Indeed Beethoven, if memory serves, makes the trombone section sit in silent self-contemplation for three movements of his Fifth Symphony, then count 364 bars of the fourth movement before issuing a brief pair of *yuck-ducka-dahs*. And that's it. No wonder the trombones are usually first down the pub and last out.

So what do trombonists do all day? They look at girls (or, more rarely, boys) and sulk. Trombones are conventionally stashed out of harm's way at the back of the orchestra, next to the percussion, behind the trumpet section. The trumpets are therefore obliged to take the full force of those sudden parps squarely on the backs of their heads. But that's all right – the trumpets can take it. Not least because they get loads of actual playing time of their own, during which they can sublimate both the parps and the hum of *sotto voce* chuntering which goes on continuously behind them in between parps. Sometimes, the chuntering breaks cover and becomes intelligible.

It is the listless summer of 1975. The Holiday Orchestra is in the final throes of rehearsing something French for the concert in the Guildhall on Sunday. We are crammed into Parkside School hall. The conductor is a guest, an eminent figure in Cambridge music circles. He is evidently very proud of a curtain of lank, middle-aged hair which falls across his face at every jerk of his artistically mobile cranium. This gives him the chance to scoop the curtain behind his ear with a flourish and then repeat the gesture every four or five seconds, whenever the curtain falls again. The trombone section decides that the conductor is too old for hair like that.

I say that we are 'rehearsing something French', but actually memory is playing tricks. Deeper reflection tells me that we are playing something Finnish. My memory wants to recall it as French partly because of the conductor's hair and partly because the composer's Christian name was French. But really we are not playing Ravel. We are playing Sibelius. A 'tone poem': a handsome airburst of Modern-Romantic harmony, banging and puffing and thinning in a way that is typical of tone poems.

As usual, there isn't much for the trombones to do – no more than a couple of passages of tempo-less chording. They probably sound good out front, these chords, but they are boring to play. We sit. We count. My attention is drawn by the distant nape of the flautist who has captured my imagination and my palpitating heart this past fortnight. The nape ducks in and out of my field of vision beyond the quills of the first trumpet's feather cut, a furrow expressing perfect unattainability. We count some more. And then it is our time. The conductor opens a fist in our direction as if to gather us up and then closes it as he brings his arm across his body in an extravagant slow arc. His hair-curtain falls. We deliver our chords with a kind of warm swell . . .

Tick tick tick.

The baton is tapped on the edge of the conductor's desk and the orchestra peters to a halt in pieces.

'Now come *on*, trombones, don't be vulgar.' The conductor shoves his hair away from his face as he whips his baton into the perpendicular position, ready for a fresh start. Are we ready? He raises an eyebrow and turns back to the main body of the orchestra. We trombones drop our wrists and blow out our spit valves, although there is no spit in our tubes, having only played three notes.

Vulgar?

Vulgar!

But wait. The conductor purses his lips and has a visible change of mind. He has not explained himself clearly enough to the trombones. He returns his gaze to the savages on the horizon. The baton is withdrawn.

'Does the score call for a swell, trombones? No. I don't believe it does. You are required to play flat, uninflected chords, so play them flat and uninflected, please, not vulgarly.' His baton twitches back to the perpendicular.

'We're playing it vulgarly because it's a *vulgar* piece of music, you wanker.'

I say this without prior consideration and take myself by surprise. I don't say it loudly, but I do say it. It just pops out, a voiced thought.

One of the chief drawbacks of thinking out loud is that, no matter how succinct or cogent your thought, it *is* out loud. And one of the worst places to think out loud is in a confined space, especially one where the confinement is created by the proximity of dozens and dozens of other bodies, none of whom are thinking out loud themselves. This means that everyone else gets to hear your thought.

And so my own surprise at hearing this *aperçu* expressed *en plein air* is only compounded by the surprise of at least 30 per cent of the entire orchestra. That means in the region of thirty players. I watch as heads turn one after another in a rippling pathway across the surface of the pool: first the trumpets, then the clarinets, oboes and flutes, then – narrowing now – a wedge of violas and a scattering of second violins, coming to a sharp point with a leading cellist, whose head rotates like a turret on a tank.

Thankfully, hers is the last rotation, and I am not sure that she knows why she is rotating, only that she must. The conductor does not register anything at all. He merely tosses his hair back and raises his baton a quivering inch or two further towards the ceiling.

Meanwhile, I lift my horn to my face as cover and prepare to begin the count once more, heat and cold rushing through my system one after another, as if pressurised. I was terribly wrong. It isn't true at all, what I said. I wish I hadn't said it. Christ, what will they think of me? Did my flautist hear what I said – sounding like a total oaf, a real village thickie?

The thing is, for all his artily conservative soft-modernism,

Sibelius is obviously great and there's nothing vulgar about him at all.

That's if vulgar is a bad thing, of course, and I'm not even sure that it is.

15

Six more weeks passed after the Baked Alaska episode without further development and then my next hospital appointment fell due.

'I wonder what they've lined up for you this time,' mused Jane. 'A few hours sitting in a corridor, maybe, followed by an offhand chat about how there's nothing much they can do, not now we've gone past the six-week mark.' She rummaged in her bag for the car keys. Looked up. 'Or maybe they'll tell you exactly what's wrong with you – what it's called, why it happened, what's going to happen to you in the future, how long you have to put up with feeling like you'd rather be dead, and then prescribe a course of action, complete with drugs, psychotherapy and rehab. Who knows. What do you think?'

I tried not to think, which was easy.

This time we sat in the corridor only for about twenty-five minutes and then an audiologist instructed me to enter her soundproof box, where I would do a hearing test.

'It's okay. There's no need,' I said gamely, waving a hand. Hearing tests had become a stupendous and oddly humiliating bore, and they always revealed the same thing: that I was deaf. 'No, really. I've done at least a dozen of these tests since it all kicked off and the results have all been all the same – I'm deaf as a post in one ear, like off-the-scale deaf, beyond measurement. There's no point in testing it again. Nothing's changed. Believe me, I have inside knowledge. But if you're interested in measuring the way my head is filled with grinding noise all the time and I can't stand up straight and my eyesight's wonky and I get tired after walking twenty-five yards and my head aches and my brain gets confused with any kind of signal-input, then point me to your laboratory and strap me in.'

'No, I'm afraid we have to test your hearing, so the doctor has all the relevant information during the consultation.'

I suppose definitions of 'relevant' are tight in a busy, target-hitting hospital department – no room for stuff that can't be measured and instantly transliterated into statistical binary. Still, we were seen half an hour or so later, which was not bad going. The doctor did not look up from his computer. It was a different guy – the ice-cream man had moved on to another hospital. The different guy continued to tap away as we sat down.

'Well, what's the story?' he said, scrolling down, amending, adjusting his mouse minutely with a single curled finger.

'I was rather hoping you were going to tell *me* what the story is,' I replied.

'You are . . . Nicholas Coleman, yes?'

And so the matey, cat-and-mouse badinage proceeded. After a minute or so I became aware of a snapping sound to my right. Jane's bag had been opened and a notebook brought down with a business-like slap on her knee.

'Right,' she said. Even in that short syllable it was possible to hear the tiny tremor at the back of her voice, an indication that her rage was towering. 'This is the story so far. My husband is a very sick man. He is only just now struggling out of bed every day after three months flat on his back, unable to move. He is profoundly deaf in one ear. He can't stand up straight. He needs sticks to get around. He gets a headache every time he staggers more than twenty-five yards. He can't see very well. He feels sick a lot of the time. He needs his head supported most of the time.

He can't stand being anywhere there's any kind of noise. He can't think because his head is full of crashing tinnitus twenty-four hours a day. He has only got better in the sense that he can now move around sufficiently to make himself feel iller than ever – granted, he couldn't do that two months ago: he could only do it lying down. And we have been given no definitive diagnosis and no form of prognosis. Nothing. It's been three months and we've been offered no help whatsoever apart from anti-vertigo medication, which doesn't work, and Temazepam to knock him out cold at night – oh, and an injection of steroids several weeks too late. We just wonder' – by now the tremor had gone – 'what is going on? What are you going to *do* about it?'

The doctor looked up from his screen at last.

'He has been on the Temazepam for three months?'

'Yes, but he is weaning himself off it . . .'

'Okay, good. And you say he is having headaches? Has he been scanned?'

'Yes.' I felt I ought to say something. 'I had an emergency MRI in August, at the time . . .'

'Right then, let's have a look.'

The doctor returned to his computer. He drummed his finger lightly on the mouse, while we all waited for the scans to appear, which they did surprisingly quickly. He looked at assorted slices of my brain, at one point twisting his own head to one side, as if the spectacle before him were too weird to contemplate the right way up. I felt a tiny movement in my chest.

'Nope. Can't see anything there. All quite good, I'd say . . .' He fell silent.

'So you have nothing to add, then.' This was Jane. 'To what we already know. Which is virtually nothing.'

'The thing is, Mrs . . . aaah . . . Mrs Coleman, sudden neuro-sensory hearing loss is . . . Let me put it this way – there is very little we can say for sure: it can have a number of causes and a wide range of effects, some of them not pleasant, I agree. But all we can do is keep an eye on it. I can book you in to our tinnitus clinic for therapy, if you like. Would you like that? I'll do that for you now.' The doctor swivelled his chair conclusively back and forth a couple of times, as if to efface everything that had gone before.

'So, then, we ought to see you again in, say . . . six months.'

As we shuffled down the corridor, Jane held up her notebook in front of my face with her free hand. The page was blank.

A week later a letter arrived informing me, apologetically, that the tinnitus clinic was in abeyance for the time being, but that they would be in touch if and when it was up and running again some time in the future. It was not possible to say when.

'Thank you for your interest.'

*

I have most of my epiphanies on the toilet. Always have done.

Without descending into Freudian cliché it's hard to explain why this might be, so perhaps you will just have to take it on trust: I am a bog visionary, a lavatorial seer. Things happen when I'm comfortably seated; they just come to me. I don't mean to brag – I certainly don't regard this capacity as a talent, more as another sort of by-product. And I really don't want to make too big a deal out of it. If truth be told, we're probably all the same: I suspect that once established on the crapper we are all a little like William Blake. It's just not something we talk about much.

I was reminded of this propensity not so long ago by my daughter, who was then nearly eight. One afternoon after school she seized my hand and addressed me in the gravest possible tones.

'Dad.'

'Yes, Beezer.'

'Something really weird happened today at school. I was on the toilet doing a poo and my brain went all funny and I started to think about what . . . about how weird . . . well, not how weird but how . . . how strange it is that I'm *me* and not *someone else* . . .'

'Uh-huh.'

'And then I started to, like, *see* me, as if I *was* someone else, but I wasn't, I was still me – and it was like really weird. I was outside myself and inside myself at the same time. Like *really* weird, you know? I was sitting there and my brain just made me do it. I didn't try to do it – it just happened. Dad,' she slumped her shoulders theatrically, 'is that . . . like, *bad*?'

'No, it's not bad. It's normal. In fact I can remember doing exactly the same thing when I was about your age, and on the toilet too. Used to happen quite a lot. I haven't forgotten what the experience was like either. I can remember the bathroom in the house where I grew up and the net curtains at the window moving in the breeze and worrying that when the edge of the curtains blew up, people on the street could see me there, exposed; and I can remember doing exactly what you did, thinking it's weird to be me and being outside and inside myself at the same time, and shivering . . .'

'Yeah, it made me shiver, too.'

'And then worrying about what it means.'

'What does it mean?'

'I haven't a clue. But I think it's probably a good thing to happen. I imagine it's to do with growing up and becoming more aware of yourself in relation to the world – that there is a difference between you and the rest of it, and that your outside might not reveal what your inside contains. I think that in those moments, and without intending to, you're forcing yourself to see yourself as the world might see you. Does that make sense? And I think it happens like that when you're doing a poo because, well, when you're doing a good one, you're partly feeling a bit vulnerable and partly really happy in a way that is completely everyday and completely comforting.'

'I *think* I know what you mean, Dad.'

The funny thing is that six or seven months prior to that early summer afternoon, not long after our third not very helpful visit to the Royal London, I found myself in my visionary position doing, for the circumstances, an acceptably good poo, and the melody of Amy Winehouse's 'You Know I'm No Good' came floating to my ear.

I joined in.

I cheated myself
Like I knew I would
I told you I was trouble
You know that I'm no good

She's not that easy to sing along with, Amy. Her melodies are elaborate, even baroque, streamed together as if to accent the lyrics in the manner of the high-sass idiom Amy aspires to speak in. They are gobby melodies and so quite hard to mimic, unless you happen to be gobby yourself, I suppose. The thing is, when Amy sings them somehow the gobby is made incredibly musical. This is how we explain her strange brilliance: although Amy Winehouse records exhibit a high level of artifice in their borrowings from old forms and in the extremity of their mannerism, there is absolute integrity in their exercise of language. Amy records are deeply, tragically authentic.

'Da-*ad*! Shu'-up! You're spoiling it!'

The Beezer was twelve feet away in my study at my computer, YouTubing every Amy Winehouse song she could find. She'd been doing it half the morning. This was a new passion; a good one, I think, despite the Winehouse tendency to legitimise the

Beezer's latent but clearly very real inclination to walk on the gobby side of the street. Then . . .

'Hey, but Dad! You're *singing*!' This was almost gasped.

The change in tone was sudden and unexpected. Eight-year-old girls can turn on a sixpence. They can flicker between little-girliness and pre-pubertal huff faster than you can register the change, as if channel-hopping personalities with a TV remote. But this was real. Her voice had gone up about half an octave and softened. I could hear the smile in it. Even though I couldn't see her I knew that her mouth was open and that she was now facing me from her feet-up position on my study chair, maybe even leaning forward, taking her feet down, swivelling. She was right. I had been singing. I had been singing unself-consciously and freely, and no doubt hideously, which meant that I must have heard Amy Winehouse's singing. In fact, yes, I could hear Amy Winehouse singing now – the tune was going up and down and in and out and all around the houses in the way her tunes do, and it sounded all right. Well, not bad. Both obstructed and clear at the same time. I couldn't hear much rhythm or harmony, but I could hear the voice. And I could follow the tune. There was indeed a monstrous, slooshing tide of white noise rising quickly in my dome as usual, but it wasn't overwhelming Amy. Amy was holding her own. She was swimming in the rising water.

I raised myself up from my visionary seat as fast as a doddery old man can, staggered into my study and caught my daughter up in my arms.

*

We cannot know how music sounds to others.

This is a truism, obviously. A thumping one. Nevertheless, however dully self-evident it is that we can have no idea precisely how bells ring in other people's heads, it doesn't stop me from wondering. I do it all the time. It's a habit.

This is not a scientific impulse. Nor am I one of those individuals who enjoys kicking at the philosophical dust in the hope of scuffing up some sexy truth or paradox. Philosophy will only take you as far as the chicken wire which marks the limits of your reasoning capacity, and my chicken wire is close, double-banked and so tall I can't see the top. I don't like going there much; makes me feel inadequate. Nevertheless, there are some things I can grasp, philosophically speaking. I know, for instance, that contrary to what instinct says, we have merely arrived at a consensus about what the colour red looks like; and we all seem to agree – those of us who aren't colour-blind – on what the word 'red' means. But I also know that there is no way of demonstrating that our minds experience redness in the same way. Not that I'm aware of. So subjectivity – how we *get* the world discretely – is to my mind the most interesting part of an individual, the one thing about a person which is authentically mysterious.

For that reason I am very happy for us all to keep our experiences close. Go on: treasure your jewels, hoard them, picket them with curses, dig them in and build ramparts around them. It's fine with me. I don't want to steal them. All I ask is that you permit me to speculate on what it's like to be you; you listening to Amy Winehouse or Sibelius or Hank Mobley or the wind chimes on porches in American films. Please? It might seem intrusive, but I promise I'll be quiet. You won't even notice I'm there . . .

I have done this ever since I listened to Nazareth with my dad. On that occasion I barely heard the record for myself; I certainly didn't enjoy it in the way I'd enjoy it later in my bedroom, on my own in the dark with the volume up and my rock 'n' roll face on. No, as we sat there on our upright chairs, *Razamanaz* punching invisible shapes out of the air dividing the green living-room carpet from the white living-room ceiling, I attempted to listen only to what my dad was hearing.

I couldn't hear anything, of course. I might as well have been deaf. I was certainly struck dumb. But there it was: the unyielding silence of the sealed unit. The unimaginable void. All I could do was speculate on what was going on in my old man's head, based on what I already knew to be true about his inner world.

What did I know to be true? I knew what he *liked*, of course. Early music, German music, sad music, music welcoming death and pretty girls in more or less equal measure. And church music. He liked those things in a solitary, contemplative way. Listening to music – as opposed to making it – was not a social thing for him. I don't suppose anyone ever witnessed my dad's most withering musical experiences for the simple reason that if anyone had been there to observe, then, by definition, the experience could not be withering. But I might be wrong about that. I just don't know. All I know is that I had in the past – at concerts and during the musical bits of church services – seen tears trickle from the corners of his eyes; and on that handful of occasions I had been smart enough even as a small child to know that something serious was going on and that attention was not to be drawn. He should be left alone.

But what else? Other than likes and dislikes? Other than 'taste'?

Let's get something straight first. We don't enjoy music only on the basis that it sounds similar to the music that we know we already like. In the digital world, that is an assumption which has taken on the solidity of a fundamental truth: music is disseminated in that dimensionless world entirely on the basis that musical taste is a linear experience, like a fairground ride, in which one piece of music inevitably leads to another in an everlasting, and therefore ever-exploitable, chain of similitude.

This is shallow stuff. We actually like the music we *really* like on the basis of the person that we are. That is an assumption I have always made and I hold it up still as an unassailable truth. (What '*really* like' means in this context is, of course, another unsayable thing – but you know what I mean by that, don't you? Of course you do.) I would never go so far as to say that our natures are shaped by the music that we like; but it is always true to say that the music that we like tells us something about our natures – not because music carries fixed meanings but because it doesn't. And on *that* basis I have to hold up my hands and say that the way into my father's inner world was a narrow way strewn with obstacles, but a straight way.

So, what obstacles? What other things were in there?

I can tell you some of the things he thought and believed. He loved his family. He disliked the professions. He despised snobbery. He had no time for unearned privilege, but considered that any sort of privilege, whether earned or not, brought with it a burden of responsibility which absolutely required enactment. He did not approve of gambling, either the sporting kind or the capitalistic sort. He enjoyed a good view and an architectural ruin. And as a kid he had a massive jones for the Woolwich ferry, which stayed with him throughout his life in echo form. Later on, as a young man, he espoused pacifism, but in a way that never quite came to anything, except in the sense that, having been drummed into the Royal Artillery for his National Service, he made a splendid hash of a bombardier's duties. He didn't like gardening much either, but he did it all the same, for hours and hours and hours.

My dad did not go in for heroes, but he was prepared to admire certain individuals, provided they were a matter of historical fact and were now dead and so not in a position to let anyone down any further than they had done already. Top of his list appeared to be Saint Jerome, the fourth-century

Church Father. If you know your Church history, you'll know that this would be unusual among Protestants of mid-to-low-church inclinations. Jerome is, after all, a saint – eeuw! – and one of the pillars of the Roman Catholic edifice, albeit one who did in real life meditate long and hard and frequently polemically on what it takes to lead an angelic life. And Jerome did translate the Vulgate version of the Bible, either from the Hebrew or the Greek, depending on your scholastic position. That is a very big deal. Jerome is therefore an all-time-great spreader of the Word, with the added bonus for my pa that Jerome was no mere zombie evangelical but a deep thinker on what the act of word-spreading means. In the iconography of saints he is usually to be found hunched over a lectern in a cave, far from the quotidian activities of mankind, accompanied by a lion: the very image of an ascetic, scholarly old git.

Regarding my pa, the cave seems more significant than the lion. My father did not find any fulfilment in his own work until the last decade of his working life, when he was made Publishing Director of the Bible and Religious Books at Cambridge University Press, and then Secretary to the Joint Committee of the Churches. In that decade he supervised the editing of the all-new, ultra-vernacular Revised English Bible (REB) and came to his real work at last.

This was a mighty undertaking, one involving a small team of distinguished chaps and the odd archbishop, with whom my dad would spend long days cracking scholarly jokes and giggling. This was the kind of thing he'd wanted to do all his life. Each weekday he'd get home from his office in town, eat supper with my mother and then spend the early evening reading the latest passage of the REB text out loud to himself in his study, to check its felicity on the tongue. By the end of the job, he'd recited the entirety of this new, demotic version of the Bible in his best lectern voice, twice – I like to think that he did it in his best Woolwich voice as well – and written copious notes, which would have impressed Jerome just a little, I feel sure. I was not around to see this undertaking unfold, because it was the decade of my twenties.

But the part of my dad's inner world I could never think about without feeling funny was the part linked to a passage of his life which ended long before I was born. It began in 1939, when he was ten, and concluded at some unspecified point during his early adolescence, before the end of the war. This was the period of his evacuation from south-east London to live in the house of a peculiar woman in Tunbridge Wells.

No one knows what happened there. It's not clear that my dad even retained much of an idea himself – he would certainly never talk about it in any detail or with any sense of having a story to tell, not even if you asked direct questions. This was not the case with the other stories of his past life (my favourites were the ones he brought back from National Service in the Libyan desert, describing remarkable feats of ineptitude in the deployment of field guns in sandy declivities). It was as if from the moment of evacuation a void opened up in his life, a sort of darkly magnetic lacuna from which nothing might escape – no stories, no memories, no feelings; not even any resentments, or at least none that he could put a finger on. He was evacuated in one sense, vacated in another.

A primary cliché of the evacuation is that the children experienced it in one of two ways: they either had the time of their lives or they endured living hell. For my dad, it seems to me that evacuation amounted to a cessation, a stoppage of experience; a sort of purgatory, I suppose. The suspension of subjectivity. This may or may not have been an act of will on his part. But to his children – thirty and forty and fifty years later – it was entirely apparent how it might have happened at the time: the little boy switching himself off for the duration, to make it so that *this is not happening*.

I do not know whether he ever got over the evacuation, not completely. Then again, that might just be me failing to settle with the idea of my ten-year-old dad being sent away from his mother, with no guarantees in his gas-mask box other than the one confirming that his parents would remain at home in south-east London without him, in mortal danger, and that things could never, ever be the same again. I can't think about it. The thought of my father being that vulnerable is literally unthinkable.

Instead I think about what marks the evacuation might have left on his subsequent life. I often wondered what used to go on in his head later on, after he became a father, during all those long hours of composting and raspberry cage-building in our chalky back garden on the toe-slopes of the Gogs. For years I used to imagine music playing in his head. But I'm not sure it was music that he was hearing.

So there we sit, he and I, listening to 'Bad Bad Boy' and I wonder what it is doing to him.

'Well I'm a bad, bad, bad, bad, bad, bad, bad, bad, bad, bad, *bad*-bad boy!' screams Dan McCafferty towards the end of the song, when all sense has left his head and the best he can do is beat with a single word against the locked and bolted door of his perturbation. 'I'm *bad*, I'm *bad*, I'm such a, such a bad-bad boy!'

Is it pissing my dad off, this racket? Does it hurt? I can imagine it might hurt. Or is he really not listening at all? Has he flipped the old switch and slipped into *this is not really happening* mode? Oblivion. His face is giving nothing away. He's not saying anything. Well, I don't suppose there's much he can say. Is he wondering why it has to be so loud? Is he wondering what I hear, what I get from this? Are we both playing the same game, listening to each other listening?

All I know is that I can't bear it. The thought of Nazareth trashing the furniture in my dad's head is a terrible one. But the thought of them not doing anything at all to him is much worse.

16

In May 1975 Led Zeppelin played five nights at Earl's Court and Yes a date at Loftus Road, Queens Park Rangers' football ground, to round off a season-long tour of the major outposts (which also included the Victoria Ground, home of Stoke City FC). Back then, when QPR were an established First Division side, the Loftus Road stadium could contain more than 30,000 spectators in the stands alone.

Lorry was poised to leave school for good. He would turn sixteen the week after the Zeppelin gigs and he was determined not to waste a further minute in the ditch pretending to be cow parsley when he could be out in the world earning money and expanding his record collection. Leaving school at the earliest opportunity was to him a simple matter of personal dignity, allied to sound economic sense. We needed to celebrate that fact. So we discussed going to Earl's Court and laid elaborate plans. I was nervous. Getting to London, then across London to the cavernous venue of the Ideal Home Exhibition, having a pint when we got there and maybe food, getting pulverised for three hours by Zeppelin's famous amplitude, and then doing the journey all over again in reverse late at night to get the last train home, followed by a night bus or cab out to the village, all during the school exam season – how much of a bastard was that going to be? And how expensive? The whole enterprise seemed rather implausible, as if such things were not meant to be accomplished by boys like me.

Then there was the question of what my parents would say. Should I ask them first or just present it as a fait accompli? I've got the ticket. I've made the arrangements. I'm *going*.

I knew I'd never get away with that stance, as I'd only just be turning fifteen that month and had Maths and English O levels to pretend to give a shit about. And on top of all the logistics and the permissions, there remained the issue of whether I could actually afford it. I was absolutely certain that I couldn't – not while continuing to have modest fun in my home town and buying records at every opportunity. I calculated that if I forked out for Earl's Court I'd be unable to afford to leave the house for the rest of the summer.

Nevertheless, Lorry sent off for the tickets and . . . heard nothing. We'd spent too long laying plans. These had been the fastest-selling concert tickets the UK market had ever known and we'd missed the boat by days. Lorry boiled with frustration, especially later on when stories began to filter back about freaks staggering out of Earl's Court at the end of the show with blood running down their necks from perforated ear-drums. Lorry loved that kind of thing. I quietly sighed with relief.

As for Yes at QPR? Couldn't be bothered. I felt I ought to go; that it was a sort of duty to the creative communion which gave shape and maybe even meaning to my life. To *not* go would be a betrayal of everything I stood for, a surrendering of the floating hillock on which I had planted my standard. But to be honest, I just couldn't face it. Perhaps the kidney infection and its torrid soundtrack had drained something from me; I could certainly think of more appetising ways of spending precious funds. Besides, the tang of old sweat had begun to gather around Yes, overpowering the traditional prog perfumes of verve and imagination. I was no longer so sure that Yes stood for lightness and originality and transport. *Relayer* had been a grind, a lonely grind. How could the many trains to Shepherd's Bush be anything but?

And anyway, I was now into Be-Bop Deluxe.

*

History has since designated 1975 the year of unspeakable bollocks. It was the year in which progressive rock went sumo – Loftus Road was Yes's fattest moment yet – while, as a mellow counterpoint to English grandiosity, Californian soft rock appeared at every freak's elbow, smirking and more sensitive than any East Anglian longhair had ever contrived to be, even in his subtlest fantasies. Girls liked the West Coast thing; they seemed to understand what these droopy, denim-clad mountebanks meant by talking quietly and carrying a big acoustic guitar. 1975 was the year rock not only got fat and sensitive but also stole your girlfriend (if you had one).

That's what history says. But I enjoyed 1975. Lots of good things happened, even if I didn't have a regular girlfriend, nor looked likely to. In fact, 1975 was a great year in which to be fifteen.

Physical Graffiti came out. So did *Young Americans*. As did *Born to Run*. And *Down by the Jetty* and *Malpractice, Blood on the Tracks, Bob Marley and the Wailers Live, The Last Record Album, Wish You Were Here, Horses, The Hissing of Summer Lawns, Another Green World, Fighting, Tomorrow Belongs to Me, HQ, Ruth Is Stranger Than Richard, Fish Rising, Fish Out of Water, Nighthawks at the Diner, The Original Soundtrack, Sunday's Child, Live at Leeds, Blow by Blow, Zuma, Maximum Darkness, Marcus Garvey, Siren, Nuthin' Fancy, For Earth Below, The Rotter's Club, Free Hand, Minstrel in the Gallery, Blues for Allah, Bongo Fury, Coney Island Baby, Katy Lied, Landed, Straight Shooter, Northern*

Lights–Southern Cross, Visions of the Emerald Beyond, The Basement Tapes, Pour Down Like Silver and *Futurama* – all records I would think were great, either at the time or later on; in some cases very many years later on. All but four of them still occupy space in my living room.

If you are of an age – and of a temperament – the preceding paragraph will reach you with a fizzing emotional spin which might remind you of poetry. This is because even though it is just a sequence of words, it is also an analogue of something lost and beautiful to do with time and your inner world. It isn't poetry; it isn't even poetic. It's just a list. But it is inexplicit and allusive and pregnant with association; it does make language into a veil, which may be lifted only by feelings already faltering within you. Some people can look at an old football programme or a tea set or a sponge cake and be similarly transported into a differently shaded state of mind, as if into a different time. We all have our madeleines.

This is quite clearly not mere nostalgia. If it were, then Proust would not be the man he is today.

Yet history, that cruelly formal accounting process, tells us that 1975 was a bum stretch; that it gave rise to a great and necessary purging: that, even measured against its own scale of values (never mind the scale belonging to the things in life we consider to be even more important than rock records), the serious-minded, semi-popular music of that year was a virulent disease requiring robust treatment, even as it scarred an entire generation of febrile young spirits. It is as if the year itself were diseased.

But it was not diseased. I was there. It was great. The UK economy might have been roiling in the pit of its Seventies slump, and the flicked feathercut might have been pre-eminent upon the skulls of the nation's youth, but, as musical years go, it was lively, stimulating, forward-looking and heartliftingly free of dogmatism. In 1975 all things were possible.

Or to put it another way . . . In the same way that the course of musical taste is only linear if you allow yourself to be made to think like that, so history does not need to be treated as a one-dimensional chain reaction, with one event inexorably leading to another in an everlasting sequence of action and reaction, cause and effect, posture and counter-posture. The fundamental problem with roller-coaster rides, in my view, is that they ride on rails: they are dully linear; what underwrites all that 'terror' is rigid predictability. Well, it might be argued that the entropic nature of 1975 – during which no posture took precedence over another, tribal relations followed the rule of mutually assured, baffled incomprehension, and order was something you placed at the bar – all that chaos and diffuseness allowed it to be one of the *great* years.

Mind you, I was fifteen. The things we experience when we are fifteen can never be repeated. They are almost toxic in their vividness. They are certainly addictive, even if the reality is that you can only be fifteen once, and nothing is ever quite the same again after you cease to be fifteen. Fifteen is when the world begins to reveal itself in passion as well as sensation, when liking becomes lust. It's when the gap begins to seem to be bridgeable between what you long for and what you might realistically claim: fifteen brings the world within reach. You can touch it, if you really want to.

I do not go in for regrets; but I have – at different times since 1975 – been visited by a notional regret that I did not turn fifteen in 1933, when Duke Ellington first came to the UK; in 1956, when Elvis became audible to the Old World; in 1959, the year of *Kind of Blue*; in 1964, when Dylan properly arrived; and, in a devastatingly near miss, 1972, when *Exile on Main St* came out. *Exile* was not a historical event; not even close to one. But how dearly I would love to have heard that record as a fifteen-year-old in the week, the day, the hour of its descent upon the Philistines.

As it is, I was fifteen just in time for . . .

But let's leave it there for the time being. I'll come back to the subject shortly, because there's a another side to the year in which I became fifteen, and it needs to be addressed first. It stands in direct contradiction to the world I've just described.

What can also be said about 1975 is that everything I wanted to be close to somehow became a little more *in*accessible. It was the year in which the perceived distance between the successful musician and his constituency of fans became an abyss. Zeppelin's week at Earl's Court confirmed this even more than Yes at QPR.

It was an abyss partly created by vanity, of course – the serious-minded mid-Seventies rock star was a creature endowed with a very special kind of self-esteem, and he had grown accustomed to doing what he liked, when he liked and to whomever he fancied. But we didn't know about that then, still less care. To the typical provincial fifteen-year-old of the period, the word 'rock' did not signify pathological ambition, mindless self-indulgence and the quasi-fascistic diminution of the lives of others. On the contrary, 'rock' expressed a kind of ontological virtue – *this* is how we make the world more agreeable, by *being* more agreeable ourselves (and yes, it may entail a little cock-faced preening, but listen: if you don't buy into the style, you won't get the substance).

To us, what separated rocker from rock fan was not the gulf of celebrity, but the kind of distance which might be calibrated the old-fashioned way, in inches, feet, yards and miles. Indeed, we all felt quite sure that were Robert Plant or Keith Richards or Be-Bop Deluxe ever to materialise in our bedrooms for a cider and a chinwag we would all get on like a house on fire, because, let's face it, we were all more or less the same person, give or take a few quid. Rock gods were not gods at all, but simply more successful and worldly versions of ourselves. They were us and we were them. In confirmation of that fact, Lorry always referred to the ones he identified most closely with by first name, while surnames were reserved for those by whom he was properly awed. Hence, 'Rick' could only mean dear old Rick Wright of the Floyd, while 'Vander' meant the terrifying Christian Vander of Magma, who saw visions of a ruined human future and then invented his own private language with which to pass on the message.

To my generational sliver of anxious junior travellers who couldn't afford to go anywhere anyway, Led Zeppelin at Earl's Court was a major bummer. A watershed. We were old enough and just about flush enough to buy the records, but not to go to the gigs. There is no escaping the irony. In 1975 Led Zeppelin made themselves available to their people and, in doing so, only confirmed that a chasm now yawned between them and us. It didn't mean Zeppelin were rubbish all of a sudden but it did mean that, rather than them coming to you, you had to go to them, like little people, to be counted. The things I wanted to do now were too big, too far away, too expensive, too centralised. Very few of the bands I really wanted to see went anywhere near the Corn Exchange.

However, in 1975 I did go to see Greenslade there, for the second time. Greenslade were a second-division prog group and I'd never really liked them much, never bought their records. But they were on, so we went. They did their tinkly thing, which included the traditional hammy drum solo in the encore, played on two bass drums with feet only, while the drummer held his sticks up high above his head in a triumphant V. And then we all trooped backstage to hang out.

Lorry, Andy, Lorry's mate Ellingham, a couple of other lugubrious fen freaks and I lined one wall of the chipboard dressing room. Greenslade lined the other. Dave Lawson, the singer and secondary keyboard player, wiped the neck of his bottle and generously offered it to his opposite number on our side.

'There you go, man.'

'Thanks.' Ellingham was the recipient. 'But I won't.' The bottle went down the line and no one took advantage of Lawson's largesse, myself included.

'Well . . . How was the show?' Lawson spread his hands on his lap, palms up. He smiled. He seemed like a nice chap. I did not get the impression that he was fishing for praise, just trying to make conversation.

'Dave.' This was Ellingham. 'I've got to say it: you're a *terrible* singer.'

Ellingham had never once minced his words in the six or seven years I'd known him. He was very bright and very contumacious. We had never been close. When we'd been ten, in what would now be called Year Five at primary school, the teacher had run a mock election to correspond with the General Election won that year by Ted Heath. Ellingham was nominated as the Tory candidate, while I stood for Labour. I am not sure what the process of selection was. What I do know is that Ellingham's Tories took the poll by a single vote, following an absolutely coruscating speech by the party leader, which proposed a variety of hard-hitting policies grounded in a clear ideological position, some of which had to do with fiscal issues, others to do with Europe. I have clear memories of Ellingham's speech and of his hand cleaving the air, but none whatsoever of my own – or even if I made one at all – which tells you all you need to know about my suitability for high office.

Five years later Dave Lawson's mouth opened and then closed again. Lorry, Andy, the fen freaks and I began to move towards the chipboard door. I had got almost all the way through it when the lead singer of Greenslade finally composed himself. I could not by then see his face, as it was obscured by everyone else's hair, but I was still close enough to hear what he said.

'Well, thank you very much,' he exhaled sadly. 'I love you, too.'

*

At fifteen I knew enough of the world to get into and out of town without falling off my bike. The hedgeless road across the prairie between our village and town was long and straight and it was punctuated only by the inverted comma shapes of those patients at the psychiatric hospital who were allowed to take the air in the world beyond the hospital gates. I would labour past them on my bike as they hunched against the wind, their pyjama trousers snapping round their ankles, and I'd think of refugees on the roads of northern Europe during the Second World War. I was capable of romanticising anything.

Above all things, I romanticised girls.

I was not sexually sophisticated. I had had my first 'full' sexual experience that year and it was so disagreeable that I resolved I would not have another one until it was completely unavoidable. So 1975 did have its blemishes, after all: hateful school, irksome exams, bungled sex, uptight parents, no money, not being able to go to Earl's Court, not wanting to go to Loftus Road . . . Awful really, when you think about it.

But I didn't think about it. I thought about Lulu.

Lulu attended the girls' grammar school over the road from my school. I could see it through the trees: a Thirties-modernist block of some structural elegance entirely full of clever, state-educated girls drawn from all layers of Cambridge society. The headmistress was a martinet of fearsome reputation; the girls were terrified of her, even as they worshipped her. My sister Becca went there, too, and tried hard not to participate in the cult.

We used to convene – the green-uniformed girls from the

High School and the purple boys from my school – in small groups in the copse of trees over the road separating the two schools' mighty playing fields. The copse was dense, but there was a point where the trees thinned sufficiently for hanging around to take place under cover. We would smoke, make leading conversation and hope that hands might brush or eyes make lodging contact. Occasionally, the more playful members of the huddle might give another member a sudden shove, so that bodies would pitch together against a tree trunk or entangle themselves in other bodies, and then giggling and hot resentment would come over the group like new weather. But not always. Mostly, the girls would maintain an atmosphere of cool superiority, or so it seemed to me. I never felt like anything other than the youngest, gauchest person in the ivy.

But then I was not particularly interested in the girls among the trees. My attention was fixed elsewhere, beyond the chain-link fence, across the car park in the endless sunny corridors of the girls' school. Lulu did not smoke. She did not come to the copse – not any more.

She had been there once in my presence, in the company of her handsome and spectacularly garrulous friend Jo, whom everyone fancied as a statutory requirement. But on that one occasion Lulu had seemed bewildered somehow and unable to join in. She had stood there gazing silently into the deeper recesses of the copse, as if the really interesting stuff were going on in there. My heart screwed itself into a tiny ball and threw itself out of my chest. It was followed by my ability to speak. I froze, and then edged away to lean coolly against a tree to have my fag. On the far side of the tree, in fact. I could not bear the thought of her seeing me close up, hearing my stupid voice uttering the pretentious things I was given to saying, and I would not countenance the possibility of being shoved against her, and then mocked.

After that solitary appearance, I had never seen her again in the copse. She was obviously above such things as cigarettes and shoving. Nevertheless, I continued to tool over the road week after week in the hope at least of seeing her on the other side of the chain-link, moving around slowly in her nimbus.

Lulu was small and knock-kneed. She wore enormous shoes like houseboats, which meant that walking seemed to be a burdensome, slightly haphazard activity for her, as if her levers had been weighted incorrectly. Nevertheless, her hair fell down in a shining torrent to her shoulders and was the colour of chestnuts. It swung in heavy curtains about the axis of her nose, which joined her forehead in a straight line without sloping in first, just like an Ancient Greek nose on an urn. What a nose. I imagined mine against hers, which also meant imagining her eyes in goggling close-up. The nose separated two vast eyes of such ineffable plangency that I felt sure that, were they ever to fasten on me and speak silently of the sadness within, I might actually faint.

She always looked either haughty or sad or bewildered, and sometimes she managed all three at the same time, even when laughing with Jo. Over the period of the awakening of my infatuation, between the summers of 1974 and 1975, I had exchanged four words with her, one after another, at Jo's party. Three of the words were mine. I was worried that they might have been enough to put her off.

'Hello.'

'Hello.'

'All right?'

Nod.

I knew where the haughtiness came from, at least. Lulu was Cambridge royalty. Her father was President of one of the major colleges and the family lived in mullioned glamour at the end of a cloister in one of the most beautiful courts in England. I had often taken a detour that year to pass the ancient timber college gates and I had seen that they were studded with iron. I did not expect ever to pass through their shadow as anything other than a sightseer. Lulu was beyond my reach in just about every way I could think of. It did not occur at the time that, to me, this may have been the point of her.

Instead, at the end of every school day, I walked the wrong way up the road to wait at the bus stop close to the girls' school rather than get on at the stop right outside my own. I'd lounge casually in the bus shelter, a prickly purple islet in a sea of green, and force myself to be natural, as if I'd come all this way in the wrong direction to increase my chances of getting a seat on the bus (that was the excuse I'd prepared, should I ever be challenged) and to demonstrate my high-minded detachment from the society of my own school. That part was easy, at least. I'd then try to breathe normally until the moment Jo and Lulu would hove round the corner, satchels swinging, hair flying, eyes rolling – the signal to my nervous system to unleash a riot of contradictory messages so incandescent I'd sometimes be unable to see for several seconds. In my paralysis, I would turn my eyes to the filaments of wire reinforcing the glass in the bus shelter and utter a silent prayer. The prayer would be that no one would laugh and point at the naked boy fizzling in a magnesium fire.

Nevertheless, I was convinced that Lulu's sadness and bewilderment were the coin of her real nature and that the haughtiness was just a protective front. I did not smile at her even once. I barely even looked at her, and if I did, it was always a casual glance, just to see which Lulu was uppermost at that moment. I would always follow her on to the bus at a distance of at least three schoolgirls, and would then either go upstairs or downstairs, depending on where she wasn't. I did not like to think that I was stalking her, even less that she might think I was.

But that didn't mean I wouldn't have welcomed her with a

warm smile if she'd come down or up the stairs to ask how I was. Of course I would have.

But I knew it wouldn't happen.

*

The young man in the picture has laboured through the clouds. He has reached the mountaintop and is standing with his back to the viewer in his greenish frock coat on an outcrop of chocolate-brown rock, looking out over creation. He sees that it is shrouded in vapour. There are other outcrops visible in the middle distance, dotted with skirmisher pines from the forest below, while, in the far distance beyond a ridge, an even taller peak looms remotely, possibly the hazy super-object of the young *Rückenfigur*'s gaze. The foreshortening created by the flat image means that the two narrowing arms of the ridge appear to join the young man's body just below the level of his shoulders. They might be wings; they might be dark radials from his heart. What they suggest to the mind behind the eye are the arms of a crucifix.

Who knows the depths of the invisible valley below and the thickness of the forest covering it? Which of us can elucidate the nature of the young man's struggle? What we know for sure is that he has endured at least two struggles. One is the inner struggle which drove him to set out from his hearth in the first place; the other is the physical effort which brought him to this peak. Our only clue is in the light of his eyes. But we cannot see his eyes. All we can see is the vastness laid out before him: the sublime mystery of creation.

I grew up with German stuff. That's partly because my family is a bit German, on both sides. I am descended from a tangle of nineteenth-century émigré German tradesmen, Hertfordshire shepherds, Cambridgeshire farmers, then London maidservants, butchers, mariners, typists, legal clerks, confectioners and civil servants. We had German books and German music in our house, the odd German picture, German instruments, German machines and, between my two sisters and father, a certain amount of German language. I am glad to say that we never owned a German car, but for some reason my mother had a German cookbook, which included a recipe for cheese in jelly. She is an excellent cook, my mother, and so she never felt the need to make cheese in jelly, but the book remained on the shelf in the kitchen as a lingering threat. Although I am far, far more English than otherwise, it is a fact that, whether by genetic default or by some subtle psychological twist of nurture, the German bit is the bit that smoulders in the dark.

A print of Caspar David Friedrich's *The Wanderer Above the Mist* did not actually hang in our house. I'm not even sure where I saw it first, although it would have certainly been in the pages of a book rather than on a gallery wall; a book either about northern-European art or about the indefatigable forest wanderings of the German soul. Wherever it was, the painting invaded my teenage mind and stayed there stubbornly, an icon of the *very interesting thing* that was German Romanticism: Goethe, the Schlegels, Heine, Schubert, Kleist, Friedrich – those guys.

Friedrich was an exact contemporary of both Constable and Turner, and I've always thought that if you ever needed a distillation of the ways in which the English differ from the Germans in their apprehension of their natural environment – and therefore a useful place to begin observing the differences between the English and the Germans – then compare Constable, Turner and Friedrich (and then lob in Goya, another contemporary, to provide another telling perspective). I am English. I think Constable, Turner and Goya are all great artists, indeed greater artists than Friedrich. Yet Friedrich is the one I have framed on my wall.

That is probably because I am given to seeing everything not as it is but as an agent of something else. Sometimes this seems to me to be a terrible failing, sometimes not.

In 1975 I bought a second-hand recording of Berg's opera *Lulu*. It was a box set, so it cost a bit, even though it was scratchy. I bought it not because I thought it might enlighten me or because I hoped for some Lulu-juju arising as a by-product of ownership, but simply because it had Lulu's name as the title. I also set out to read the 'Lulu' plays by Wedekind. Wedekind was, after all, German. But the plays weren't in the school library, so I ended up reading the first twenty pages of the first one in an alcove at Heffer's bookshop one afternoon. Wedekind's Lulu didn't seem remotely like my Lulu, except in the sense that she was desirable and misunderstood and an obvious victim of society. Meanwhile, the fiercely dissonant Berg opera made my heart go to sleep, even as I longed to find in the music traces of the kind of Luluness I might get next to. I solemnly played it all the way through once, then traded it in.

My smouldering inner German achieved very little in the way of bringing Lulu closer. In fact, it seemed only to lengthen the distance and intensify the mountainousness of the topography which separated her soul from mine. Fortunately, Stevie Wonder came back to me at this point, more than two years after his first appearance. He came this time not as a pale-faced and Spandex-clad yob-superhero but as an agent of love.

It may or may not have been forgotten what Stevie Wonder meant to ordinary white English people in the middle 1970s. By that I mean two things. One is that even if we have lost a collective memory of Stevie Wonder's particular station in the order of things in 1975, then I am pretty sure that as individuals every one of us who was around at the time can dredge up something of the impact he had on our private minds; minds which were basically geared, in the popular realm, towards the adulation of Rod Stewart. Secondly, by 'ordinary white English people' I mean the kind of people I knew.

Here's the thing. Stevie Wonder's penetration of everyday life was so seamlessly pleasurable and so essentially warm, so universal in its appeal yet so strong in its purchase on the individual psyche, that no one actually noticed themselves falling in love. Wonder simply entered British life and made himself comfortable, as if he'd always been there and we just hadn't noticed before how nice it was to have him around: a black American in a kaftan and heavy shades singing about the lives of black Americans as if they were exactly the same lives, in essence, as the ones lived on King's Parade in town or in the badlands of Six Mile Bottom. 'Get in that cell, nigger' and all.

Girls adored Stevie Wonder. I don't think I knew a single fanciable girl who didn't profess to liking Stevie Wonder, and profess it with total and believable conviction. You just knew they were telling the truth and not simply trying to be cool; neither were they all Smoothies sticking to the letter of convention. I knew plenty of non-Smoothie girls who liked Stevie Wonder almost as much as I liked Be-Bop Deluxe.

The string of Stevie Wonder hits running from 'Superstition' in 1973, through 'You Are the Sunshine of My Life', 'Higher Ground', 'Living for the City', 'He's Misstra Know It All' and 'You Haven't Done Nothing' to his one success in 1975, 'Boogie On Reggae Woman', constitutes a mini-canon of almost ineffable brilliance and lovability. It was wonderful simply to be alive for the duration. A privilege. Through time, the songs uncoiled a ribbon of warmth; in space, they made listeners feel as if they were participating in a discourse which spoke truly of the world and its iniquities, yet offered a resolution to all of that unpleasantness in the intelligent exercise of compassion, gentleness, sensualism and melody. Plus several of the songs were funky as all hell. In Stevie Wonder I perceived a way to get close to Lulu.

I bought *Innervisions*.

Innervisions actually came out in 1973. 1974's *Fulfillingness'
First Finale* was the latest work and a very fine thing in its own
right, but I knew that *Innervisions* was the one. Outwardly, it
wore beautiful geometrical Afro art on its gatefold, showing the
physically blind Stevie seeing all kinds of extraordinary things
on a higher plane, while on the inside it quacked with rhythm.
I brought it home on the bus from the marketplace with the
same trembling that had accompanied *Razamanaz* two years
before, only this time I had an idea as to what would be the
outcome.

I did not *know* that Lulu liked Stevie Wonder, but I was willing
to bet that she did. All girls of substance liked Stevie Wonder.
My conviction was that if I listened to the thing with the kind
of attention that Lulu was bound to bring to the same activity
in her boudoir, then communion would surely result – not actual
communication, obviously (what do you think I am? Naive?),
but some sort of co-eventual emotion, some unanimity of inner
vision. A co-habitation of thought and feeling. I imagined her,
sad as ever, solitary and prone on cushions in her hammer-beamed
bedroom in the eaves of the President's Lodge, listening to 'All
in Love is Fair' in a trance of concentration. I watched the yellow
Motown label revolve on my awful stereo . . .

And so Stevie Wonder displaced my inner German and stood
in for girls. In fact, it's broadly true to say that, for a few
months in 1975, Stevie Wonder was my girlfriend.

*

It was late in the summer of 1975 that I first heard a Stevie
Wonder joke.

That summer was my cricketing *annus mirabilis*. I played an
entire season for the county schoolboys team; I made my first

break into the middle order of the school First XI; and I was signed up to add youthful flair to the rather aged village side. 'Young Bradman,' the village team captain called me – not, I thought, without a hint of sarcasm. One thing was sure, though. That year I couldn't help scoring runs. Even though my hair was halfway down my back and I was obliged to wear an elastic headband just to see out, that didn't prohibit my thin-wristed cuts and drives and pull-shots from bobbling over the fen turf to the boundary with monotonous frequency.

One Sunday the village eleven were struggling on a sticky dog at some outpost located in a bog several feet below sea level. No batsman could get in. Everyone was getting out. I couldn't hit the ball off the square; indeed, I could barely hit the ball at all. And I was facing the obligatory fen fast bowler, whose legs were as bandy as his chest was broad. He was not in the least tall, but he was getting the ball to swing in the rancid air and then bite out of the sticky dog's back as if he were a new incarnation of Geoff 'Horse' Arnold.

He was boiling. I'd played fruitlessly at four consecutive deliveries outside the off stump and missed the last one by inches, not millimetres.

'Gaaaaah!' yelled the fast bowler, throwing his hands above his head very much as he'd seen Horse do on telly. And then his hands descended to his hips and he glared down the pitch.

'Jesus fuckin' Chroist, Stevie Wonder – yer s'poosed to *hit* the cunt!'

17

'So no one at the hospital suggested that you be sent to see a specialist?'

Nope.

'They just offered you sessions at a tinnitus clinic which turned out not to exist?'

Yes.

'And they said they'd see you again in six months – when you can't even stand up straight?'

They did say that, yes.

'That doesn't seem very helpful somehow, does it?'

No, not really.

This was a friend speaking at another friend's party. I'd forced myself to put in an appearance, partly to lend support – it was a book launch – and partly because I wanted to see how I got on in such an environment, even though I knew it would be excruciating. Maybe I wanted to show off a bit, too. You know: I may need two sticks and a beautiful woman on my arm to get around, but check out my pluck! That sort of thing. And anyway, if I can get to the Arsenal, then I can get to the Design Museum.

Of course, it was torture.

It was bad enough standing there, leaning my head at a stupid angle against the glass doors on the museum terrace, trying to sublimate the overwhelming electrical interference in my brain and not look stricken, while kind people asked after my well-being. That was bad enough. But getting over the threshold in the first place had not been without its difficulties.

I'd dressed up for the occasion: squeezed into my wedding suit, waistcoat and all, shaved my chin, moisturised my dome and pinched my cheeks in the bathroom mirror to try to make myself look less like a corpse. Even, slowly, put on proper shoes. Jane had then driven through east London as darkness fell, while I closed my eyes against the lights, which jerked and flickered all around. We had parked in the back streets around Butler's Wharf. After dark, everything around there is coloured an even sodium orange.

We walked to the museum at funereal pace, Jane's hand hooked lightly into the crook of my elbow, more as a moral support than an actual one. My sticks clicked faintly on the tarmac. Everything was so orange; orange as sin and nausea. The din of early evening traffic heading towards Jamaica Road was far enough behind us to stimulate no more than a sclerotic hum in my brain. But everything was orange . . .

'I'm going orange! I'm orange as HELL!'

This was what my father-in-law used to cry as he sensed the onset of a diabetes meltdown, more often than not following an extended session with a bottle. His insulin levels would then drop to 'orange' levels. *I'm orange as all hell,* he'd splutter drowningly to anyone within earshot, and quite often when no one else was in the room – he could sometimes be heard bellowing away on his own from the other end of the house. He had been stopped from saying that he was orange by his death eleven months previously. Jane was still in mourning.

Geoffrey had not been a happy man. His abiding truculence and fondness for several drinks too many were born out of a combination of blindness, grinding diabetes and, at bottom, the frustrations of an unfulfilled musical life. I think that if he'd been able to pursue that life then the diabetes and the blindness might have been coped with. As a young man he had been a good enough clarinettist to aspire to the ranks of the professional soloist, but found his ambitions thwarted by his inability to see anything much at all apart from movement and light, unless the object he was trying to eyeball was held up against the side of his nose. Instead of playing clarinet quintets at Wigmore Hall, he'd become a clarinet technician, looking after the instruments of the great and good of the clarinet world, including, for a while, Acker Bilk's. He was proud of that, at least. He even invented a new keying option for the instrument, which had been universally adopted as the 'Geoffrey Acton System'. He was, in his way, a distinguished man. But he was also a very angry man and the last few years of his life had been a torture for all concerned, including Geoffrey.

I always got on reasonably well with him, despite his foibles. Following my acquiescence to his Benny Goodman lecture in front of the stove in the cobwebbed house in Suffolk in the winter of 1992, we'd settled for a neutral relationship conducted through music talk. Some men sublimate their social anxieties by talking only about football; we would talk about Mozart and Count Basie, and he'd tell me about Acker Bilk and Jack Brymer and Gervase De Peyer, each of whom he'd known. He would always have Radio Three on in the room, and we'd discuss whatever was playing and what we liked and didn't like, and why. And every Christmas I'd make him a compilation tape of modern jazz I thought he might enjoy. He received the tapes with mustered grace, although I was never entirely convinced he didn't feel slightly resentful about it. I suspect that he suspected me of patronising him. Nevertheless, I got the impression he developed a taste for Art Pepper because of it, which was both apt and satisfying.

And then he'd do or say something I couldn't stand and I wouldn't know what to say or do in response. He was my wife's dad. He was old and blind and disappointed and vulnerable and buggered and his anger was to be understood; absorbed, maybe. I could say nothing. I don't think I was ever the object of his rage – not that I knew of anyway – but he was sometimes the cause of mine. I suppressed it, of course. And when he died I felt both sadness and a sense of relief on his behalf, as well as everyone else's. No more anger. No more discomfort. No more orange.

Yet less than a year later Jane found herself helping another dependent old git around, another old git with orange issues. The new one was now using the pair of sticks which had once supported the lately deceased one (he'd turned down the offer of Geoff's Zimmer frame out of sheer vanity) and he was just as slow-moving and bent over in more or less the same unsteady configuration. Jane did not draw my attention to the repetitious cruelty of life, nor dwell openly on her misfortune at being surrounded by gits, and I was grateful for that. But I did often wonder how much more stomach she had for us all.

This may or may not have been the cause of the panic which began to rise through my body as we approached the entrance to the museum. I asked Jane to pause for a minute, while I gathered myself. I told her it was because of dizziness, and this was partly true – when I start to panic I feel dizzy. But actually it was only panic which made me run aground at the Wharf, as it had been panic of a much more thorough kind which deposited me in a heap on the pavement outside the GP's surgery on the day I was first struck down.

On that occasion I shouldn't have been anywhere near the surgery. I should have been in hospital. But we'd made the mistake of ringing NHS Direct, who had told Jane in no uncertain terms that – given that it was eight o'clock in the morning – we should go to the GP's surgery when it opened in an hour. Instinct had told us to do something else, but we obeyed the command. By the time Jane had forked me into the car and driven the few hundred yards up the road to the doctor's, I was almost completely sightless, choking back vomit and so deprived of balance function that I'd been compelled to clamp my head against the front-seat headrest with my own two hands. Worse still, the children were in the back of the car.

Much of what occurred that morning has gone now. It is completely lost to memory, apart from a few flashes. One of the flashes makes me feel sick still. It is of my gradual descent down the lower shaft of a lamp post outside the surgery, while I cry like a baby, unable to walk, see, speak or stand, completely overwhelmed with panic and horror. I can still hear the sound of my own whinnying, distorted and shut inside my head.

It fell to my children, then aged ten and seven, to help Jane half-carry, half-walk my violently shaking frame the remaining fifteen yards to the surgery threshold, where help materialised.

It is perhaps not such a strange thing that a memory like this is almost literally unbearable. It is not within a father's natural compass to expose his vulnerability to his children in such a way, or in any other way for that matter. This is not machismo. I do not feel that my manhood was compromised by my slide down the lamp post. It was not a failure of testosterone supply that caused me to beseech my daughter to hold my head as tightly and steadily as she possibly could. But the slide certainly left me with a compromised sense of fatherhood. How could it not? I let the children down: I exposed them to a vision of one of the two most frightening things they can imagine.

The children seem all right, though – children are resilient, as we all know – and they are hugely sensitive to my condition and their roles in accommodating it, which I am really impressed by: but I do not want them to be party to anything like that morning's events ever again, at least not until they are adults and I am on my very last legs. The Beezer has already forgotten the episode, at the conscious level at least, which is convenient. Thank you, Beezer-brain. But I do worry about what residue of horror remains inside both their sealed units. It is out of such dregs that hauntings are made.

And it is that anxiety which feeds the panic which rises in me sometimes and, on this occasion, began to bubble like magma in my chimneys and flues on our slow walk to the Design Museum.

We stopped.

I breathed deeply for a minute, felt the magma cool and subside a little, and then we went into the museum foyer, where hubbub reigned and a funk DJ did his thing, albeit at a literary level of amplitude.

Yoiks.

Imagine your brain being stirred with spoons. Not one spoon, but several; maybe a dozen, stirring this way and that. And the spooning is being done not only by a funk DJ but by a lot of people who think they're being nice to you – in fact they *are* being nice to you – and who only want to make you feel better by asking after your well-being, discussing your condition, speculating on possible causes, making jokes about your suit, admiring your pluck . . . Yet the more they stir, the faster you crumble into flakes of consciousness whirling in an irregular downward spiral to the floor and the longed-for possibility of total silence. *Take me DOWN!* your mind screams, and your body does its best to oblige.

In response I could only grin and nod, as I had done at Arsenal, and try not to betray anything with my face. But I imagine I just looked mad. Within five minutes I was slurring my words. Within twenty-five I had to leave. As we quit the terrace I got wedged in the doorway with an acqaintance I hadn't seen in a couple of years. There was no way out of this one for either of us.

'Good heavens . . . *Nick!*' she said, surprise and shock etched over her features. It was clear she hadn't immediately recognised the hunched and pallid old geezer in front of her as the ruggedly charismatic Clark Gable figure of previous encounters.

'Er, how are you doing? Gosh, I'd heard you hadn't been well . . .' And she trailed off. Poor thing. We didn't know each other well enough to be able to shift through the gears of sick-person protocol with easy companionability. She still looked shocked after about a minute of toing and froing and was quite unable to get into a conversational rhythm. But I was grateful. She was in no position to give my brains a good stir, and so I was able to mumble something soothing and then push off with maximum celerity. People who are obviously ill enjoy massive social advantages.

But it was another friend, Sarah, who asked the direct and not at all confusing questions which began this chapter. She is brisk, but in a good way. Talking to her is never like having one's brains stirred with a spoon; more like being bopped on the head with one.

'So what are you going to do about it then?' she said.

'I suppose I could go back to my GP and see if I can get another referral . . .'

'Tell you what,' said Sarah. 'Why don't you get in touch with my friend Theo in Gray's Inn Road . . .'

*

And so it was that a couple of months later I found myself attending a clinic at the Royal National Throat, Nose and Ear Hospital in King's Cross.

The Royal National does not bear comparison with the Royal London in Whitechapel, partly because it is a specialist hospital. The queues are long, but they move purposefully. The floors and walls are obviously, rather than technically, clean. The entrails of the building do not hang out of holes in the building's ceilings.

I was seen first by a junior doctor who made an initial assessment before I was sent further up the line to be examined by more senior figures, among them Theo himself, who is eminent but not feudal in his manner. In due course I found myself sitting in a room with three senior bods, Theo included (he was obviously unaware that the slightly mad-eyed man in front of him was the fellow sent to him by his old friend Sarah), all of them listening intently, thinking about what I had to say, and responding as if what lay before them was a problem which needed addressing, not a statistic to be processed as quickly as possible.

And even if they were equally unable to give me an account of precise causes and offer a comprehensive diagnosis, they did give some indication of what to anticipate over the coming year. They explained more about the electrical processes currently going on in my brain. They also told me firmly that there was no reason to expect further calamity, notwithstanding the certainty that my hearing had gone for good. It was interesting to be told that. No one had said anything like as much before. They then took me through the likely story of what had happened to me, neurologically and audiologically speaking, and they explained how the adaptive properties of the brain were such that 'I'd be very surprised if you don't feel rather better in a year's time.' They sorted out hearing therapy to address the tinnitus, physiotherapy to help with the balance; they said that they'd like to conduct further tests to establish the extent of the damage and the severity of my handicap; and they said they'd like me to consider the possibility of being fitted with a Bone-Anchored Hearing Aid.

I couldn't keep an idiotic smirk from spreading like jam all over my face. This was great. Someone was taking me seriously at last. They were making positive noises. They were offering something like a prognosis. They were even offering me the opportunity to have a hole drilled in my skull so that a device might be implanted in there to pick up vibrations on the dark side of my sealed unit. I felt so pleased about this that I made an admiring comment about the way Theo's ears went up and down when he smiled. He did not seem hugely charmed by this and I am not surprised. But I couldn't help it.

For the first time in six months I felt slightly different. Not physically better as such, but more solidly human in my crappiness, as if made of bones and flesh as well as faltering electrical charge. It was only as I flumped down on to the disabled seat at the front of the bus home that I realised what the difference was. I didn't feel frightened.

18

I joined the Rolling Stones on lead guitar in 1975.

The mellifluous Mick Taylor had left the band in December 1974 to widespread consternation and it was unclear for the first part of the following year who would be his replacement, if indeed he was to be replaced at all. There were dark rumours going round that the Stones might even take the nuclear option and engage a session player on a pay-as-he-plays basis. You know: a hack.

Happily, they settled on me as Taylor's natural successor.

I don't remember much about the selection process. Memory places me in a succession of chintzy palaces, dressing rooms and low-ceilinged rehearsal spaces being treated to the full repertory of Keith Richards' mood swings, from charming hipster via dishevelled incompetent to playground bully. I got the cold shoulder a lot, as I recall, especially from Jagger. Charlie was all right. Bill? Hardly noticed him at all. I just hung in there and did my best. I knew, as the modern affirmation has it, that I really, really wanted this.

Of course I was a different kind of guitarist to Taylor. He was a high-romantic melodist; a beautiful, Gibsonian, singing player, whose lines vaulted across the Stones' chuggy rhythms like a Gospel tenor. I could not claim such eloquence. I was percussive not mellifluous, passionate rather than fluent, romantic but endowed with the astringent romanticism of the fen, rather than the flighty kind you get in Welwyn Garden City, which was where Mick Taylor came from. Naturally I played a Fender rather than a Gibson. I was different but, God, I was good.

But was I, really?

The sequence of dreams which installed me in the Stones continues to this day: I'm still in the band. Although, amazingly, I remain a total newbie in the other Stones' eyes, forever on trial, nervous, unsure of myself, prone to anxiety attacks and frequently kept waiting at rehearsal by other band members, who plainly do not share my view that being late is an unsubtle way to show your contempt for those you're being late for. Or maybe they do share it. Still, the dreams persist, now at a rate of about one a year at most. Oddly, I never see Ronnie Wood in them.

One factor remains constant, other than the cold-shouldering. At the outset of each and every dream it is entirely unclear whether or not I can play. I show up with my guitar, I hang around a lot being ignored; occasionally Mick or Keith, but mostly Keith, mutter something that might be construed as instructions, sometimes accompanied by a brotherly wink, and we walk up a ramp and plug in, usually in front of a baying audience. There are always girls with their elbows on the stage apron. I seldom see drugs and I never find myself in a position to take them. And nine times out of ten I wake up at the point of revelation. Keith counts it off and . . . Hands turn to wood. The plank on a strap around my neck remains a plank. My eyes widen.

I can't play! I am a fraud.

I've had the acting dream many times, too – the one where you walk on stage and can't remember your lines. I have some-times not even known what play I'm in. And, of course, I have sat in examination rooms and not had a clue what to put down on paper – a dream which has cleaved more closely to dreary reality than I care to think about. But the fraudulence dream I have endured most in my life is the Stones one. I'm fond of it, partly because . . . well, because it's me joining the Stones, innit? And partly I'm fond of it because it comes with a lottery ticket.

I say that nine times out of ten I wake up at the point where my fraud is exposed, but actually those odds aren't quite right. It's closer to nineteen times out of twenty. The twentieth is the winning number on the lottery ticket. Every twentieth Stones dream, Keith Richards plays the uncoiling introduction to 'Tumbling Dice' and . . . I *can* play! Don't know why or how, but I can. And it is an exquisite feeling; a dream feeling within a dream. I float into the music, I join the current, pulling out of the flow to leap off the back of the downbeat. My hands fly. The plank is a voice. The song is a magnificent calling river and I ride it like a fish.

On those occasions, I wake up in a state of ecstasy.

Happy.

But pretty soon I start wondering what on earth I thought I was doing. Who do I think I am? Just how infantilisingly delusional can an adult male get? Guitar playing of that fluency is hard; it doesn't *just happen*. You have to work and work and work and even then, still, if you don't have the jam in you, the doughnut of a fulfilling life goes unfilled. Talent is meaningless without labour, but talent does not arise from labour. It is something you either have or you don't.

I once even joined Led Zeppelin, but on that occasion found there was no room in the group for both Jimmy Page and me. Talent needs space to live in too.

*

It is important to understand that these are English dreams. They are not American ones. They are the sort of dream you dream when you are asleep; they are not the thrusting aspirations of a conscious mind. It has never been a 'dream' of mine to become a rock star.

Well, I say that; and I'm pretty sure that it's true up to a point – I think I'd remember if I'd spent long years harbouring an unfulfilled longing. I remember all the other longings quite clearly. But I must have contemplated the idea at some level once upon a time, because it remains one of my mother's favourite stories to tell about her occasionally daft but fundamentally sensible son, that she found me weeping silently in my bedroom one afternoon when I was fifteen. 1975 again.

'What,' she wondered, 'seems to be the trouble?'

Oh, I whispered, barely able to raise a breath: oh, nothing – it's just that I have come to the horrible realisation that not only will I never be a rock musician, but also I will never play cricket for England.

In my *annus mirabilis*, too.

It doesn't do to be too forensic about such things, especially when mothers are involved. But I do have a watery memory of this event, if not of every detail of the sequence of insights which brought me to this epiphany. One part of the memory is clear, though. I experienced the epiphany after a cricket match played for Cambridgeshire Schoolboys against mighty Surrey, who were mighty not only in ability but also in physique – their shortest player was taller than our tallest. Could they really be Under-16s? Or do they just have better genes in Surrey?

Whatever, they steamrollered the fen spindlies in short order and I was out for three, caught in the gulley fending off a throatball. It had been the first delivery I'd seen. And the whole dismal experience confirmed what I already knew in my cricketing bones: that when faced with extreme fast bowling I was crap. Just couldn't see the ball; had no time in which to move. Probably looked scared of it, too. Which was no good at all as I had a thing about getting into line, as all earnest batsmen do. The upshot was that, against exceptional pace, I'd expend all my psychic energy on the counter-intuitive effort of getting my skinny bod into what I presumed to be the line of the hurtling invisible orb and then, unable to react cogently, I'd just get hit. *Zonk. Doof.* Embarrassing.

It hurt in more ways than one. At fifteen I'd found the limit of my batting talent. And it was that episode which precipitated the collapse of morale in my bedroom. I think the failed-rocker lamentation just got chucked in for good measure, to bring richer colour to the picture of despair. After all, I already sensed that the path to rock 'n' roll superstardom was strewn with drawing pins and that, frankly, I'd rather put my feet up and play records.

But I did quite like doing it. Being in a band. Making the noise. Listening out for the river's call. Oh yes, I was in bands.

The first one I was in rehearsed in a real garage, although it actually amounted to less than half a garage. It was so small and so full of stuff that once the metal up 'n' over door squeaked down there was no room left inside for movement of any kind. We'd huddle together among the crates in the jittering glare of a single fluorescent tube and feel the sharp ends of each other's guitars. As lead singer I felt obliged at least to jiggle around a bit, but even nominal jiggling was out of the question, not least because any exaggerated movement would trigger the garage door's release mechanism and the door would then fly up in a rush leaving the four of us exposed, frozen in stop-frame, to the gaze of passing locals. Nevertheless, I'd stoically wedge one shoulder against the ridged aluminium of the garage door, allow the other shoulder to be repetitiously whanged by the lead guitarist's headstock, and console myself with the thought that Eric Burdon must have started in conditions not unlike these, surely. And then we'd stumble out into the cruel brightness of a Saturday morning in Sawston and know that we were not the soul of rhythm and blues reborn in a metropolitan back-street lock-up, but a bunch of talentless provincial schoolboys in somebody's dad's shed.

To be fair, only three of the four of us regarded ourselves as useless, and this was reflected in the band name we settled on by majority vote, the witty and *echt* Lost Cause. Chris the bass player was in no sense deluded about his abilities, and Chris the drummer couldn't play for toffee. And I still to this day regard it as a cosmic tragedy that my genuinely serviceable boy treble had been replaced at the climax of puberty by a textureless English baritone of no range whatsoever and even less flexibility. Still, at least my name wasn't Chris.

Chris the guitarist thought he was God, though – or at least God in his manifestation as Rory Gallagher – and his self-belief carried us through to our one and only gig, at a farm on village open day in Sawston. The other two Chrises and I were perhaps not quite as grateful for Chris's commitment as we ought to have been – but that would possibly be because of his unremitting self-regard, which blanketed everything within range like ash. Still, there we were in Sawston, nervous as lambs on a stage set fashioned in a barn from an arrangement of haybales. We then twitched and lurched through a short set of songs by The Faces, the Animals, the Stones and, at some length, Rory Gallagher, and people clapped and laughed as if this were a small but amusing diversion at a village fete rather than the first rays of rock 'n' roll's new dawn. Afterwards, Chris the guitarist's disgust was such that he was unable to speak and he stalked off to be alone.

My other teen band was a bit better than Lost Cause, although it, too, only lasted for one performance and I have no recollection of what it was called.

Once more I took the role of lead singer, more out of

deference to the other guitarists' greater technical ability than from any great desire to prance around in a hooped T-shirt with an Indian scarf tied around my waist in the face of what I knew would be an audience of slavering sceptics.

This time the gig was mounted on a proper stage at the sixth form college which was beginning the process of evolution out of the boys' County High School, the one once attended by Syd and Roger of the Floyd and, now, by Andy Peacock. It had lights and everything. Even space for me to prance around in, if I wanted to.

Did I feel the burden of their presence – Syd and Roger's, I mean – as I minced out in front of the sceptics? I did not. I felt only the roar of the twin guitarists' 'Jumpin' Jack Flash' and the surge of adrenalin which would never be quite enough to counter bowling of the highest pace, but was always sufficient to get one's feet moving in the direction of girls.

This time we even had a couple of orginal songs at our disposal. I had written some caustic anti-materialist lyrics to fit Tony the rhythm guitarist's elegant funk licks, and I was determined to make them connect. One verse concerned the inevitable loss of identity which arises from the mindless daily round of consumer avarice. I sought to dramatise this theme by enacting a gradual 'disappearance' offstage, reversing inch by inch into the wings as the song went on and its message hit home. This'll get 'em, I thought.

Instead, as I made my exit, backside first, I caught sight of a familiar rotund and greasy figure in the front row, and he was laughing.

Val Widdowson was a Cambridge face. If, in 1975/6, I liked to think of myself possessing a certain Keith Richardsy air, Val Widdowson cultivated a Falstaffian stench. He was three or four years older than me and had recently left the High School. He was now busying himself both acting and directing at one of the Cambridge theatres and doing his reputation a power of good about town. He was a coming man, no question, and commendably weird. I quite liked him. I had exchanged oaths with him before at parties and enjoyed being patronised offhandedly by him. He was fat, unwashed, unkempt and unruly. And now he was laughing at me. Worse, he was mouthing something.

By this stage of the song it had been my intention to have disappeared altogether from view, leaving only my hand and the microphone visible to the audience – a relatively incisive dramatic metaphor, I thought, for what I was trying to say. But I didn't want to let Val out of my sight. I wanted to know what he was mouthing, so I left my head protruding from the wings, along with the microphone and my hand, while I tried to read Val's lips. I decided that his message was 'Coleman, you are a wanker.'

The song reached its thunderous conclusion and I marched back centre stage and shoved the microphone into the slot in its stand. I planted both my hands on my hips.

'Right.'

I pointed at Widdowson and his cronies ten feet away.

'*Right.*'

Val's eyebrows went up.

'Okay. Right. If you don't like it, you know what you can do.'

The eyebrows kept on going.

'All right? Okay, there's the door, you can . . . There it is, over there. If you don't like it, you can *fuck off.*'

And then Val's right hand came down on his thigh like a thunderclap and he put back his head and roared.

He died about three years ago, of an intestinal haemorrhage, which made me sad. He never really got out of Cambridge. Not properly. He was often homeless during his life, sometimes imprisoned. He was certainly very talented. And he was the reason that I did not – even for a minute beyond that night – think that I might like to become a real rock 'n' roller.

I remain grateful. Lots of them are real tossers.

19

We stood at the top of our little hill and surveyed the carnage. The light had dissipated almost completely by now, but it was still possible to see in the gloom the bodies strewn across every square yard of the hillside and to sense their movements, although by this time of night – perhaps ten o'clock, ten-thirty – there was not much movement at all beyond a barely perceptible, irregular twitching of the surface, as if the hillside were dead meat and the thousands of burrowing forms on top of it were maggots. After the tumult of the day the quiet was eerie.

There were four of us under our small stand of trees. We said very little. Me, Thompson, Thompson's far-out elder sister Alex and Alex's friend. It had been a long day and a hot one. Hard hot. Cloudy hot with heat that clamped around the temples like a metal hat. We had been grateful for the shade of our trees and we had fought hard all day long to avoid being shifted from our position by the press of bodies flooding on to the field from behind.

On arrival that morning we had deployed ourselves around our hamper like an infantry square and dug in our heels, and then watched the day's events unfold with, for me, that strange mingling of thwarted excitement, physical discomfort and edginess that I have ever since associated with music festivals, and that has ever since kept me away from them.

Knebworth Fair in late August 1976 ought to have been one of the highlights of my short life. At last I was going to see my favourite band play live. The Stones. In East Anglia, just about. Yet the day had dragged and dragged to the point where I just wanted it all to end.

The bill had treacled before the multitude in a slow parade of remote mediocrity. The Don Harrison Band (no, me neither), Hot Tuna, Todd Rundgren's Utopia, Lynyrd Skynyrd and 10cc had struggled and failed to project themselves from the scarlet, vaguely gob-shaped stage, and the sound, relayed on rickety towers, had established only a tenuous purchase on the hanging heat of the day. Despite the stillness, the music seemed to swirl and eddy. Individual instruments and voices would suddenly project themselves out of the flux and then disappear back into it as arbitrarily as they had emerged. Every note was slippery, every beat contingent. It was like listening for fish. I knew the Lynyrd Skynyrd songbook pretty well and it was fun trying to connect song titles to out-of-phase guitar riffs. Fun for a while. But there were no buildings in this music, nothing solid you might climb inside and settle into.

In fact, only two exciting things had occurred all day: the hippie who had fallen on me out of a tree and a short-haired man in bright blue jeans and shiny black shoes who had enquired in a deep voice whether I'd 'like to score, lad?' (it is just possible that the 'lad' was appended by me afterwards to make the story better; but if it was added on, then it has stood the test of time far more tenaciously in my memory than Hot Tuna). Besides, by ten in the evening I had still not recovered from a late-afternoon trip to the toilets. These were huge round green-painted tin tubs, about the size of a giant garden paddling pool, subdivided into triangular segments at the top but not subdivided at all at sump level. By late afternoon the sump was full and, as I'd lowered myself nervously into position in my segment, something had tapped my backside quickly and gently, almost apologetically. I did not turn around to look. Whatever it was, it wasn't one of mine.

And then 10cc had gone on and on and after them there was an hour and a half wait as the sun went down, so that the Stones might hit the gob-shaped stage in an ejaculation of nocturnal excitement. By the time they appeared – tiny, distant figures in a moderate blaze of light, 'Satisfaction' snatching at the ear like a dying radio signal – Alex's friend had gone to sleep and so had my hormones. The Stones might well have been at the top of their game, but from where we were standing there was no way of telling.

'Want to get in with me?' said Alex eventually from inside her sleeping bag.

'Not 'alf,' I said, slipping into Alan Freemanese because I wanted to sound blithe.

And so I did. It was nice in there with her. It really was. Warm and tense and unexpected and tired. Nevertheless, I was unable to tell whether Alex shared my dominant emotion as we snuggled up: that the day's events marked not the beginning of something but the end.

*

Punk approached Cambridge – as it approached all provincial centres – as an idea, without much form and even less heft. To begin with, there was no sound at all, only words and pictures in the music press. What noise it did make was of the rhetorical sort.

By the summer of 1976 my disenchantment with all things prog was not yet complete, but it was certainly entrenched. This was not through any great ideological turnabout; more the simple exercise of taste, which can act as decisively as any outlaw widowmaker, but more often acts as soft soap. Taste is partly the art of self-flattery and I was entirely impressed with my own recent excitement over Stevie Wonder, Dr Feelgood, Bob Marley and Be-Bop Deluxe, not to mention Miles Davis. I could sense the subtle evolvement of a new me, a sharpened, socialised, more eventful, less prolix me; one who lived in the world as it really is, rather than as he thinks it ought to be. My enthusiasm for the Stones and Zeppelin remained undimmed, but poor old Yes, Genesis and Pink Floyd now had the exhausted look of yesterday's progressives.

Lorry was disgusted. He took the view that my gradual opting out of the prog project amounted to a slow act of betrayal, slow being the worst kind of betrayal – the sort grounded not in burning conviction but in a weak-willed desire to swim with the tides of fashion (as magnetised by the pages of *NME* and *Sounds*). He did not quote Johnson on the subject of chasing the new-blown bubbles of the day but he did resort to poetry of another kind.

'This is all just pretentious, trendy wank,' he spluttered. 'Be-Bop Deluxe are weak as gnat's piss – just another bunch of art-school arseholes with a David Bowie hang-up and no balls. Bowie did this shit years ago and much better. And who the fuck is Jean Cocteau anyway? As for Bob Marley – since when have you lived in a ghetto? What the fuck do you know about the lives of Jamaicans? Come on, let's have it – what is the ever-so-special meaning of Jah to a white East Anglian schoolboy doing his O levels in a purple uniform at a school full of priv-ileged tosspots? Who, for that matter, *is* fucking Jah?' He stared venomously at the wall as if Jah were reclining on his brother's bed in the room next door. 'It's just bullshit tourism, is what it is. Bullshit tourism for white middle-class arseholes who've given up the fight on their own turf and gone off on holiday with their fashionable mates. Besides, all reggae is shit. Come on. It's the same thing played slowly over and over again, getting slower and slower until everyone dies of boredom. Listen to it. The keyboards aren't even in tune with the guitars . . .'

And on he'd go, pausing only to lower the needle on to his latest acquisition, which in 1976 would have been Magma, Can or Little Feat. Magma and Can were Lorry's leading edge, Little Feat what he did for a good time. He knew better than to bring Frank Zappa into the argument.

The worst of it was that I kind of saw Lorry's point, even as I felt the urge to disagree with him. What *was* I doing? Was I really a trendy middle-class arsehole?

How exciting!

By the fullness of that most ferocious of all summers, Lorry had been earning money for more than half a year pushing paper at the Examination Syndicate in town. It made me shudder to think that he might know my O level results before I did. But still. Our paths were slightly divergent now. He was already up to his waist in the world of work, wading through piles of cash and empty pint pots, while I continued to follow the middle-class arsehole's road to a proper education. Separately, we were making new friends.

At school, my relationship with the smartarse renegade Thompson had evolved into a tactical social bloc. We were outlanders; two boys straight out of Ursula Le Guin. We stood back to back, metaphorically speaking, and held our outlander ground. We did not spend much time explaining our inner worlds to each other or hatching plots to bring down the state or even moaning – for such a smartarse renegade, Thompson was always indefatigably sunny – but we did take elaborate care over the contents of our inner worlds, which we guarded jeal-ously. What gave us confidence was our superior sense of taste. No rugby-tackling straight was going to get even a fingernail's purchase on what we had stashed.

As it happened, we didn't actually like the same music; not entirely – not at the foundation anyway. Whereas my taste was English in bias, his was American. He had done the prog thing up to a point, because one was obliged to in the early 1970s, if only out of intellectual curiosity. But his real preference was for wiggy American guitars. He liked Johnny Winter and the Allman Brothers and Mountain and Hendrix and the Mahavishnu Orchestra. He claimed that he'd 'been into' the Allmans since primary school. Yeah, right, Thompson – and I've been into Miles Davis since I was in my mummy's tummy. But there was a certain credibility to his breezy hipnitude, a credibility founded not only in his own wishful thinking, but in the curious textures of his family background. He was from Leeds, his sister was inexpressibly far out, his mum was a left-wing lesbian, his dad was a bank manager.

Thompson was much cleverer than me, but neither of us seemed to mind. What seemed important was that we both liked Harlan Ellison, M. John Harrison, Michael Moorcock, Le Guin and the rest of the SF awkward squad, and we both liked art lessons, because the art room was the only place in the entire school where conformity was officially disdained. It was Thompson who introduced me to Bob Marley. It was with Thompson that I got into Be-Bop Deluxe and, soon after, Dr Feelgood. Our friendship was a matter of uncomplicated vector convergence.

And there was another vector coming out of left field. Straight out of Five Alpha, in fact.

Bevington was tall, stick-thin, pale, freckly and always unmoved. This was because he was just too hip for most things and so most things were a disappointment to him – especially those things which seemed on the surface to be hip but actually weren't, such as the music enjoyed by other people. His standard response to just about any proposition was to turn his mouth down at the corners, jut his lower mandible and snort, with a small disdaining backward jerk of the head. Approval, if it ever came, came equally wordlessly, in the shape of an eyebrow-elevating smirk accompanied by a decisive sequence of short nods. The nods were rare and golden because, generally speaking, the Bevington visage was home to no recognisable form of emotion other than contempt or contemptuous amusement. He didn't even frown.

Both Thompson and I liked him, though. He wasn't in our class at school, but he certainly had qualities which set him apart from the rest of our year, not the least of them being his strange, ironic, flappy yet extraordinarily rapid walk, which somehow mocked the very idea of athletic poise. The other thing he had was an elder brother further up the school who was a rock 'n' roll sage.

Perhaps as a result of having a sagacious bruv, Bevington was a neo-fundamentalist and a convert to boot, which explained his fanaticism. Not so long ago he had been a Smoothie. He had worn Oxford bags and bracelets. But now he liked the Flamin' Groovies, a besuited San Franciscan garage band who, from scratchy beginnings in 1965, had somehow etched a needle-narrow career path out of a trove of half-decent riffs, some tidy power-pop harmonies and a wicked way with a cover version (especially if the original was by the Rolling Stones). As a rule, the cover versions were incorruptibly faithful to the spirit of their source material, yet gleaming with dew. The Groovies were believers. Bevington was a believer. What both appeared to believe in was the necessity to make new.

Yet, although he never actually said as much, it was clear from the angle of his mouth that Bevington considered the self-consciously 'new' Be-Bop Deluxe to be the sort of overweening art-school twerps who give novelty a bad name. 'Make new' was not the same thing at all as 'make novel'. Make new meant 'make *real* again'.

This was how punk first found me, in Bevington's ex-Smoothie sneer.

*

A lot of shorthand myths have gathered over the years in the minds of my generation about the coming of punk. But then we were sixteen at the time. We were not only vulnerable to lively rhetoric, but also concerned to invest our lives with stories worth telling. Most of the myths describe Damascene conversions in the annihilating glare of a fluorescent tube in an amphetamine toilet in a suburb somewhere.

The tube flickers and . . .

My hair must go. My flares must go. My Led Zeppelin records must go. My expectations, and indeed my expectorations, must be reformed. I am rotten to the core, as are all things.

The flickering stops.

I am born again!

According to this shorthand, punk was an epileptic fit experienced, individually or in small groups, by thousands of teenagers up and down the country over the year between the summers of 1976 and 1977. And if not an epileptic fit, then an ecstatic vision, which amounts to pretty much the same thing . . . Oops, there goes another one: another teenager taken in the jittering fluorescence, falling down, jerking in the floor-wet, frothing, cursing, unlearning everything, then standing up with tautened sinews to clear his passageways with a good, hard flob at whichever cipher of authority happens to be standing nearest in the moment following the flash of transformation.

Made new.

I can see why such shorthand became necessary. After all, how tedious would it be to have to recall the real story every time? The real story, as Sir Joshua Reynolds would surely recognise, was laborious and involved a lot of fat talk and posturing and embarrassment and inconvenience.

The inconvenience was the important part of the process; that was where you had to make a real commitment. The talk and posturing were easy. The embarrassment, too, up to a point.

Lorry and I had spent the past three years arguing about everything, from politics to religion to who was the better guitarist – Gilmour or Page – so there was a natural contiguity to our new arrangement, which was to argue about the bankruptcy of dinosaur rock as set against trendy bullshit wank. And posturing always came easy to me, provided I could do it with sufficient playfulness to allow me to yank the ripcord any time I felt I was plummeting too quickly into earnestness. The embarrassment? Ach. What embarrasses sixteen year olds? Parents and losing face in front of girls, and both can be avoided. Keep the posturing and the arguing out of sight and embarrassment ceases to be a factor.

But the inconvenience . . . Inconvenience is a much more serious issue.

What must always be borne in mind about the subculture tribalism of the Sixties and Seventies is that, however preferable it might be for anthropologists to perceive those subcultures as self-sealing, unadulterated, pure and resolute to the core – in other words, a punk is all punk, a hippie all hippie, a mod all mod and so on, in much the same way that a banana is a banana all the way through – it is always the case that a punk is always only ever a punk in degree and, no matter how vigorous his protestations to the contrary, is *never* a punk all the way through. Sorry. That's just the way it is in consumer economies. It's just the way it is with people, who are not made the same way as bananas.

Nevertheless, it is a feature of standard histories of the period that the most reviled figure in the punk movement was the 'part-time punk', who brought real punks into disrepute by giving himself days off from being punky. The creep. Well, I have to say that, at the time, I never saw a full-time punk, not once, not even in London (the committed, photogenic, bumbagged, 'full-time' punk emerged later as punk became a marketable lifestyle vocation, following the death of 'Sid'), so I was ill-equipped to judge the precise point at which committed mendicant purity gave way to partial corruption. In my experience, punks were punky only as far as they could comfortably manage, and some were so part-time that they declined to refer to themselves as punks at all, even if they did rip all their clothes into streamers at the weekend and bought records by the Ruts. Right from the start this was the Cambridge way, where the overdoing of anything was met with scorn, but the overdoing of personal style got you laughed right out of town and back to the Home Counties suburb where you belonged.

In Cambridge, the small 'punk' contingent was drawn from the lower-middle- and middle-middle-class constituencies of the state schools of the area (both secondary modern and grammar) and was about as true to the punk ideal as is convenient in a town like that. The opposition, against which all 'punks', part-time punks and quasi-punks stood in union, was, of course, the traditional one – the one historically despised by hippies too: high capitalism and its cohorts, which included rock star princelings, bourgeois consumers, right-wing politicians, local councillors, parents, straights, Smoothies; plus, obviously, plod, parkies, traffic wardens and college porters. Hippies were, in their turn, despised by punks because they had woolly taste and long hair and because they lacked 'energy' and tended to be 'bland' in temperament, which was a reliable indication of having fallen under the yoke of the system at last.

Having said that, I do not for a minute imagine that irony and idleness were confined to the streets of Cambridge. I imagine that they abounded everywhere else, too, apart from Bromley

– although, of course, I have no way of demonstrating that. But in Cambridge, as in most places, the punk idea was interrogated, tried on for size, adopted conditionally and finally accepted as a good thing once it had been established that no one was obliged to get carried away or start behaving in a foolish or embarrassing manner. To trendy arseholes, punk's onset was as irresistible as morning, but that didn't mean you had to leap out of bed and start doing the exercises. That *would* have been inconvenient.

There was nothing inconvenient about the music, though. The building blocks of a brand-new aesthetic were already in place. Dr Feelgood had made SHORT and SHARP aesthetically desirable; Patti Smith had made expressionistic gutter-romanticism sexy; the Stooges, the Dolls and the Groovies had, over the course of a few years' semi-obscurity, made coarse exciting. But for a long time – oh, *months* – before the Damned and then the Pistols sounded like anything at all, the Ramones had sounded like the incarnation of all perfection. Pith in a nutshell. I'd heard them on the *Alan Freeman Show* one summer Saturday afternoon, of all places, and they had then colonised my bedroom and most of my non-sexual waking thoughts for the remainder of the year, giving rise to a whole new realm of speculation and conjecture.

Much less convenient was unpicking the seam on my favourite flares, scissoring out a triangular wedge of material, then sewing up the tube again. My mum was very obliging about this. She made technical suggestions, but did not embarrass me by offering to do the needlework herself. She further covered my dignity by announcing that this strategy was not actually being adopted to spare me embarrassment, but because she can't stand sewing. I nodded along. I wondered whether a mother and teenage son have ever been so happily in accord over anything.

But the drainpipes were only a preliminary gesture. Hair, footwear, jackets, shirts, socks and pants would certainly come, but could surely wait, as they were raiment only to the body and offered little to the soul, which, in my case, was reborn in a much more satisfying way. For me – Knebworth notwithstanding – the boiling summer of 1976 was actually a season of incontinent joy.

This was because it had been agreed that I would leave the school to do A levels elsewhere, the most thrilling part of it being that 'elsewhere' meant the girls' school over the road, where Lulu went. It had only been at the start of the preceding academic year that the Cambridgeshire High School for Girls had begun the gradual process of transformation into a co-ed sixth-form college, leaving a dwindling tail of green-uniformed girls to carry the spirit of the old grammar into eternity (my sister Becca remained in the bottom class throughout her secondary-school career, all the way through to the upper sixth form, at which point, for the first time ever, she enjoyed the privilege of feeling older and wiser than the juniors in the year below for three whole terms – she is now a teacher of the most passionate and committed kind). By the time of my acceptance into the new fold, the dozen or so boys who had been a part of that first pioneering generation of male sixth-formers were easily distinguished around town by their shit-eating grins. And now I was going to join their number, swelling the total number of boys in a student body of more than five hundred to, oh, nearly forty.

I wasn't the only one to depart in a hoopla of rejoicing, either. Thompson jigged off to Cambridge Technical College to do his A levels. He had fixed on semantics as his ultimate higher-education discipline – who'da thunk it? – but then got the heebies over the summer about whether our school was the right place in which to equip himself for such a future (the headmaster insisted he should be preparing to read law at Oxford), but by then he had left it far too late to find a place at a sixth-form college.

Bevington came with me over the road to the girls' school. He didn't do hoopla, of course, but I could tell he was pleased to be there, too. He actually smiled on the first day and shook my hand. Well, he touched it briefly, when I held mine out.

20

In May of last year, the fine and witty novelist David Lodge published a novel about a man going deaf. It was called *Deaf Sentence*, and if the title itself weren't warning enough, the review carried in the pages of the *Observer* was sufficient to guarantee that I would never, ever read it.

It was a broadly complimentary review. It opened with a quote from the text: 'Deafness is comic, as blindness is tragic'. It then went on to list some of the ways in which encroaching silence makes a monkey out of the book's protagonist, Desmond Bates. 'Am I half in love with easeful deaf?' he maunders happily as he mishears everything anyone says to him at parties, including a book recommendation. He heads out to buy the book, which is called *Being Deaf*, only to find on arrival at Waterstones that, actually, its title is *Being Dead*. Naturally, Desmond Bates is a retired professor of linguistics. Puns shower like ticker tape.

Comedy? Tragedy? Error of judgement? Errors of judgement are essential to both comedy and tragedy, of course.

Hmm.

All I know is I will never read the bloody thing, not if it were the last book on earth. I like Lodge's novels, the couple I've read; obviously I feel for his incipient hearing loss. But I cannot bring myself to titter complicitly along with his story, despite its clear relevance to my own life. Here's the thing: I understand why Lodge says deafness is inherently comedic, as blindness is tragic.

I hear what he's saying, I really do. The trouble is that I happen to be deaf, too – and not the one making the jokes.

How do I know that deafness is comic? Well, I have walked into a lamp post because I'm partially deaf. It was one of those hollow metal ones and it went *guh-doing* when I hit it. I heard that much. But how, I sense you wondering, does a deaf man walk into a lamp post? Lamp posts are the destiny of blind men. Deaf men get run over by buses, because they can't hear them coming; they get trampled by herds of cattle, because they do not heed the farmer's shout, the thunder of hooves or the klaxon moo. Deaf men don't walk into lamp posts.

Oh, but they do. This one does, anyway. As to the reasons why, I shall leave you to speculate. Besides, lamp posts are the thin end of the wedge, as well as the slapstick end of comedy. There are much, much duller ways in which we deafies invoke the mojo of the laughing mask. For example, on a number of occasions – in perfectly dreary circumstances at the greengrocers, on the bus, in the school playground, at the barber favoured by my son – I have managed to get completely the wrong end of the conversational stick, with mildly amusing consequences. Furthermore, because I have no directional hearing whatsoever, I have also spun round and round on the spot in the street, like a toddler who's lost his mum, while searching frantically for the source of a friendly call. It turned out not to be someone calling my name, but someone yelling 'shit' into a mobile phone.

Then there's the pratfalls. I have overbalanced comically on buses, on kerbs, on staircases, getting into and out of cars, on escalators in John Lewis, getting into and out of the bath, getting into and out of bed, bending down to stroke a hamster, and once even helping my mother-in-law up from a chair. That episode resulted in multiple losses of dignity and much hilarity.

There's more. I also cup my ear with my hand, to help with the scooping up of sound. Am I showing off by doing this? Am

I drawing attention to my handicap to elicit sympathy in others? No, I'm not. If you have two ears you won't be aware of just how much difference the act of cupping makes to the way sounds reach the brain through a single ear. But take it from me, it does. The tiny Jodrell Bank-style adjustment of a cupping palm can make all the difference between 'Nick' and 'shit', so it's always worth taking the extra trouble. Yes, I know: a Dickensian ear trumpet would be much more stylish, but you just can't get them in the shops these days. Ear-cupping – plus its physical ancillary, craning – isn't rib-crackingly funny, I grant, but as a social spectacle it does play for the comedy team rather than the other lot.

We can go lower. Not even as amusing as the ear-cupping is the do-si-do I have to perform with folk when walking side by side with them down a street. In public space it is not possible for me to hear what is being said by anyone stationed on my starboard side, so I am obliged to manoeuvre companions on to my left-hand flank at the earliest possible opportunity, before I miss something important (I often miss important things, and I imagine that for a period after I've done so my face is a picture of perfect idiocy as I try to work out, politely and from residual clues, what it is I've missed and then react appropriately – I am forever playing conversational catch-up). At first I was bashful about all this shunting around, especially with people I'm not on touching terms with. But I do loathe having to explain in full about only having one useful ear, so I make a small verbal gesture – 'Erm, would you mind if . . . ?' – and then perform a crab-like foot shuffle and a figure-of-eight gesture with the hands, followed by an apologetic ear-point, which is met with a puzzled look in return and then the dawning of what the gesture actually means and the consequent hurried rearrangement of positions, accompanied by crashing shoulders and stifled, considerate chortling, because no one wants to make a big deal out of it . . .

The manoeuvring is not comical as such, of course. But there is unease in it: disorientation and unease, the sort that belongs in comedy rather than tragedy; the sort that comes in a job lot with parcels of embarrassment and self-consciousness loosely packed to leave lots of room for misunderstanding – the basic conditions for comedy. But it isn't funny, not like when you mistake the word 'shit' for your name or make a sudden turn into a lamp post because you've got your auditory bearings all wrong.

And that's all right. I don't mind being a bit comical. And there is nothing tragic about my condition; not properly tragic. It's no one's fault my life has changed irrevocably. There has been no error of judgement (except in the ways certain Health Service protocols are set out). But equally, just because I feel the need to maintain a sense of perspective, it does not follow that I am saintly. In fact, I am more than capable of petty resentment. And this is where Lodge's *Deaf Sentence* really cops it.

Petty resentment of the most putrid kind is the real reason the book is so unattractive to me. Resentment and envy. I envy Desmond Bates – and, by extension, I suppose I envy David Lodge. I have actually read two reviews of *Deaf Sentence* and both lead me to believe that Desmond Bates is not deaf like I'm deaf; they lead me to believe that Desmond's incipient hearing loss requires him to sink quietly, and amusingly, into a warm bath of silence. Mmmm. Lovely. I accept that the bath also brims with social alienation and, for all I know, authentic despair, as well as the hush in which those things float. But it's a bath, nevertheless. It is quiet and warm. It is not a breaker's yard.

I would do anything for silence.

*

At the Royal National in King's Cross they had me doing some fun things.

One of them involved sitting in a spaceman's chair, which moved smoothly in total darkness, while tiny points of red light jumped and dodged in front of my groping eyes. Another one had me gazing unsteadily at a tropical horizon while strapped into a harness, my feet planted on a split footplate, the two halves of which gently tilted beneath my feet until I lost my balance. The harness ensured that, if worst came to worst, instead of falling I'd merely dangle. Less fun was the episode which involved the pouring of warm fluid into my ear to disrupt what little balance function I have left, while more winky lights jiggled and spun. Nasty.

But great really. It was wonderful to be given attention and to be actually doing something, even if it did all feel a little like playing party games after the party has ended. There was more talk of a Bone-Anchored Hearing Aid (BAHA), which would counterfeit the effect of binaural hearing by picking up vibrations in the bone behind my dead right ear through a special sensor drilled into the skull. I'd have a permanent socket fitted, about the size of a five-pence piece, into which I'd plug a small amplifier on a short stalk. The amp would be the size of a square Licorice Allsort and come in a range of colours including silver and matt black. It would surely go well with the polished dome of my cranium – it's the sci-fi robot look, baby: plug me in! I'd then be in a position to pick up sound from both sides of my head, not to mimic the effects of stereo hearing, but certainly allowing me to register in the good ear what's going on on the 'blind' side. To give some indication of what an installed BAHA might be like, they fixed me up with a behind-both-ears, double hearing-aid rig, complete with wire connecting one unit to the other in a dangly curve, like a smile on the back of my head. But I didn't take to it. The results were artificial and unpleasant in the ear, even slightly confusing, the amplified vibrations from the starboard side compromising the integrity of my port-side hearing. More distortion.

I got physiotherapy, too, from a very pretty physiotherapist, who blushed every time she looked into my eyes, as her job obliged her to do over and over again while I stood on one leg in front of her, waved my arms about and blinked, hopped and teetered around her clinic like a drunk. Presumably she could see my pupils dilating with a snap every time I was required to return her greenish elven gaze. (I should add that, despite the blush, her pupils remained steadfastly undilated.) Meanwhile, back at home, I did low-intensity calisthenics and experienced no difficulty at all in persuading my son to walk round me in a circle while throwing tennis balls at my head from strange angles. I was supposed to catch them. I also performed eccentric exercises with my eyeballs, picking out a distant object and then flicking my gaze back and forth between it and an object much nearer at hand, while walking heel-to-toe in a straight line down the street. I began to feel much more stable. I seldom felt nausea. And I felt quite comfortable nodding expansively when they told me that all of these activities were improving my eye-brain co-ordination hand over fist; that my brain, in all its plasticity, was now working of its own accord to compensate by subtle new means for my lost balance function. Well, some of it at least. The exercises certainly made me feel purposeful. For the first time in my life I obeyed instructions to the letter and without taking liberties, and for the first time in eight months I began to feel that things might be getting better in actuality as well as in theory.

But silence was not mine. The breaker's yard inside my head persisted in its roaring trade, its jackhammers and metal-crushers and steam hydraulics continuing to grind away, night and day, as if working to overthrow the world. The hissing was sometimes unbearable.

*

There is silence and there is silence.

When I say that I would give anything for silence, I mean, of course, the kind of silence you can hear, not the silence of no hearing at all.

There have been very few occasions in my life when I have heard it, though – the good kind of silence, I mean. This is because ever since I can remember I have had music playing in my head, at all hours and in most circumstances. It's like a jukebox in here. Or a concert hall. But perhaps most like an old-fashioned record shop, where music of every type plays continuously, whether you like it or not, and people talk about music in agued recognition of the fact that life – real life, as it exists outside the heftless realm of rhythm and tonality – is hard. The shop's racks are well stocked, albeit contaminated by the occasional shocker. The sound system is good. The rulings of taste are continuously being evaluated and then, if not found wanting, observed.

In fact, I sometimes think that I have never had a thoroughly thought-through thought because of it. Or at least I have never had a proper thought that hasn't come with soundtrack music attached – music which eventually becomes the subject of the thought. Where most people have a mind, I have nice music playing.

However there have been occasions when the music has stopped.

My dad died in 2002 to end a long struggle with cancer. The night he departed I heard nothing. No Elgar, no Marvin, no Bach or Booker Ervin. No Girls Aloud. Just unmerciful silence.

I watched him go. I was with my mum at the hospital after midnight when he took his four last breaths and died. It had been an epic struggle. He left one grey eye open and I watched its clouded depths clear as the minutes turned into an hour and then into another one as his wife made her last addresses. We then went back to their house – her house now – and sat up until the sky went peacock blue after dawn. Eventually I went to bed and lay there and there was no music at all. Nor sleep.

At the memorial service a talented local tenor sang 'Never Weather-Beaten Sail' by Thomas Campion, my dad's favourite Tudor lute song. It describes a longing for death as a release from labour and weariness, and the reward to follow in glory. As a small boy treble I used to sing it to his piano accompaniment, and I think it used to make him happy to hear me do it.

> Never weather-beaten sail more willing bent to shore,
> Never tired pilgrim's limbs affected slumber more,
> Than my weary sprite now longs to fly out of my troubled
>   breast.
> Oh, come quickly, oh come quickly, oh come quickly,
>   sweetest Lord
> And take my soul to rest.

The melody is as longing as any blues and as familiar as my family's faces, but I did not hear it at the memorial service. I have no memory of it even being sung, although I have been told it was sung beautifully. I can, however, remember singing it and him playing it.

Grief is not an emotion. It is a new universe, forming itself in silence.

21

I'm-a leaving outta Babylon, I'm-a leaving outta Rome,
I'm-a leaving outta Israel. This place could never be a home . . .

The room is small and dark, perhaps twenty feet long by
fifteen wide. Two narrow pillars in the middle of the floor
support the ceiling, which is low. There is a tiny bar in one
corner at which a gassy, sweet, strong 'malt liquor' in an ice-blue
can is dispensed cheaply and without a great deal of enthusiasm.
This concoction is called Breaker and it's what you drink.
Illumination is provided by three feeble wall-spots, a couple of
them fitted with coloured bulbs. Their job is to shine on the
space in the centre of the room and define it as a dancefloor.
The two pillars, which also occupy that space, do their intransi-
gent best to obstruct movement; dancers need to retain some
level of sobriety just to avoid crashing into them. All night long
the pillars take a hammering.

But not everyone is moving. On the very edge of the illu-
minated area a dark shape is defining stillness in a new way
– stillness as a gesture of defiance, of aggressive reserve, perhaps
of strangulated embarrassment. It is a stillness that will not
answer. The shape is as broad as a shed and dark as the mouth
of a cave. It wears a long black coat and its feet are planted
as intractably on the floor as the feet of the two pillars. It
clutches a can of Breaker in a big fist. The shape is Lorry, and

Gregory Isaacs' 'The Border' shall touch neither his body nor his soul.

No more, no more will I roam . . . in-a Babylon!

I haven't been seeing Lorry so much over the past eighteen months or so, not since he started his second year in his job at the exam syndicate and I went into the sixth form. We have both spent much less time than we used to in the village, preferring instead to hang out with new friends in town: me with my quasi-punk acquaintances, he with mates from work. But there is a small overlap in our circles: Lambert.

Lambert is an opaque, would-be hard nut with a granite jaw who works with Lorry but likes to do the latest thing, particularly at the Midland Tavern. And tonight the two circles have intersected at the Midland for the first time. Lorry has been persuaded that it would only be a creative thing if he were to come out for once to Cambridge's premier – and indeed only – reggae club. It has been put to him that, were he to cross the threshold at last, how much stronger would be his position to judge whether reggae is fatuous or not? Come on, mate. You might be surprised. You may think you don't like the music but you've never heard it in the context it was designed for. Come on, you'll have a great time. Promise.

It is never actually said that what makes Lorry uncomfortable is less the music than the pretensions of the small handful of playful white boys and girls who shamble around to the Rockers beat in respectful imitation of their poker-faced Jamaican brethren, who mostly line the walls, presumably until the white boys and girls have finished. It isn't said, but I know it's true.

And so the posse has tanked itself up at the Kingston Arms on the other side of Mill Road, consumed a swift spliff en route

(Lorry not included), and descended lightly upon the Midland's back room, where entrance is free provided you are seen to buy cans of Breaker, and where the Jamaicans whose club it is are grace personified, given what they have to put up with.

There is only one turntable and a single microphone on a short lead. The console is manned by two DJs in tams and an MC, whose job it is to toast over the brief silence while the twelve-inch discomix on the turntable is flipped by one of the DJs, then needled by the other. Cambridge does not number the new incarnation of U-Roy among its tiny black population. Nevertheless, the whole operation is conducted with eminent smoothness, provided you don't object to the MC's limitations. 'Seh natty in-a huptown Cambridge' is his stock phrase. Sometimes it's his only phrase.

Gregory's 'The Border' is the prime cut all summer long – nine minutes-plus of floating, dauntless rhythm, as hypnotically compelling in the spliffed mind as the prospect of another spliff; 'The Border' backed with its magical flipside dub and toast by the mighty U-Brown, which flows like the River Jordan in spate and contains the most poetic, meta-historical lamentation in popular cultural history. 'Roman soldier a trifle brutalise I,' bawls U-Brown, as if the welts are fresh upon his back. We dance on in our leathers and drainpipes. It is hard to tell whether the spectacle of the prancing punks is found to be an amusing one by the assembled dreads and their womenfolk; it is certainly a cause for anxiety in the minds of the assembled punks when the stratospherically high Lambert begins his circling descent upon the prettiest of the womenfolk. Round and round he goes in his lumbering gyre. It is to him a simple matter of masculine honour that he should do so. The rest of us skank on and pretend that we have never seen Lambert before in our lives.

At a time like this you gotta wash your soul
Seh, what about the half thatta never been tol'?

Booma-booma-booma-boooom . . . Lorry does not move. His can of Breaker is being crushed slowly, not by his fist but by the psychic force exerted in his determination to hold himself aloof. This is not his scene.

Afterwards he attempts to be gracious. 'Look, man,' he says, clapping me on the shoulder with one of his hams. 'I have a completely reggaeless soul. I just don't get it. It's kind of bemusing to me what you see in it. And no, I didn't feel like dancing. I wasn't *trying* not to dance, I was just *not dancing.*'

Later on when a few more pints have gone south, he becomes a little more forthright.

'Reggae?' he grunts. 'Fucking load of old shit.'

I am not in a position by then to explain to Lorry why I now regard roots reggae as the Solomon of all musical forms, because, at the time, I am not entirely sure myself. I am also unable to speak. All I know is that, in the vaulted grip of the mighty drum and bass, I am both at home and leaving home. I feel the music's weight and its seriousness and the liturgical cadence of its wording; I get the language and the rhythm gets me. It's like being in church again.

I can't say that to Lorry, of course.

*

But where the hell is Lulu?

I have spent a year at the same school as her, yards, sometimes mere feet from her lovely person, yet she might as well be a ghost for all the meaningful contact I've had with her. It is as if she only exists to be just out of reach. I usually see her in morning assembly, of course – and it's frustrating how often I snatch glimpses of her haughty profile three rows in front, only to lose it again as she turns her head and another rank of chairs is swarmed by incoming greenies. I begin to register Lulu not as an individual to whom I am distantly, unavailingly linked, but as a composite of tiny gestures, like a disassembled jigsaw: fragmentary visions of tossed hair and fleeting quarter-smiles; of raised eyebrows and kissing knees; hands which seem to hang in resignation at something to which I am not privy. I never hear her laugh, because there is always too much other noise going on. I never face her; I always see her from an angle. And now that I find that somehow I have acquired a girlfriend – well, *I* think she's my girlfriend – the ghost of Lulu is gently dispersing, as if blown apart by a subtle breeze. She is fading.

Meanwhile, I busy myself with the effort of self-reinvention. It is a gradual process, accomplished slowly and haphazardly, brushstroke by brushstroke rather than in a frenzy of concentrated self-making. To make new is not to make novel.

My new favourite rock group is Television, the New York art-punk amalgam of the Byrds and John Coltrane. My new jacket is a leather biker one. And by the spring of 1977 I have cut my hair back to a punk-acceptable mop – off my collar for the first time in five or six years, but crucially not exposing the tops of my goblin-like ears. I am beginning to wonder whether an earring might not serve.

The Clash have brought out their first album and so Bevington and I monopolise the sixth-form common-room record player. I dash out of school one lunchtime and come back with 'Complete Control', hot off the stamper, which is the best record ever made for a week or two. It is lent extreme cachet by the fact that it is produced by the eccentric Jamaican knob-twiddler Lee 'Scratch' Perry – not that you can tell by listening to it – and it becomes the duty of every student in the common room to suck up its perilous thrusts along with the contents of their lunch boxes. Most of them just ignore it.

Since autumn 1976 Cambridge has had its own punk band, too – although it is only punk by affinity. Being a Cambridge band they cannot afford to be seen to be suburbanly modish and so, rather than come off like bandwagon-jumpers, The Users accept the immutability of their local psychedelic heritage and model themselves on the look, sound and vibe of those obscure American 'garage' groups of the 1960s which it has been their privilege to have heard of in mid-1970s East Anglia. Plus the Stooges and the Stones and the Dolls. Through a punk filter. Spiky barnets, tight clothes, emptied-out faces, Gibson SG slashed at rather than played. They're nice guys, for the most part, and their 'Louie Louie' is as exemplary as either the Kingsmen's or Iggy's. They are one of the first dozen or so punk bands in the country to get a record out. Its title is 'Sick of You'. One day Bevington joins The Users on bass.

But Lulu does not go to the Scout Hut off Elizabeth Way to see punk bands, or Alex Wood Hall down Norfolk Street. She is never seen at the Corn Exchange. And the Alma, the Zebra and the Clarendon are notable for her absence; which is perhaps no bad thing, since the landlord of the Clarendon's idea of a joke is to put Wayne County and the Electric Chairs' 'Fuck Off' on the jukebox under F75, the co-ordinates for 'Sailing' by Rod Stewart. We all think this is a tremendous joke – as indeed it is – but I would not like to have been caught tittering at it by Lulu. Christ, no.

So where the hell is she? In her hammer-beamed bower snogging other boys, I shouldn't wonder. Probably more than snogging. Lulu is occasionally glimpsed through the window of a bubblicious coffee bar in Trinity Street, but it's not the kind of place I can go without arousing suspicion – it is a girls' coffee bar, with a girl's name spelled out in chubby letters over the front window, and a solitary boy might just as well hang an I AM STALKING YOU placard around his neck as cross its threshold to buy a bun. Lulu has almost completely disappeared from my life.

It is as if she had never been in it in the first place.

*

That summer, my mother colludes with an old college friend in persuading their two sons to go hitchhiking together in France. Presumably, the mothers are sick of the boys lying about their respective houses, clogging up the works, playing records, generating a pall. The mothers even offer financial easement, should it be needed. But what's to pay for, other than the ferry and subsistence and the price of a bed in a youth hostel? And I have been working in the kitchens at one of the lesser colleges and have a little dough saved. We can do it, can't we, Simon? I don't know Simon all that well, but I've always got on pretty well with him, and our socio-political differences surely need not stand in the way of a convivial week schlepping down the Loire in the backs of other people's Renaults. Hell, yes, it's what one's seventeenth summer was made for.

We go.

We have a perfectly jovial time, getting lost, making no progress and dodging chateaux on the grounds that we can't be bothered to go the extra three kilometres in the heat and dust. And after a stifling week on the road in each other's company, speaking schoolboy French to French people, drinking red wine out of plastic bottles and not sharing the same views about the higher procedures of life, we've just about had enough. We crawl back into Chartres and dissolve ourselves in the nastiest bottle of red yet. We become maudlin – we are probably homesick. We get so drunk that we confess to each other that we are broken by love.

I have never spoken before to a living soul about Lulu, and I don't say much now, apart from mentioning her hair and her eyes, her nose and her haughtiness. I explain how the haughtiness is almost certainly a veil to conceal her inner sadness. Simon is similarly heartsore, although I am not convinced that he is as heartsore as I am. He does, however, evince a more get-up-and-go attitude to both the specifics of the issue and to life in general, and before we have soaked up the last dregs from the ridged and crackling litre bottle, he has persuaded me that action is what is called for: action and follow-up action. There and then, drunk as we are, we write postcards to our respective beloveds, telling them exactly how we feel and laying down a barrage of billowing words behind which we might at some unspecified near-future date steal to within touching distance.

'We've got to back this up,' says Simon. 'It's important. Promise me that by the end of the summer holidays you'll have done something about it; I mean *really* done something about it, face to face. It's no good just saying stuff. You have got to ask her out. She doesn't have to accept, but you have to ask. Okay? *Okay?*

As ever, it takes forty-five minutes to locate *La Poste* in Chartres – although it would probably have taken only ten if we'd been able to see where we were going – and as the yellow flap in the post-box snaps shut I feel an equivalently sudden, hard, unanswerable constriction snap tight all over my body.

I cannot unsay the words now.

No.

No, no, no, no, no, no!

*

And then I find myself standing in front of the ancient iron-studded timber gate. There is a postern in it, which is closed but evidently not bolted. I have just watched an academic figure emerge and pat all his pockets, one by one. In search of what? In search of bicycle clips, of course. Two weeks have passed since Chartres and sufficient time has elapsed for the postcard to have arrived, provided it survived the French post office's legendary proclivity for heaping English postcards into mounds and then burning them. The morning sun is shining with rare intensity and there is not a cloud in the sky. I feel sick.

I am going to do it.

Aren't I?

Yes, I am.

I push gently against the wood and step through the postern. I do not glance into the Porter's Lodge – to look would be to invite scrutiny – but march straight through the gatehouse and into the first court, which opens out in front of me like a film set, a space conceived and designed to frame extraordinary acts by remarkable people. Again, I do not pause to look but walk on. If I do everything with conviction then surely I will get away with it; I will be mistaken by passing college members for a student – a young and rock 'n' rolly one for sure, but then they do take them young these days; young and brilliant and no doubt as dashingly romantic as I look today in my leather jacket and carefully ironed and then dishevelled white shirt and brothel creepers. And if I'm challenged then I am Cambridge man enough to bluster my way out of any trouble. Besides, what kind of trouble could I possibly get into? I am paying a legitimate call on the daughter of the college President. Where's the problem? How can they do me for that? I don't have to tell them I am in love with her, do I? I am not obliged to reveal everything. I won't stammer and blush and lose my train of thought, will I?

A young man rushes towards me in the black-and-white uniform of a college servant. The sun illuminates his bush of sandy hair as if it were a halo. He is carrying something heavy in a large cardboard box.

'Good morning,' he says.

'A lovely one,' I reply, my insides flipping like a fish on a river bank.

He carries on rushing.

And before I know it I am through the second gatehouse and into another court. This one might do as a set for *Cyrano de Bergerac*. Across a sward of perfect grass a cloister supports a double-decked and timbered range of mullioned windows as ravishing as the stern galleries of a capital galleon. It is a breath-taking spectacle. The weight of the sight of it is close to unbearable. My temples pound, my fingers tingle. I head for the shadows of the cloister and continue my progress with faltering swagger – I am beginning to feel, even hope, that the search for the President's Lodge will prove fruitless. After all, this could go on all morning, until either hopeless disorientation or sheer embarrassment overtake me and I am forced to retrace my steps and stumble out through the postern again into free air. The college seems to go on and on and on – I know without having to look that it extends over a famous bridge on to the far side of the river, where there is even more of it, modern and sprawling and grandly involuted. And besides, how will I recognise the President's Lodge when I get there? They're hardly going to advertise the location of the most prestigious front door in the joint . . .

And it's as I am resigning myself to this, and thinking that perhaps I really should call the whole thing off and go home, that the words THE PRESIDENT leap out of the shadows in tongues of flame.

They are, in fact, tongues of polished brass, but the impact of the words is biblical. I stand for perhaps twenty seconds in a shaft of sunlight in the corner of the cloister and I do nothing. I am shaken. I am here. I am nowhere else. I do not take a steadying breath, because I am not breathing. I knock. And then, for what seems like several minutes, I listen to the sound of footsteps approaching over creaking floorboards and stretches of carpet and tiles and flagstones and more floorboards. Finally, the footsteps stop and bolts and chains are withdrawn, keys turn, the heavy black door swings open and I swallow hard. It is a tall, pleasant-looking middle-aged woman who addresses me with a smile from the doorstep.

The first thing I do is tell a lie.

'Hello. I'm a friend of Lulu's, from school.'

And since I am already lying, I decide to carry on.

'And I was just passing – is she in?'

Lulu is summoned. She appears in the framing darkness of the doorway. Her face is subtly lit by stone-reflected cloister light. Her face registers . . . what? Haughtiness? Sadness? Bewilderment? Disdain? Pity? Utter lack of interest? It is very hard to say which, if any of them, it is. She does not smile or speak.

I open my mouth.

*

Perhaps four minutes later I stumble out through the postern and into free air again. I am not gasping, at least not out loud. I am in control. I simply drink oxygen in, slowly and carefully, like a man who has entered a vacuum, quickly traversed the void and then come out the other side. It is now time to breathe again. My ribcage expands and contracts. I lean between two bicycles against the ancient outer walls of the college and feel my shoulder blades grate on stone. It is only then that I start to punch myself in the face.

22

It is decision time in Springfield. The decision sure is a big one. But who is man enough to make it?

'Don't go with your gut, Homey,' says Marge Simpson. 'Why not go with your *brain* for a change?'

Homer looks worried.

'Go on, *try* it!'

Homer utters the whimper of a man suddenly, unexpectedly troubled, raises one finger to his mouth, rotates his eyeballs in a northerly direction and the camera zooms in to reveal the contents of his brain, as if through a porthole. Inside Homer's brain we see a donkey in a hat playing a ukelele.

My family insist that I share many characteristics with the Mage of Springfield, but the brain-donkey is the only one I accept. And even then only up to a point. I don't have a donkey in my brain playing a ukelele – nothing so shallow and cartoonish. But I do have an ear-worm. Always have done. I take him as much for granted as I do my hands and feet.

There is a neurological explanation, of sorts, for ear-worms – how they get in there, what they're made of, the way in which they serve the greater good of humankind. Oliver Sacks writes about them extensively in *Musicophilia*, and I heartily recommend that you read the book for that and for many other reasons. My interest on this occasion, however, is not the science of ear-worms but the subjective experience of them.

I assume that you, like everyone else, from time to time get a tune on the brain. My wife Jane, for instance, who is a pretty normal woman in most senses of the word, gets them on average a couple of times a week – sometimes more, sometimes less. They mostly last an hour or two. There is no pattern to her worms. The tunes she gets stuck with are as likely to be ones she likes as ones she can't stand. Sometimes it's a snatch, sometimes an entire melody. Always it's melody rather than harmony or rhythm. A particularly tenacious worm can last a morning, a day and sometimes a few consecutive days, but seldom as long as that. 'Go com-*pare*!' she'll bellow, suddenly, while emptying the food recycling bucket. She does not regard her ear-worms as anything other than an incidental irritant in her life.

Unlike Jane, I have an ear-worm all the time – literally all the time – from the moment I wake up to the moment I zonk out; and then, for all I know, throughout the night, except, of course, that I can't hear it when I'm asleep. I don't see it as incidental at all; I see it as part of the permanent fabric of life. That it is rarely irritating for me has to do with the fact that I am entirely accustomed to the little horror – and to the fact that I can usually get rid of a bad one by thinking hard about a more tasteful alternative, which then takes over. Have I got one now, as I write? You bet. Want to know what it is? No? Well, I'm going to tell you anyway, because it's a great piece of music and it might do you some good if you were to get it in your brain, too.

Harold Melvin and the Blue Notes' 'The Love I Lost'.

There you go. Great song. Superb Gamble and Huff arrangement. Heartbreaking voices. Enjoy.

Why do I have it going on a loop in here? It's because I listened to the original Philly International recording the other day after the Blue Notes' Teddy Pendergrass died and, through the hissy fog, it moved me – another great brick-breaking soul voice gone for ever. Yet the song stuck fast and it won't go away. The good news for me is that, in addition to it being an excellent song, it displaced something much less edifying. Another small triumph for Taste.

But here's a rum thing: I can hear 'The Love I Lost' almost as effectively in the ear-worm version as in the ambient one. The worm one is not at all distorted and only slightly clouded by noise and, furthermore, crucially, it doesn't make the tinnitus any worse than it is already. A considerable advantage. But there is one key problem. It is vestigial, as is the way of all ear-worms. I get it (get it? somehow the verb 'to hear' isn't quite the right one) in fragmentary form. In bits. Yes, with a little work I can organise those bits: I can summon the beautiful stepping Rhodes chords which open the song, and the guitar part, which ties a pretty bow on them; and with a real effort of will I can isolate Teddy Pendergrass's voice from the proto-disco chassis on which it rides, and then, for a while, go along with the groove of the thing, as if it's really there, ploughing its furrow in real space, moving air around. But the process involves work and is never what I want. It's not like *listening* to music. It's more like music listening to me, sounding me out, ringing my bell; a sort of invisible biograph testing my circuitry; a winking internal LCD telling me that I'm switched on. It is not *out there*, in the world of the night train where I'd like it to be.

The ear-worm version of 'The Love I Lost' – in other words the song as it imposes itself on me rather than as I choose to listen to it – is a series of musical cues which circulate in my head in a sort of randomised constellation: Teddy's dog barks, the guitar lick, the Blue Notes' chorusing ('We loved each othe-e-er, we *jerrrst* couldn'geddalong!' and, wonderfully, 'I lawst it; sorry, I *lawst* it'), the train-like locomotion of the rhythm and, above all, a certain passage of the string arrangement, which skims through my inner space like a thin bird above water – they whirl around continuously in there, diving in and out of focus, moving to the foreground and then away again, lit, then unlit, like some kind of weird kinetic, cubist installation expressing something to do with the relationship between Music, Time and Space – a bit like the best kind of Jamaican dub music, in fact, only without the repeat-echo and the colly weed. And it doesn't stop. If I want respite, I have to distract myself. It would be thrilling if it weren't so hard to control and, ultimately, so mocking.

So I try not to take it as mockery, and I remember what Oliver Sacks told me about how the memory of music amounts to more or less the same thing, in electroencephalographic terms, as the experience of listening to music. I look at what I have left to work with and I am forced to concede that what I do now is blur the distinction between the two, between listening and remembering. Between ear-worm and real music, between inside and out. In fact, music and its memory have joined together and become pretty much interdependent in my head. If I can *remember* a piece of music, then I stand a much better chance of enjoying it when I hear it again.

It's a funny sort of progress, but it is progress.

After all, for the six to eight months immediately following my calamity I was quite unable to listen to music for pleasure. Music no longer belonged to that category of things in life I associate with pleasure. Well, it wouldn't. How could it? Music did not make reliable sense any more and it hurt in a peculiar way. (Want to know what the 'hurt' was like? It's not easy to describe. But try this. First organise a stress headache, then see if you can contrive to burn your hand viciously on a hot baking tray: *zing!* That feeling. Not the burnt-hand pain, but the crawly shock in the rest of your body – the big neural shake-down which will bend you double and make you shudder if you don't exercise self-control.)

I thought then that I'd had my musical oats. And since there was little difference, neurologically speaking, between my experience of a scrunched crisp packet and my experience of music, I imagined that silence would have to become the supervening goal in life, as happiness used to be. Jane and I talked about moving to an estuary in Suffolk we know where the only noise you ever hear, apart from the mewing of seabirds, is the occasional chug of a boat motor skulking through the deeper water.

But eight or nine months on, Amy Winehouse appeared to me in an auditory vision and indicated that I was capable of getting pleasure from music, so long as I didn't think about it too much, and so long as I didn't try to hear too much *of* it. A bit of melody was clearly permissible, as was a neat bass line and an elegant arpeggio, certainly a beautiful voice; and God knows I have a terrible weakness for a harmonic suspension, so I'm allowed to indulge that as well, briefly – it comes and it goes, which is in the nature of harmonic suspensions anyway. But I'm not to get clever; I musn't count on getting all these things at once or being able to organise them together. I can't expect to hear the big picture. I mustn't get *greedy*.

In other words, so long as I am prepared to take music as it comes to me – in small, deconstructed, incidental fragments rather than as a complete apparatus, serendipitously rather than through my own effort of will – then there is every chance I might get a little something out of it in passing: music overheard as casually as chit-chat on the bus, as unsought as birdsong, as involuntarily as an ear-worm. Music in bits. Music without mind.

And I can live with that, if I have to. At least it *is* music on the outside.

*

My father's dust lies under turf in the Camary Garden in the lee of the south transept at Wells Cathedral. I try to visit at least once a year, more if possible. I go there and sit on a bench which is conveniently situated right next to his patch of grass, and I generally look up, not down. When I look up I see the angle of the transept roof, its lead work, its lichens, and beyond that the sky. I generally sit there for twenty minutes or so and allow the silence to envelop me. Or rather, I allow myself to envelop silence. I don't talk to my dad as a rule and I'm careful not to mutter to myself. I don't really notice what's going on around and about either, not that there is ever much activity in the Camary Garden. It is a lovely, lonely place, dedicated to the resting of old bones. And it is the only place I ever hear the silence of the breaker's yard with no music in it. I have no explanation for this. I sit down and quite quickly the music in my head just stops. The Blue Notes zip it and tiptoe away.

But to get to the garden you have to pass through the cathedral, and if there's one environment in which my brain struggles more than any other, it's high-ceilinged, reverberant spaces where a busy hush prevails. Hush with echo. Art galleries and big museums are a bloody nightmare; much worse than football grounds. And capacious public toilets of the kind you get in motorway service stations and airports are just awful. But cathedrals are the worst.

We walked one day last year – my wife, children, mother and I – into the cathedral with a view to showing the kids the Camary Garden for the first time: this is where your grandpa is, and so on. They had been asking. But just inside the door we'd been stopped in our tracks. *Paff!* By a wall of sound.

'Uh-oh,' said my mum, much louder than she normally would in cathedrals. She cast me a sidelong look and exaggerated her elocution. 'I don't suppose you brought your earplug, either. Do you want to rush on ahead?'

'No, I'll be fine. In fact, I'd quite like to have a listen. You go on if you want . . .'

Paff! Paff! Paff!

I didn't recognise it at first. It was big, that was obvious. And maybe British. *Paff! Sloosh!* I walked round a pillar and there they all were, stacked up in rows around the chancel steps: it looked like a large orchestra and a big choir – in fact, a massive choir. A double chorus with soloists.

I know what this is!

It's . . . it's . . .

I picked up a leaflet from a pile at the rear of the nave.

It's *The Dream of Gerontius* by Ted Elgar. I knew it! Well, I think I did. Hard to be confident when it's also a physical assault. But there it was: a rehearsal for a concert the following day with the Birmingham Philharmonic, the Frome Festival Chorus plus four soloists giving it the full treatment, as you safely may in rehearsal when performance tension is not an issue and there is still time to get the cock-ups out of your system.

'Mum!' I yelled. 'I'd quite like to stick around and listen for a while, if you don't mind. You know, test it out. If you and Jane fancy taking the kids through to see the old man, I'll catch up with you in ten.'

Paff! Paff! Paff!

I allowed myself to be pinned to the flagstones for a while, and then I began to walk towards it.

The Dream of Gerontius is an odd thing. It was composed in 1900 for the Birmingham Music Festival: an English oratorio, yet a setting of verses written by the Roman Catholic Cardinal Newman about the flight of a pious soul from deathbed to purgatory. There are angels and demons in it, and, of course, a priest. Lots of theological cog-grinding; lots of crashing metaphysical gears. Not my kind of thing at all. Give me Finzi, Traherne and *Dies Natalis* any bright morning. Or J.S. Bach. Or the Swan Silvertones.

I got halfway up the nave before caving in to the pain and

blocking my good ear, which I tried to do casually with one finger, as if having a scratch. This was only good manners. Imagine you're the mezzo-soprano standing on a box in front of that lot in a nearly empty cathedral, giving it some, and you're just getting your lovely voice attuned to the space when some weird-looking bloke starts crabbing towards you up the central aisle, white as a sheet, agony scrawled across his features and his fingers in his ears. You wouldn't thank him, would you? So I rummaged away distractedly with my finger as I drew closer and then hooked a sharp left around the side of the orchestra to a position behind and to the left of the harpist. I was now close enough to touch, if I wanted. I'd only have to take three small steps to interfere with the thing that was hurting me.

As I stood there I felt my brains begin to liquify. Electric soup. Colours. I imagined the soup issuing from my ears like lava and trickling down my neck. Fortunately, the harpist was stationed right in front of a pillar, and so I hung on to it, the side of my head, my shoulder, my hip, an ankle and foot all pressing into the stone. I leaned in and let the music crash into me, tried to feel the exhilaration of it, as if I were a rock and it were the sea. Come on, motherfucker, come *on*: you can wear me down but you won't shift me! You can eat away at the sand on which I stand, but I'm not going anywhere. The sand can take me with it. But I won't walk. I *like* what you're doing to me.

My vision began to go. It became slotty and blurred around the edges. I began to shake. I thought, 'I'm going to have to move after all, otherwise I might go over. I might slide down this pillar like I slid down the lamp post outside the GP's surgery.'

'Rouse thee, my fainting soul!' bawled Gerontius to a swoop of early twentieth-century English strings.

I laughed.

And that got me moving. But instead of moving away I moved closer; two, maybe three steps closer, and having got close enough to put a finger on the great scroll of the harp, I began to move laterally around the orchestra, skirting its fringes, as if skirting a curtain of sparks from a vast welding operation.

PAFF! PAFF! PAFF!

But I felt no heat – only cold; a chill crawling all over my skin and into my flesh. I was inside the music now. Right inside its pocket of shifting air, as if in a blizzard, a cold storm torrential enough to pound my own noise into powder. And even if the neural shakedown were now all-consuming and my legs weakening and my heart rate whipped to a lick, at least I had no need for directional hearing or for three-dimensional stereo effects. The music was in my bones and cavities, scraping my strings directly, pushing and pulling in every chamber. My body had become a vessel. The music was playing me.

I walked shakily right round the back of the choir, through the chancel, back up the south aisle and re-entered the storm on the other side of the orchestra, behind the double basses. I stood for a while, scooped up their sawing, swallowed their chugging, gulped it in like oxygen. Stood there for I know not how long, trying hard not to let the moment get lost in its own confusion. And, after a while, I felt a shove from behind and my daughter's face appeared like a spare head in the crook of my elbow. She looked up. I looked down.

'Daddy?' she mouthed, concern and amusement jostling for control of her features. The orchestra ploughed on. She reached up and caught some of the tears falling from the end of my nose and held them in the bowl of her palm as if cupping snow while it melts.

23

'I think,' said the consultant, 'that you may have had a migraine so bad that it sent a blood vessel between your brain and your inner ear into spasm, and the spasm lasted long enough to kill the cilia off on that side and leave you with the mess inside your head. I say "may" because it is a may.' She looked at me intently and then went on. 'There is no way of proving anything. I know it has been referred to before as a kind of stroke, and you can think of it as a kind of stroke if it's easier to do that, but it isn't really what we mean by stroke. It's migraine; it's your brain chemistry – it's what's been given to you by your family's genes. I do think, on balance, given what you tell me about your family history and the length of time you've been having headaches and visual phenomena, that this is probably what happened.'

I sat on the swivel chair in her consulting room and swivelled a bit.

'And even if the damage to your hearing was, in fact, done by a virus – which I think we have reason to doubt – that doesn't alter the fact that you have what we call a hypersensitive nervous system, something you've had from birth which has been exacerbated by the chemical changes which every middle-aged body is subject to.' She paused for a beat. 'That hypersensitivity underlies everything. The extreme neurological reaction you've had to the hearing loss is certainly a result of that. Now, tell me a little more about what happens when your eyesight goes, as you put it, *funny* . . .'

A migraine! It was a bloody headache what done it. Furthermore, it was always going to happen, given the way the genetic cards were stacked. Or should we think of genes as loaded dice? No, stacked cards. And while I'm in the mood for trite wordplay, I might as well compose my own middle-market screamer headline: 'HEADS YOU LOSE! Big-eared man's migraine a life-and-deaf time bomb, experts say.' Frankly, I'd much rather it had been a proper stroke, an embolism or even a frigging virus. How about a stress-related aneurysm? Or bird flu? Anything, anything, ANYTHING but a sodding migraine.

And it gets worse. Apparently, I have a 'hypersensitive nervous system'. How great is that? Why not go all the way to Memphis and add that I am also anxious about hoodies and that I have weak ankles? And then broadcast it on Radio Five. 'Big-eared man's migraine a life-and-deaf time bomb, experts say – but it's all his own fault for being such a great big girl's frilly blouse.' Christ, I'll never be able to show my face at the Mildmay Working Men's Club again. Nicky Wise and his brothers will be laughing their Pringle knitwear off.

I swivelled some more and tried not to look disappointed.

And then I decided to be mature about it. Perhaps there is more to be learned from this. After all, a 'hypersensitive nervous system' may not explain why quarks stick to protons, but it might shed some light on why I went mental on the beach in Thurlestone in 1971, giving rise to another of my mother's favourite anecdotes about the peculiarity of her firstborn. It was always her contention that I went mental that day because of the sea.

'You went a funny colour and collapsed in a heap,' she has explained more than once, as if I had been somewhere else at the time. 'And then you came to and were exhausted for a while. All floppy and absent. Very strange. Anyway, I've always said it was the rhythm of the sea and the smallness of the bay. You and the girls were collecting cowrie shells with your backs to the water, and the sound of the breakers was booming repetitively off the cliffs and reverberating around the tiny little bay like cannon shot. It was incredibly loud. You were about ten or eleven, skinny as a stick like Tom is now, and I was watching you fill a bucket and you suddenly looked up, uttered something incomprehensible like "Guh-duh!" and turned a ghastly shade of green . . .'

It was the sea all right. The sea resounded in the tiled chambers of my cranium that grey afternoon like the worst kind of banging techno slowed down to an infernal, mid-paced slam. I vividly remember thinking 'The sea, the sea!', rather as Iris Murdoch must have done once, and then my patch of pebbles became a slot of pebbles; it loomed and retreated . . . and then came up to meet my face.

This 'hypersensitivity' would probably go some way to explaining quite a lot of things, actually, not all of them behavioural anomalies: from strange lapses of cognition as an adolescent – happened twice in my first term at university – to the incessant headaches, bizarre visual phenomena and the utterly screwed digestive system which have scarred the past two decades of my existence; all of which were put down at one time or another to the stresses of working with diminishing enthusiasm in an unwell newspaper industry. Then there's my lifelong inability to drink alcohol in any quantity, my longstanding failure to get on with most recreational drugs and, above all, my abiding hatred of parties. I am an incredibly boring person and now I know why.

And then there's music. What about music?

The consultant was still talking.

' . . . which might explain why you have always placed such importance in your life on music. It's only a "might", mind you. But if you are always having to find ways to sort out or distract or deflect from the overloading of your nervous system, then music would be a very good way of doing it. When you're getting overwhelmed by too much input, as people like you tend to, then to focus everything on music might well make real sense – emotional sense as well as neural and intellectual. Such involvement would drown out the other noises, obviously. And it would distract. But also, there's a chance it would reprogramme your sensibilities by taking over the chaos you're experiencing and returning you to a basic state of simple functionality. It would be a bit like rebooting your system . . .'

*

This is not definitive. I know it isn't anything like definitive. It is speculation and conjecture. But it does have a certain logic to it. Music has always – as far back as I can remember – been a prerequisite of any situation I might find myself in where nerviness is an issue. Nerviness or anxiety or insecurity or uncertainty or confusion. Or, more often, just too much information.

For instance, it has been my habit all my life, when moving house, to fix up the music first, before there's even a chair to sit down on or a bed to lie in or a kettle to boil for tea. And when Jane declared that yes, she would, after all, like to have some music in the delivery room when she gives birth – and would I care to make some suitable tapes? – my sigh of relief was indecent. Jane no doubt imagines that all those hours of Coltrane, Marvin, Luther, Prefab Sprout, Underworld, Miles Davis, Nick Drake, Massive Attack and Lee 'Scratch' Perry were scrupulously spliced together for her benefit and for the child's natal edification. But actually, for the duration of both births, it was me who clung on to 'Equinox' and 'Let's Get It On' like a despairing, naked creature in *The Raft of the Medusa*; holding on and flapping at the horizon for all I was worth, desperate to reach dry land again. Jane only had to swear a bit and push.

Then, after being told that my father might not survive the weekend during the early days of 2001, I found myself rummaging frantically in cardboard boxes under the spare bed and in the boot of the car for the only pair of tapes I could countenance playing in the car stereo on the four-hour westward journey to Taunton Hospital. They were tapes of music I didn't like at all, made for me by two separate friends who'd both had the independent thought that it was high time I got my head round the Grateful Dead. 'It's *live* stuff, Nick. Much the best way to hear the Dead. You'll love it.' Both tapes were getting on for a decade old and, following cursory dismissal at the time on the grounds that the music said everything that needed to be said about hippie prolixity, they had been discarded to languish unattended in rattling obscurity, which is the place all cassette tapes used to go to expire. But now I had to hear them.

'What's going on?' said Jane, as I emerged from under the spare bed swiping dust off the flaps of a cardboard box.

'Oh, just looking for something for the journey,' I replied blithely, probably correct in my assumption that further explanation would only muddy the water. What could I say? That I couldn't bear the thought of driving off to witness my father's death to the sound of music that I *liked*? Or worse, *in silence*, with my body and mind clattering like trains passing each other in opposite directions over the same set of points? No, the Grateful Dead had a job to do: to distract me with endless, circular, cadenceless improvisations which stood for life against death and didn't stop for anyone, let alone my finely pointed sense of taste. Furthermore, forced contemplation of the Dead's live corpus might yet lead me to a place I'd never been before, and that could only mean one thing. Art! Whichever way it went – distraction, insanity or art – it was the only viable way of completing the journey.

And so for four hours straight I listened to the Grateful Dead, and then for four hours on the return journey the following afternoon I did it again, and by the end of it I did indeed love the Dead, not least because my dad survived the weekend and then another sixty weekends beyond that. I still love the Grateful Dead, although I am alone in the household in that respect.

So, yes. My nervous system and I share a relationship not unlike that enjoyed by the princess and the pea. Music is my pile of mattresses. Stack 'em high, my sensibilities cry, and there's a chance I won't feel a thing. Actually, hang on – that's not nearly enough mattresses. Give me more. More, more, more! One way or another, comfort *shall* be mine, eventually – and, to extend the metaphor so that it touches on the realm of taste, so shall beauty sleep.

It's a theory, as far as it goes. It certainly explains why, until two years ago, I found it difficult to do anything in the world without having music to hand, if not acting like a mattress then as a sponge to sop up the neural chaos (betablockers do that job now); and it makes a credible account of strange events such as Thurlestone, childbirth and the Grateful Dead. It is especially good at explaining why I have, all my life, been unable to bear overhearing other people's music – that is, music which is not subject to my will and control and is therefore only an irritant, an agent of further chaos.

But, actually, I think the theory only really goes so far as to address the ear-wormery. It offers a hint of an explanation of what music *may do* for me neurologically. It does not explain what music means.

24

The door opened. It was a white door set into the brickwork of a 1920s semi under a small, functional porch supported by a single metal perpendicular. She stood a couple of feet back from the threshold, shrouded in the darkness of the hallway, one hand resting on the edge of the door.

'Hello.'

'Hello.'

Her face was hard to read. Haughtiness? Sadness? Bewilderment? Utter lack of interest?

I smiled. She smiled back, just about, but it was not the longest smile ever seen.

'Come in.'

Memory, like grief, is strange and unreliable. Nevertheless, it had brought me quite efficiently to her door again, although it was a different door in a different century. What memory could not do was furnish me with the telling detail, and that was my reason for being there again on Lulu's doorstep.

I could remember getting in to the secret heart of the college thirty-one years previously, and I could remember getting out again, exiting the postern in the knowledge that Lulu would never be mine; and I could remember leaning up against the college stonework afterwards like a scraggy mop soaking up a bucket of self-disgust. Yes. I could even remember the sensation of landing a couple of solid-ish rights on my own face – until the idiocy of the act began to outweigh the satisfying pain in my cheek, at which point the pain became less satisfying. But of the nubby content of my visit I had no recall whatsoever.

The fact is, I had not really thought about my little expedition to the President's Lodge at any time since that day. Not at all. That same morning, walking back through town in lustrous sunshine, my cheek smarting, my heart a ruin, I had effaced the memory for good. *Zzzchoom!* Gone. How could I have gone back to school for my final year otherwise?

And as things panned out, I barely saw Lulu that following year and after that not at all – except once, walking down the other side of Mill Road the summer after my first year at university. I'd waved and she'd half-smiled back, probably because I was wearing a ridiculous hat. It was as if whatever had passed between us in the cloister had been drowned out in the white noise of A levels and the frantic gathering of new relationships; then by a year working for the owner of the record stall on the market (who had by now established a highly successful chain of shops across the Anglian region); then by moving out of the family home to live with Lorry and Lambert in a haunted dump on the edge of town; and then by pissing off to a northern university, where I might rewrite the co-ordinates of my existence from scratch and no one would be any the wiser. Did Malvolio get the opportunity to skip town following the yellow-cross-gartered-stocking incident, and do it on a government grant? I doubt it. Of all the fools in history I was surely among the best served by time, circumstance and prevailing socio-economic conditions.

But what *had* I said to her in the cloister?

Why did I need to know?

I looked her up. Google did not reveal her to be working a tramp steamer in the Essex roads, but there was a Lulu of her surname (now with an additional barrel) working for a charity in Cambridge. The tiny 'corporate' portrait looked right. The nose. The eyes. She appeared to have gone ash blonde.

I emailed the charity.

'I know this is an inappropriate usage of your email resource. I'm sorry. But I'm writing a book about Cambridge in the 1970s and I'm very keen to talk to a member of your staff, who I was at school with . . .'

The next day: *'Nick, nice to hear from you. How are you? I'd be a rubbish person to interview. I have a terrible memory. I don't think I'd be much use to you really.'*

'Are you sure I can't persuade you? I've only got a couple of questions, very specific ones. If you can't answer them, I'd quite understand; but I think you might be able to. It'd take 20 minutes and then I'd be gone.'

'Oh all right then. Since you ask so nicely.'

I recognised the address as being on the southern side of the city, quite near our old school. Wasn't that road a bit posh? Trees, grass verges with a footpath down the middle, proper drives leading to houses set fully thirty feet back from the road. I pictured her as the chatelaine of a rambling Cambridge villa, filling antique vases with flowers in breaks between sessions on her biting novel of donnish life, plus yoga and work at the charity, while her husband did important research at Downing and the kids made their way jumpily through the jungle of early adolescence.

But no. It didn't look that way. Not from the doorstep – not now I was standing on it. This was the other end of the avenue from the rambling villas with drives. The avenue was long and straight and appeared to modulate demographically as it drew closer to Cherry Hinton. This was much less intimidating.

'Come in.'

It was a beautiful spring day. We went out into the garden through a small conservatory full of little pots full of little green

shoots. Lulu, it transpired, is married to a Buddhist psychotherapist and the garden is the sort you'd expect a Buddhist
psychotherapist to have. Productive. Green. Little terracotta
Buddhas here and there. For some reason I made the assumption
that Lulu did the potting.

'So tell me about what happened to your hearing.'

She sat in the sun, one flip-flop sole very gently clapping
against her heel. I parked myself on a metal chair under the thin
shade of a tree; tipped the chair back and felt the back legs sink
into the turf a little. Sat up straight again. The noise in my head
from the journey was startling and I did not want to boil over.
I looked at her and tried to recall what it had once been like to
be unable to do so. She was as unreadable now as at any stage
during the 1970s. She did not blink and her head remained still,
erect, so that she looked ever so slightly down her nose. Did she
really want to hear about my hearing or was she just making
polite conversation – keen to observe form until a decent, caring
amount of time has passed and baldy over there under the tree
could be on his way?

'Well, I won't bore you,' I said, and then did so for about five
minutes. It's very difficult to explain about my hearing in less
than five minutes, unless you opt for the perfunctory version,
which takes about five seconds. 'I'm deaf. Got bad noise in my
head. My balance is fucked.' But that seems abrasive somehow,
and a little bit bitter. People do seem interested to hear the fuller
version, though, so I have got it honed pretty well now, so as
not to be too tedious, for me as well as them.

Lulu barely shifted on her seat. She seemed gentle, thoughtful
and sadly empathetic – albeit at a distance. Recessed rather than
haughty. If she was bewildered then she did a very good job of
hiding it. Once I'd finished explaining about my calamity, I
asked questions about the path her life had taken since 1977
and about her family. She has two teenage daughters, now more

or less the same age the two of us had been when last we'd seen each other. She works for the charity part-time; been married twenty years and back in Cambridge for most of that time. And while I listened to her answers I tried to see this situation as she must see it. Spring morning. Garden. Sunlight. Invalid revenant from a part of her past which had been of no significance to her whatsoever. Small talk. All things considered, she had every right to be bewildered.

'Anyway,' I said, 'I don't want to use up all of your day. I said I had a couple of questions for the book, and I really have only got a couple. Honestly. I'll be as straightforward as I can.'

I transferred my gaze from the sole of her flip-flop, which was now quite still, to her eyes and then back again.

'Were you aware at the time that I had a massive crush on you, and that it lasted for three or four years?'

I forced myself to meet her gaze again. Her eyes seemed greyer than they used to. I remembered them being darker than that. But then again, from my position in the shade under the tree seven feet away, I wasn't anything like close enough to really tell – no closer than I had been in the copse in 1974. Perhaps I had never known the real colour of them. She smiled briefly and scratched her head, as if to embark on hard but not especially painful thought.

'I had no idea.'

'I'm sorry. I don't mean to be embarrassing and I know it is a bit . . .'

'Well, a bit, yes . . .'

'But I've got to a point in the book where I'm thinking about the big and little things I did and didn't manage to do when I was a teenager. The things that seemed immensely important at the time. You know, the things that played the big tunes. The things which reveal character, I suppose. At the time, those things were . . . they just were what they were – the most important and only things in the world. They didn't mean anything, but they *were* everything. The point being that . . .'

I looked up and saw that she wasn't really bothered what the point was.

' . . . Well, never mind what the point was. The fact is that I have this hole in my memory where something important used to be, and I really, really want to find out what the missing thing is. Don't know why.' I looked up again. Tried to swallow without being seen to. 'So you had no idea that I was stupid about you all that time?'

'Well, I don't suppose you'd have sent that postcard if you hadn't been . . . had a crush on me.'

'So you remember the postcard. Oh God. Do you also remember me turning up on your doorstep?'

'Of course.'

'That's the thing I can't remember. Well, I remember turning up, of course, and you standing on the step and the look in your eye, but I haven't got a clue what I said to you or what you said back or how I got out of there. I'm sorry . . .'

I stopped because I thought she was going to say something. But she didn't. She opened her mouth slightly, then shut it again. She was obviously thinking about how best to phrase whatever it was.

I began again: 'There's no reason why you should . . .' just as she said, 'It wasn't a step.'

'A step?'

'There wasn't a doorstep. It was flat flagstones which went straight out into the cloister from the hallway. There wasn't a step.'

'That's funny, because I remember looking *up* at your mum. And then when you came . . .'

'My mum was quite tall when she was younger.'

'But you were a titch.'

'I was.'

'And you had knock knees. I loved your knees.'

She laughed for the second time, a little more freely this time. And it sounded even more like her. When it was over there was a beat's silence. Then she spoke.

'I can remember being a little embarrassed and surprised when you turned up – although not that surprised, I suppose, since you'd already sent me the postcard. And I can remember thinking that you were very brave. That was the surprise, I suppose.' This time she smiled. 'How patronising does that sound? But it *was* brave. Really brave. All I can remember you saying was sorry. You apologised for sending the postcard and explained that you'd been really drunk. And then you disappeared up the cloister. I think that was it.'

'That was all?' Oh no. Oh no.

'I think so. If I can remember that much, I'm pretty sure I'd remember if you'd said anything else. It was a nice apology.'

I opened my mouth to fill the space. But nothing came.

'I don't know what to say.'

And I didn't. I hadn't a clue. I stared at the grass, and then at Lulu and then at a Buddha. He did not offer inspiration.

'Did you,' I mumbled eventually, 'think that I was a brave but bumbling fool who had bottled the major part of his commission, which was to ask you out?'

'Look, I was madly in love with a Chilean refugee who was in the process of dumping me. It was a bad time. I don't think I was capable of any kind of thought or consideration. Nothing worth remembering. I'm sorry. I really have no idea what I thought.'

She looked at me steadily. This time I tipped the chair and did not feel guilty about the sinking feeling, not for a few seconds anyway. I needed some time to assimilate the horrible truth of my moral cowardice. I looked up at the sky and made an airy 'mmmm' sound. Scratched my cheek. Tipped the chair back on to four legs again.

What a blow. But at least I had the truth of it at last, even if it wasn't terribly edifying. Here's what I'd done. I'd done the hard part and then bottled the *really* hard part – and that's why I'd ditched the memory. Shame. Sheer, unadulterated shame. Christ. Still, there were compensations: at least I didn't lose out by bottling it. It was obvious that she wouldn't have been interested in me anyway. That was something at least – I didn't have to swallow the mortifying rejection that would have certainly ensued had I possessed the balls to stand on her doorstep at the President's Lodge and ask her out. I, a mere village boy. Spotty de Bergerac in brothel creepers. An apologist for myself. A living, breathing apology of a boy.

'But it was very brave of you,' Lulu was saying, 'and I'm sure I thought that at the time.'

Kind woman. She's trying to make me feel better. But I'm not going to let myself off the hook, not this time.

'Well, that's nice of you to say so. Perhaps one day I'll wake up in the morning with the memory fully restored in the mono version of Dolby Stereo and I'll be able to relive the agony in all its hilariousness all over again. But I hope not. Eeeurgh. Hah.' That's right. Let it go. Toss it lightly away. You are, after all, a man in his late forties. 'The other one of my couple of questions is about the postcard. I have even less memory of that, because I wrote it when I was off my face. I can remember posting it but not writing it. I dread to think what I said . . . So go on, finish me off. What did I say? Please try and remember, if you can.'

She uncrossed her legs and put both flip-flops flat on the ground. It was the first time she'd moved since we sat down half an hour before. She exhaled through her nose and I realised with a gust of relief that there was no possibility she'd have the slightest recall of the contents of a gauche postcard sent to her in the mid-Seventies by a village-boy suitor amid the scorching embers of the first great love of her life. She's trying to think of an unhurtful way of saying that, because, well, because she's a nice woman.

'Actually,' she said, 'I don't have to remember. Hang on a minute.'

And she got up and went into the house and returned a few seconds later with a card in her hand. She handed it to me, picture-side up. The west door of Chartres Cathedral, photographed slightly wonkily. One corner of the card was bent, but otherwise it was well-preserved. Brown. Dull. A cathedral door.

'It's been in a box all this time with . . . well, with other things like that. Keep it.'

I did not turn it over to read what I'd written. And I did not know what to say for the second time in as many minutes. I put the card on the garden table, where it lay word-side down.

'I'll read it later,' I said. 'When I get home.'

'So what's this book all about?' she said, moving swiftly on. 'If it's partly about Cambridge in the Seventies, why am I in it? I know I was there at the time, but not in your bit of it. Not much, anyway. And if it's partly about going deaf, why am I in it? And if it's about music, why am I in it? In fact, why am I in it?'

'That's a very good question,' I said, enjoying the fact that it was now her turn to ask the questions and the fact that Lulu was turning out to be funny. 'You're in it because it wouldn't be the same without you in it.'

'But what's it *about*?'

'Well, I suppose it's about music and about going deaf and about what it's like to lose something that you not only care passionately about, but also take for granted. But then I suppose it's also about what it's like to lose something that you care passionately

about that you *don't* take for granted, and which, on closer examination, is revealed to be something you never possessed in the first
place, even if you wished you did. It's about that as much as it
is about the other thing, so I suppose you could also say that it's
about delusion and ownership – and how the experience of all of
it is contingent and fluid and difficult and, actually, lovely. And I
suppose it's about the fact that loss is inevitable and that you start
the losing process quite early in life, despite what people who need
life to be about winning think. Life is as much about loss as death
is – as well as having babies and longing for things you can't have.
And I think I'd better stop there before you start wishing you'd
never asked.'

Whatever Lulu then said was lost to me, because at that moment
a light aircraft passed low overhead. Low-flying light aircraft and I
don't get on. I slapped my fists over my ears and bent double. Don't
know why I had to bend, but I always used to when assailed by
noise, although I can manage much better now – with more dignity
anyway. And being a light aircraft, it took a couple of minutes for
the drone to die away as the plane headed towards the Gogs. Then
I sat up again. Waited for my head to clear. I looked at Lulu. She
was looking at me, impassive as ever.

'Ouch,' she said.

'Hmmm,' I replied.

Then she pointed to the bottom of the garden and away
beyond the stitch of trees which hemmed it.

'See the back of that house there?' she said. 'I think that's the
one. But if not that one, then one of those in that row. That's
where Syd Barrett lived – with his mum, I believe, until she
died. He died recently, didn't he, Syd Barrett?'

'Yeah,' I said. 'A couple of years ago. Me and my great friend
Lorry used to have arguments about Syd that would last for two
or three hours at a stretch. We'd go on and on and on, and
neither of us would give in. We'd often have to end the

argument by just walking away, and then it'd all start up as soon as we saw each other again. The weird thing is I have no idea now what it was we used to argue about. Not precisely. I can only remember the feeling of being in the argument. Stretched. Scratchy. Syd was Lorry's great hero and I had nothing against him, either as a musician or as an acid casualty. Nothing at all. He just . . . wasn't my taste.'

The plane did a turn in the distance and began the return flight to Marshall's airport. The drone began to grow again.

'But I think it was as important to Lorry that Syd *should* be my taste as it was important to me that he *wasn't*, and neither of us was going to give an inch. If either of us had been violent boys we would certainly have whacked each other. But there you go. We weren't, thank goodness.

'Poor old Syd. He was very important to us. He was important to everyone we knew. He was a kind of little god, a local little god. He conferred something special on us by being around – but invisibly around. The magic thing was to see him. Everyone wanted to spot him on his bike going to the off-licence in Cherry Hinton Road, and then they'd brag about it to everyone they knew. He was quite fat by then, Syd, or so it was always said, and the only way to tell it was him was if he was wearing his Yogi Bear suit.

'I never saw him, though.'

*

Halfway down Long Road I pulled the car over into the gateway of our old sixth-form college, the girls' High School as was. Lulu's daughters are recent alumnae, too. Fished the postcard out of my pocket. It came out picture-side up again. I turned it over. The handwriting was shocking, but legible.

As I sit here in this dingy ill-lit garret, the only thing that prevents me from sinking rusty needles into my veins, or turning consumptive, is the memory of you posing in your green and white rugby shirt for my crappy drawing. It's amazing what art lessons can do.
With much unrequited love,
Nick Coleman

I put it back in my pocket.

'I like the rusty needles,' I thought, as I pulled back out into the traffic. Rusty needles indeed. 'Ill-lit', too. But, all things considered, I'm not all that ashamed. I can live with that. Yes, I can live with that.

No need to apologise, after all.

25

There lurks in my son Tom's bedroom cupboard an ancient Grundig reel-to-reel tape recorder, complete with stubby microphone and brown tapes in a plastic bag, all of it manufactured in the 1960s. All still in working order. Well, it is a Grundig. It was my dad's. It was passed to me for safe keeping after he died. He used to record his compositions on it, and the musical groups he ran. Most of all he liked to record his children playing music.

Not so long ago I thought I might sort the tapes out, although the impulse was really an excuse. What I really wanted to do was find a tape with Brass A Capella on it.

Brass A Capella was a small brass ensemble I used to play with in Cambridge when I was fifteen, which often used to rehearse at our house. The six of us just about squeezed into the living room in a tight half-circle. Trombones, trumpets, a French horn on occasion (which was not strictly right for the repertoire). We played late-Renaissance brass music, as honked in the grander churches of sixteenth- and seventeenth-century Europe. The Gabrielis, Scheidt, Schutz. Good stuff.

Brass A Capella were pretty good, too. Renaissance church music is great music to play because it is so strong-boned and, yes, so extraordinarily architectural, and we played it with real passion. It remains the only musical thing I've ever been involved with that I thought was any good. Music with magnificent spaces in it. We did one memorable gig in Great Saint Mary's church in town, put on in conjunction with the Open University, no less, where I actually sat there in the middle of the ensemble, trombone between my knees, while some academic lectured the assembly of nice old ladies and ardent young men on the complexities and simplicities of the polyphonic idiom, and I thought, 'Yes, *this* is what it is to be a musician.'

And now, thirty-three years later, I really wanted to listen to Brass A Capella again, insofar as I can listen to anything these days, just to . . . well, you know, just to see whether we were *really* any good. So I settled down on Tom's bedroom floor with the Grundig and the pile of tapes, plugged the thing in and unclipped the lid.

There was a tape already spooled on to the machine.

How long has that been there? What's it *doing* on there? This must have been the last thing my dad listened to on the machine. But when was that exactly, because he'd made far greater use of his ghetto blaster over the last ten years of his life? The reel-to-reel was by then a relic from another time. I switched the knob to 'play' – it engaged with the same satisfying German clunk it had always done – and the tape began to wind.

Hiss. Scuff. Whisper. More hiss.

Then the slightly hesitant plunking of a piano introduction. Something Victorian by the sound of it. Then the sound of a boy's voice. Not a big or bright boy's voice, but a boy's voice hitting all the notes smack in the middle and not dragging or driving sharp or warbling.

'Oh, for the wings, for the *wiiiings* of a dove . . .'

The sort of thing that my gran regarded as proper music. Refined, bourgeois, improving. Wonder if this recording was done for my gran's benefit or out of some subtle irony for our own? Did we laugh afterwards or were we solemn? I must have been ten then, no more: long before I knew what taste was, let alone had any. But I could sing.

'Far a-way, far away wou-ould I rove . . .'

Mendelssohn. Prissy German Romanticism-lite for the upholstered domestic market. Soupy chromatic harmony. My dad all thumbs. Me lifting off and taking flight over the tops of the trees like a white bird symbolising peace and happiness and rescue, flying west into the setting sun. The place we all want to go – *deserve* to go if we're good.

'In the wilderness build me a nest, and forever remain there at rest.'

Tosh. Unremitting tosh.

Nice voice, though. I wasn't bad, you know.

I found myself listening hard. Really hard. In between the notes. To the space around the notes. To the air. The molecules. I listened through the hiss of the tape and the clunk of my dad's feet on the pedals. I listened to the room we were in, him sitting, me standing at his shoulder, the green carpet under our feet and the German guitar hung on the wall over the piano, and the piles of music on the top of the piano and the radiogram in the corner with its under-belly speaker and bakelite knobs and the recorders in the piano stool and the snare drum stashed under the Ladderax bookcase screwed into the wall, where it periodically gave voice to a deathly rattle for no apparent reason. His hands on the keys. Mine in my pockets.

I listened hard to that old, dead, unresonant room with my one remaining ear, listened as hard as I ever listened to anything. The music was flat in my head, of course, as flat as an architectural drawing.

But wouldn't it be great, I thought, if, in between the notes, I heard the faint passing sigh of the train to Peterborough, making its way into the distance?

EPILOGUE: SIXES AND SEVENS AND NINES

In the summer of 2010 – three years after I lost my hearing – I agreed to write a modest piece for a Sunday newspaper on the subject of the Rolling Stones' *Exile on Main St*, which was coming out again in remastered form with a cohort of previously unreleased cuts from the sessions, plus a film all about the album's making.

I didn't want to write a modest piece. I wanted to do the full ticker-tape parade – three thousand words-plus on the record's place in history, its legend, its myth, its mystery, its historiography, its strange way of expressing a certain kind of post-war Englishness through the medium of American music, its even stranger way of expressing excitement as an adjunct of heat-stroke, self-indulgence and disease. I wanted to write about how, even though you can't decipher many of the lyrics, the songs stimulate a range of feelings which make an irrelevance of the dull conventions of verbal intelligibility. I wanted to describe how *Exile*'s very resistance to interpretation made it one of the most telling cultural artefacts of its time.

But the paper said, no, we don't want the parade: we'd like a modest piece on what the album means to you personally. You know, five hundred words max on what it was like to grow up thinking *Exile* was, like, the best thing ever.

Fair enough. Cookies crumble. Who is to say which is the best way?

But I couldn't for the life of me think of anything pithy to say about what *Exile* meant to me. Or at least, every time I tried to write something amusing and/or edifying about my relationship with it, I found that I'd used up my allocation of words without actually saying anything at all. Lifelong relationships with odd artefacts cannot be distilled into the sort of solution you dispense with a pipette. You need space and time to explore stuff like that, much as you need space and time to do the research – a lifetime's worth. Because relationships like that are subtle, contingent, qualified, grey, unreliable, potentially mutable, certainly fraught. No, my close personal relationship with *Exile* is not for sharing through the medium of showbiz-style anecdote; it's far too serious for that, as well as being of no significance or amusement whatsoever to anyone else but me.

But I needed the work, so I had to come up with something – so, what?

Well, I decided that before I attempt to be clever with the editor I had better do what twenty-five years of writing about music have taught me always to do first. Listen to the music. Listen to it uncritically. Listen to it for pleasure, and if any pleasure arises from the experience, ask why. And how. And what the 'why' and 'how' might mean. Then listen to it again, but imagine I'm somebody else listening to it. Then, if I enjoyed that, listen to it again with my own ears and enjoy it all over again as myself. Then, having done that, listen to it again while doing something else – it is remarkable how listening to music while cooking or driving or chiselling children's bogies off the underside of a kitchen table can reveal fresh nuances.

After that, I might think about having a serious go at picking the bones out of the music musicologically. And then – and not before – I might feel ready to form thoughts about what this music might have to say, where its value might lie, and what its place is in the greater scheme. I might also be ready to let go of it forever without another thought.

Where *Exile on Main St* is concerned, I will never let go – and I never need a second invitation to listen. In theory, you just have to say the word: I'll get next to it any time you like. It's *the* default art experience for me – it's what I revert to. Sure, over the thirty-two years which separated 1975 from 2007, I listened to *Exile* less and less. By 2000 I can't have been addressing myself to it properly more than once a year, and then only to reconfirm what I already knew to be true. But that thinning out in no sense diminished my sense of intimate connection with the funny old thing, nor my incontinent love for it, nor my pride in having put in the hard yards when it counted, back in the days of my sixteenth and seventeenth years.

In 1976, for instance, I listened to at least part and sometimes the whole of *Exile* every single day of the six months which passed between my birthday and the unforgettable autumn night during my first term at sixth form college when I didn't go home at all. When I rolled back into the house early the next morning, unannounced, I was met on the stairs by a mother radiating like a breached nuclear reactor, and I knew I'd been inconsiderate. But it was in the nature of teenage bio-chemistry that I would actually feel more guilt over busting my run of votive daily listens to *Exile* than over what a sleepless night of worrying might have done to my mum.

By 2010, though, one or two things had changed. For a start, I was now fifty years old. I was also three years into a process of adaptation to a new way of living life, which involved an awful lot of stoic reasoning and getting by with what I had left. This was very different. Reasoning? Getting by? Where once I used to live life as a matter of course – exemplarily so when I was sixteen – instead of *just doing it*, I now found I had to *make the most of it*. It's what people are supposed to do when they're old, not middle-aged.

Progress had been made, though, on several fronts. I found I could ride a bike again – a bit nervously but pretty well, provided I didn't go fast or look too abruptly over my shoulder. I found also that I could stand far more in the way of everyday ambient noise, like kettles and diesels and crisps, and that I was much less prone to those bouts of enervation which would dump me into bed like a corpse into a mortuary drawer. I was more resistant, less vulnerable, more likely to last the course, provided the course itself lasted no longer than an hour or so and was conducted in library quiet. The brain is a weird but impressive organ, because it will just get on with its rewiring work without fuss, demanding in return only gallons of Earl Grey tea and plenty of genteel admiration; and it will do so without submitting an enormous bill at the end of a day's labour. The brain is the ideal electrician, really.

I'd also embraced the art of Mindful Meditation, thanks to the perseverance of my lovely Hearing Therapist, Jo. The meditation didn't fix the tinnitus, but it did improve my relationship with it. I could now do stuff without having simultaneously to fight a distracting (and losing) battle on another front – although reading still has to be done in virtual silence: text makes only scrambly sense to me if examined in a rowdy environment. I'd also discovered that the daily ingestion of a small dose of the betablocker Propranolol helped subdue the migraines, which would spring up automatically following any real-world activity involving even the tiniest amounts of noise-stress or strain.

But one threshold had not been examined properly, let alone crossed.

If you've read the rest of this story, you'll know that from the outset I was determined to try to get music back – or at least to reconnect with it in such a way that, even if the musical experience itself was compromised, the emotional and intellectual benefits of being exposed to music would be in some worthwhile part restored. I wanted to *feel* music again and to be able to think viably about it, too. I was desperately committed to the idea that a breakthrough would, must, *will* come. I wanted it as I imagined a buried miner wants to feel sun on his cheeks. So from the word go I'd maintained a steady input, a persistent drip of harmony, rhythm and tune, increasing the intensity and volume in due proportion to my sense of well-being, doing what I could get away with. Chiselling at the rock face.

The weird and terrifying 'disassembled' effect, exemplified by the *The Song Remains the Same* experience described in chapter three, in which the separated parts of 'Black Dog' would arrive through my cognitive letter box at different times and in various states of decomposition, was the first unpleasantness to be resolved. It took about six months to get the last of that nonsense out of my system. This, said the authorities, had been the result of the auditory cortex in my brain going into shock, losing its composure.

In due course I got back to writing about music, too, as far as I could. It meant changing the parameters of what I did and it meant accepting that my musical scope had narrowed, possibly for ever; not to a fine point, but certainly to the point where I would never need another excuse to duck Frank Zappa or Rammstein.

Nevertheless, as those three years passed I found I could get increasing pleasure out of more and more stuff, provided the music reached me in relatively compressed form at low volume, or at higher volume provided I was prepared to accept the three or four days of migraine and enervation that would inevitably follow. I listened to a lot of country music and folk and jazz and old reggae – in other words, music where form is a given, not an issue, and so content can be accessed at a stroke – and I began to feel that I was being spoken to.

This was exciting. It came neither as epiphany, nor as revelation, but as a creeping sensation. This was a qualitatively different experience to Amy Winehouse taking me by surprise on the toilet. There was more mind involved, less serendipity and no household products. I'd find that I'd come away from an encounter with a Roy Orbison retrospective boxset with the feeling that I'd been *visited*. Not haunted, just visited. I can't put it more precisely than that. It was a nice feeling, if a nebulous one. It had very little to do with architecture.

Exile, though . . .

I'd listened to 'Tumbling Dice' as an experiment the previous year and come away from that experience without horror, but with a lot of sadness. 'Tumbling Dice' is the default song in my default art experience: it had never previously failed to make me feel happy. In fact, it represents happiness to me. It does this in lots of ways, but chiefly in its unimaginable push and pull – especially its delayed shove on the One ('Tumbling Dice' is James Brown slowed down and spread out by white boys to form a whole new picnic) – as well as in its riverine dynamics, its evasive, essentially sordid throwaway metaphors about the excitement implicit in the turn of a card, and in the wiggy stroll of the thing, which corresponds so precisely with an image I have in my mind of the true physicality of exultation. The song and the feelings it contains are in my bones and muscles and fat, as well as in my brain: I can't help it. I walked back down the aisle on my wedding day, my beautiful wife on my arm, and 'Tumbling Dice' filled me to every corner, pushing and pulling . . . 'Got to roll me' . . . and I found I had to restrain myself quite consciously from strolling wiggily. If I am brutally, sentimentally honest, 'Tumbling Dice' is my favourite piece of music ever.

But then I am ruled by sentiment. And the prospect of listening again to the rest of *Exile* with half an ear and a head full of steam presses was not a good one. For the first time in my life I really *didn't* want to get next to it. Got to do it, though. For money if not for love.

So I ducked into it casually, having it on in the kitchen while chiselling or cooking, in the car while going to Sainsbury's, and in my head in between – just in there, spooling away, song by song by lick by groan, as impervious as ever to intellectual penetration, but totally permeable in every other way. I couldn't play it very loudly or for very long stretches, but I kept plugging away, allowing it to seep back into me as I seeped into it, like drizzle going into porous rock. 'Shake Your Hips', 'Ventilator Blues', 'Turd on the Run', 'Rocks Off', 'Let it Loose' – a bunch of songs, but also the climax of an effort to scour a world war and its aftermath from the corners of the mind: the house party as serious work. And by degrees, as I relaxed into the process and rode the unpleasantness, hanging on less like a rodeo buck than a small child on a large pony at a church fete, I found I could hear it perfectly well. That actually, I could hear it better than ever before; although what 'better' meant in this context was hard to say – 'better' in this context is a very confused concept. But I could see that this much at least was true: the strange illusion of better hearing signified that I had learned a new way to listen.

Hearing and listening are different things, of course. To listen is to involve one's mind in the process of hearing. Listening is itself 'better' than hearing, because of that very fact. So I suspect that the illusion of better hearing stimulated by the act of listening to *Exile* in all my trepidation had a lot to do with the quality of my listening: I was hearing better because I was listening better. I was, after all, not merely listening for pleasure, but for the touch of sun on my cheeks.

And, of course, I was listening to something I not only know as well as my children, but also love uncontrollably. There it was in my mind, pre-formed in all its jolie laide shapeliness – not architectural, but certainly articulate and alive and pressingly cogent and absolutely overflowing with content: the rip of Jagger's voice in its fight for air, compressed in between sedimentary layers of guitars, themselves recorded airlessly not in a digital vacuum but in the concrete sub-basement of a mansion on the sweltering Côte, where the ventilation unit on the wall is bust and everyone involved is to a greater or lesser extent angry or resentful or depressed or alienated or frightened about one thing or another, but also, in a whole other way, having a great time, because them's the rules. Music about the fight for air.

What? Of course it hurt. Everything hurts. It gave me a headache and then some, because I was playing it too loud, too often and for too long. Playing it at all. And yet, in its journey through the fuzzy pink canal of my one remaining ear, garnished with *pffffffs* and flat as a pancake, *Exile* sounded starkly beautiful, as it always used to. Music hasn't changed after all, and I do still have access to it. It's just that I get to it through unpleasantness now, not pleasure; and without the benefit of architecture.

We adapt in any way we can.

Funnily enough, though, I didn't write about that for the Sunday newspaper. Instead I wrote five hundred words about the rather odd, singular sound of *Exile on Main St* – its peculiar temperature, its unreadability, its ugly beauty – and why a single (quite possibly misheard) line in 'Rocks Off' stands as a summary of the entire thematic thrust of the album: 'Plug in, flush out and fight and fuck and feed'; and how, when it comes down to it, that is all we can ever require rock 'n' roll to say. After all, it isn't what rock says that really counts; it's how it says it. (Just ask Little Richard.)

But the big upshot for me was that the effort of listening – and loving the listening despite the effort – had caused the floodgates to swing open at last; and in it all came, an inundation of all the things I thought I'd lost to pain and despair, but now found I could embrace once more, only this time in pain and exultation. Coltrane, Marvin, Bach, Booker Ervin, Howlin' Wolf, the Marvelettes, Gregory Isaacs, Al Green, Fairport Convention, Richard and Linda, Jackie McLean, Aretha, Joni, Bob, Bob, Bob and Earl, Bobby Bland, Television, Miles, Amy Winehouse, Ronnie Lane, Peter Warlock, Giovanni Gabrieli, Tiburtio Massaino, the Ramones, Chuck Berry, U-Roy, U-Brown, Dennis Brown, Ann Peebles, Eric Dolphy, Mott the Hoople, Nic Jones, George Jones, Rickie Lee Jones, David Bowie, Tom Waits, Ella Fitzgerald, Prefab Sprout, Schubert, Elgar, Stravinsky, Elvis, Patti Smith, Dusty Springfield, Free, Heinrich Schutz, Danny Wilson, the Clash, Junior Byles, Bootsy Collins, Burning Spear, Led Zeppelin, Justin Townes Earle, Bill Frisell, Aimee Mann, Hank Mobley, Mahalia Jackson, Gerald Finzi, John Martyn, Dr Feelgood, Wilson Pickett, Allison Moorer, Mingus, Lee Perry, Sonny Clark, George Clinton, Steely Dan, (early) Genesis, Bobby Womack, Flying Burrito Brothers, Emmylou Harris, Jean Sibelius, Herbie Hancock, Wilco, Weather Report, Austin Lucas, Prince, Bruce Springsteen, Lal Waterson & Oliver Knight, Marry Waterson & Oliver Knight, Sly Stone, the Band, Mary Margaret O'Hara, the Grateful Dead, Louis Armstrong, Iggy, Jerry Lee Lewis, Laura Marling, Poulenc, Fauré, Messiaen, Bill Evans, Gil Evans, Chic, Roxy Music, the Sensational Alex Harvey Band, the Swan Silvertones, the Miracles (and Smokey Robinson), Little Richard, Southside Johnny & the Asbury Jukes, Bon Iver, Christian Wallumrød, Lew Lewis Reformer, Horace Silver, Graham Parker (and the Rumour), Charlie Christian, Harold Land, James Brown, the Isley Brothers, Tom

Petty, Jim Moray, T. Rex, the Meters, Laura Veirs, Can, Robert Wyatt, the Temptations, Little Walter, M. Ward, Be-Bop Deluxe, Billie Holiday, PiL, Sonny Boy Williamson, Toots, Richard Strauss, the Be-Good Tanyas, Otis Redding, Irma Thomas, Nirvana, the Pretenders, Donald Byrd, the Soul Stirrers, Art Pepper, David Sylvian, Hank Williams, Solomon Burke, Solveig Slettahjell, Belshazzar's Feast, Patsy Cline, the Upsetters, Tinariwen, Frank Sinatra, Gillian Welch and Dave Rawlings, G.F. Handel, Radiohead, the Moonglows, Monteverdi, Joe Tex, Lynyrd Skynyrd, Roy Orbison, the Four Tops, Gladys Knight (and the Pips), Harold Melvin & the Bluenotes, Dexy's Midnight Runners, the Righteous Brothers, the Shangri-Las, Ray Charles, Van Morrison, the Everly Brothers, Stevie Wonder, John Lee Hooker, Pink Floyd, Yes, Booker T. (& the M.G.s), Jimmy Smith, Billy Lee Riley, Israel Vibration, Wayne Shorter, Lester Young, Muddy Waters, Etta James, the Chi-Lites, the Chiffons, Big Youth, John Fahey, Defunkt, Aswad, the Specials, Allen Toussaint, The Who, Earth Wind & Fire, Thin Lizzy, Alicia Keys, Randy Newman, Robert Johnson, Bruckner, Björk, Big Star, Massive Attack, Charlie Parker, Roscoe Gordon, Dexter Gordon, ZZ Top, Tomasz Stańko, Duke Ellington, The Faces, the Sundays, Kimberley Rew (and the original Waves), the Bible, Harold Darke, Benjamin Britten, Captain Beefheart, Sam & Dave, the Drifters, the O'Jays, Creedence Clearwater Revival, Thelonious Monk, the Jamaicans, the Melodians, the Paragons, Curtis Mayfield, Beethoven, Pergolesi, Count Basie, Sun Ra, Louis Jordan, the Abyssinians, Paul Simon, Trammps, Nick Drake, Luther Vandross, Prince Far I, the Velvet Underground, Charlie Rich, Arve Henriksen, Misty-in-Roots, Jimi Hendrix, Thomas Campion and Nazareth, all of whose music, in some seized, lightning-bolt moment in the past, has sounded to me like the best thing I've ever heard.

On reflection, the world is full of beautiful music.

ACKNOWLEDGEMENTS

I would like to extend warm thanks to a number of people and for a variety of reasons. It's a long list but a lot of people have been very kind, one way and another.

To Laurie Staff, Andy Peacock, Mary Coleman, Becca Coleman, Deb Coleman, Pam Peacock, Linda Keller, Miranda Willers, Geoff Peacock, Bill Thompson, Alex Brockhurst, Pete Bevington, Adrian Cuthbert, Emma Perry, Oliver Sacks, Daniel Levitin, Sarah Lowry, Virginia Bovell, Helen Acton, Robert Webb, David Ellingham, Ian Blackaby, Caroline Stacey, Angus MacKinnon, Phil Johnson, Jo Blaquiere, Lee Sargent, Becky Gardiner, Nick Hornby, Amanda Posey, Derek Chapman, Ginny Clee, Simon Edwards and Lulu, who turned out to be neither haughty nor sad and is entitled to her bewilderment.

To Jenny Hewson and Peter Straus at Rogers, Coleridge and White, and Dan Franklin and his team at Cape.

Above all to Jane, Tom and Berry, whose love is all I need to get by.

GUN IN HIS HAND

Although Web Scott had tried to live a good and honest life, the brand of his father was upon him. For Mort Scott had been in prison for ten years for rustling and murder, and everywhere Web went he was pointed out as a jailbird's son. But now Mort, about to die, was protesting his innocence. Furthermore, he was laying the blame on Cole Tillotson, Web's uncle, who owned a big spread in Tomahawk Valley and who had brought Web up when the youngster had been left without a father to raise him.

And Web did not know whether to believe the parent he had grown to resent and to hate for ruining his life, or the relative who had taken him in and had taught him to live by the gun in his hand.

GUN IN HIS HAND

Wayne C. Lee

GUNSMOKE

First published in the UK by Hale

This hardback edition 2007
by BBC Audiobooks Ltd
by arrangement with
Golden West Literary Agency

ISBN 978 1 405 68176 6

British Library Cataloguing in Publication Data available.

Printed and bound in Great Britain by
Antony Rowe Ltd., Chippenham, Wiltshire

Wayne C. Lee was born to pioneering homesteaders near Lamar, Nebraska. His parents were old when he was born and it was an unwritten law since the days of the frontier that it was expected that the youngest child would care for the parents in old age. Having grown up reading novels by Zane Grey and William MacLeod Raine, Lee wanted to write Western stories himself. His best teachers were his parents. They might not be able to remember what happened last week by the time Lee had reached his majority, but they shared with him their very clear memories of the pioneer days. In fact they talked so much about that period that it sometimes seemed to Lee he had lived through it himself. Lee wrote a short story and let his mother read it. She encouraged him to submit it to a magazine and said she would pay the postage. It was accepted and appeared as *Death Waits at Paradise Pass* in *Lariat Story Magazine*. In the many Western novels that he has written since, violence has never been his primary focus, no matter what title a publisher might give one of his stories, but rather the interrelationships between the characters and within their communities. These are the dominant characteristics in all of Lee's Western fiction and create the ambiance so memorable in such diverse narratives as *The Gun Tamer* (1963), *Petticoat Wagon Train* (1972), and *Arikaree War Cry* (1992). In the truest sense Wayne C. Lee's Western fiction is an outgrowth of his impulse to create imaginary social fabrics on the frontier and his stories are intended primarily to entertain a reader at the same time as to articulate what it was about these pioneering men and women that makes them so unique and intriguing to later generations. His pacing, graceful style, natural sense of humor, and the genuine liking he feels toward the majority of his characters, combined with a commitment to the reality and power of romance between men and women as a decisive factor in making it possible for them to have a better life together than they could ever hope to have apart, are what most distinguish his contributions to the Western story. His latest novel is *Edge of Nowhere* (1996).

GUN IN HIS HAND

I

The heavy iron gates of the prison slammed shut behind Web Scott, and he followed the uniformed guard across the open space to the building that housed the warden's office.

"The warden will be mighty glad to see you," the guard said.

Scott didn't say anything. There was an oppressiveness about this place that disheartened him. It had been nine years since he had been here, and he had promised himself then that he would never come again. But that promise to himself, like so many that others had made to him, had proved to be only hollow words.

The guard opened the door into the warden's office and motioned Scott inside. The warden, a heavy-set, almost bald man, looked up from his desk.

"Webster Scott?" he asked.

Scott nodded. "They tell me you've been looking for me."

"For some time now," the warden said, coming out from behind his desk. "Your father has been asking for you."

"Why?" Scott asked bitterly. "Does he want to see for himself what a good job he has done of ruining my life?"

"It won't hurt you to see him," the warden said sharply. "He says it is very important that he talk to you now. According to him, your last visit here was nine years ago. That's a long time."

"Not long enough," Scott said.

"He's in the prison hospital," the warden said, frowning. "He'll never walk out of it. Go talk to him."

The warden nodded to the guard to open the door. Scott turned through the door, knowing the warden must think him the hardest-hearted man who ever wore boots. But the warden couldn't know all that had happened in the last ten years since Mort Scott had been sent to prison, ten years in which Web Scott had been branded the son of a jailbird everywhere he went. He might as well have rustled those cattle and pulled the trigger on Mike Hammond himself.

Scott followed the guard, barely noting his surroundings. At the far end of the big prison yard, the guard directed him into the prison hospital.

There were at least twenty men on the cots that lined either wall along the narrow room. Scott was led the entire length of the long room, while men in varying stages of illness or injury stared listlessly at him. On a cot at the far end of the room lay an emaciated man, his blue eyes blazing from sunken sockets. Scott barely recognized him.

"Web!" Mort Scott's voice was weak but filled with excitement. "I was hoping they'd find you before it was too late. Why haven't you come to see me?"

Web Scott, looking down at the shriveled, wasted form of his father, couldn't bring himself to answer. Mort Scott ought to know without asking. He should have known ten years ago, when he was sentenced to life imprisonment, what life would be like for Web, the son of a jailbird.

As long as Web had stayed with his uncle, Cole Tillotson, he'd had a good job and a good place to live. But he had worn the brand of a jailbird's son, a man nobody would trust.

Then he had struck out on his own, going far away where no one knew him. He had gotten a job and had built a decent reputation. He had found a girl, the right girl for him, he had been sure. They had picked the ranch they wanted to own not far from the town where she lived and had planned to buy it. Then the roof had caved in on Scott again.

The morning that he went to the bank to get the loan to buy the ranch, word of Scott's past reached town. The son of a jailbird! The bank refused to loan him the money. The girl was shocked to find that her husband-to-be had a father in prison. She broke off the engagement and told Scott not to come to see her any more.

And then had come the call from the warden saying that Mort Scott wanted to see Web in prison. He had come, the hate in his heart so big that it crowded out everything else. If it hadn't been for Mort Scott's crime, Web would be happily married now, building up his own ranch.

"I've been mighty busy," Scott said finally.

"I've been busy, too," Mort said. "Busy dying. I had to see you, Web, before they sent me home in a box. You've been cheated."

Web frowned. Nobody needed to tell him that he had been cheated. He'd been cheated from the day he was born, having a father like Mort Scott.

"Where is Cole now?" Mort asked finally.

"I haven't seen Cole for two years," Web said. "I hear he's got a big spread over in Tomahawk Valley."

"Never heard of it," Mort said. "He cheated you, Web."

Anger surged up in Web, overriding the pity he felt for the sick man. "Cole cheated me? That's not the way I figure it. You were the one who always told me I should live without violence. Then you rustled cattle and killed the man who caught you."

Pain worked across the pinched face of the man on the cot. "Is that what you really believe?"

"What else can I believe?" Web said. "You preached

no violence, yet you robbed and killed. The courts proved that. It was Cole who always told me that if I wanted to get out of life what I had coming, I'd have to take it with a gun in my hand."

"And you believed him?"

"I didn't when you were home. You know that. But after what you did, what else could I believe?"

Mort turned his face to the wall. "I should have known Cole would work on you till he changed you to his way of thinking. Why aren't you with him now?"

"I had to make it on my own. Everywhere I went with Cole, I was pointed out as the son of a jailbird. A man can't get anywhere with that brand on him."

Mort looked back at Web, the pain deeper in his eyes. "You hate me, don't you?"

Web shook his head. "I reckon I don't hate you. But you sure didn't leave me much room to like you, either."

"I've got to straighten you out, Web. I don't know what sickness I've got, but I'm not going to walk away from it. Take a dying man's word for it, Web. I didn't kill Mike Hammond. I didn't steal his cattle, either."

"The testimony at the trial said different."

Mort Scott nodded. "The evidence was strong, all right. But it was wrong."

"Why didn't you say so then?" Web studied Mort's face, wondering if Mort's sickness had reached his brain. Surely no innocent man would allow himself to be sentenced to prison without declaring his innocence.

"It wouldn't have helped anything," Mort said. "The evidence was all on their side. I couldn't prove anything. And if I'd tried, I would just have hurt your mother."

"How could you have hurt Mom more than you did? Letting the world believe you were a rustler and a killer hurt her more than anything."

Mort shook his head. "She never believed I did it. And nothing I could have said at the trial would have changed what the jury thought. I would only have torn down her faith in the one person she had left to depend on: her brother."

"Cole?" Web exclaimed. "Do you claim that he had something to do with that killing?"

"He had everything to do with it," Mort said positively. "But I couldn't prove it. If I'd told the court what I knew but couldn't prove, it wouldn't have helped my case any, but it would have destroyed your mother's **faith in her brother.**"

Web Scott studied the sunken cheeks and bright blue eyes of the sick man. How could he believe what Mort Scott was saying? Yet how could he doubt the truth in those eyes?

"I suppose you think Cole shot Mike Hammond," Web said.

Mort nodded. "Either Cole or that gunman friend of his, Johnny Russo. I wasn't sure at the time. But when Cole stole the Crossed S from you and sold it, it convinced me that he'd had that in mind all the time.

Getting me framed for Hammond's murder was just part of the scheme."

Web leaned over the cot. "What do you mean—Cole stole the Crossed S from me? I never owned any part of that ranch. It belonged to you and Cole together."

"That's where you're wrong, Web. Cole never owned any part of it. I let him pretend to be a partner to please your mother. But he didn't own an inch of the land."

"But he claimed he owned half of it, and Mom signed over the other half just before she died."

"Did he ever make such a claim while she was living?"

Web considered, then slowly shook his head. "No, I don't think he did. What difference would that have made?"

"He wouldn't have dared say anything like that while she was living. She would have put him in his place. The papers on the ranch were all in my name. It was to go to you, all of it."

"But Cole said Mom signed over the papers," Web objected.

"How could she sign over something she never had? Those papers were forgeries, Web. Cole stole the Crossed S from you. What did he get for it?"

"Ten thousand dollars, I heard. He never told me exactly."

"Then he owes you ten thousand dollars," Mort said with finality.

Web studied the sick man's face. There was no look of irrationality there; just the fervent desire to be believed. Could he be right?

"You still think I'm lying," Mort said when Web remained silent. "There is a little box under my cot. Look in it. You'll find a little packet of letters your mother wrote to me. You were only seventeen when she died. I'd been in here only two years. I didn't find out until a long time afterward that Cole had sold the Crossed S. I've been trying to get the warden to find you ever since. Until I was put in the hospital and the warden knew I wasn't going to get out, he wouldn't make much effort."

From under the cot, Web pulled out a little box that held the few personal belongings of his father. Digging into it, he found the package of letters neatly tied into a bundle and handed them to the sick man.

Mort tried to loosen the string holding them together, but his feeble efforts couldn't untie the knot.

"You'll have to do it," he said. "It will be the top letter, the last one she wrote me before she died. I want you to read it. You'll believe me then."

Web found the letter and took it out of its worn envelope. He recognized his mother's writing.

" 'I want to come down and see you next month,' " Web read. " 'I've been pretty poorly lately. Don't know what is wrong. But I must talk to you about signing the ranch over to Web. Cole has been trying to get me to sign the ranch over to him so that he can have a free hand in running it. He says he can make it pay off much better than it is doing now. I've told him my name isn't even on the deed, so I can't sign anything legally. But he won't listen. Since you can't be here to take care of this, I think you should sign it over to Web so that he can manage it. He is seventeen now and near enough a man to take care of it, I'm sure.' "

"Convinced?" Mort asked when Web dropped the letter in his lap.

Web nodded.

"Cole owes me ten thousand dollars," he said slowly. "But he owes you a lot more. If he did frame you for that murder, he owes you ten years of life."

"He can't repay that," Mort said wearily. "But he can pay you the ten thousand—with interest."

Web looked down at his father and saw the blaze in his eyes. "You always preached against violence."

"That was before I spent ten years of my life in this hole for something I didn't do. Any kind of violence that you use on Cole Tillotson will be too good for him!"

Web nodded grimly. "I'll get my ten thousand dollars from him. And I'll make him clear your name of murder and me of being the son of a jailbird. He taught me to use a gun. Maybe now he'll find out how well I learned my lessson."

"Promise you'll make Cole square things," Mort said,

fighting the weariness that seemed suddenly to over-whelm him.

"I promise," Web said grimly.

He turned and started down the long aisle toward the door at the far end of the building.

II

During the last day of riding before getting to Tomahawk Valley, Scott pushed his horse harder than usual. The time had come to face Tillotson and demand an accounting, and Scott found it hard to wait.

Scott came to Tomahawk Valley from the east. The valley was little more than a depression in the rolling plain, running northwest to southeast, a small creek cutting through its center. To the south, sand hills rolled away to the horizon, while to the north, the ground rose in long low swells, leaving no clearly marked rim to the valley.

To Scott's left was the little town. That would be Tomahawk. It didn't look like much of a place, but Scott reined that way. Information would be there, and he needed that before he faced Tillotson.

As he dropped down off the hills, his ranching eyes noticed the rich grass. This was a paradise for cattle, and there didn't seem to be enough cattle to keep the grass short. No wonder Cole Tillotson had selected this place to build his ranch.

Scott came into the town from the north and rode down the main street, noting the weathered buildings, none of which had been painted. One of the first buildings he came to housed the deputy sheriff's office, with a jail in the back. Then he rode past a block of buildings that included a hotel, saloon, hardware store and blacksmith shop. He had his eye on the livery stable down at the end of the street next to the creek. His horse had had a long trip, and Scott's first concern was for its care.

He swung down in front of the long barn, noting that the corral behind the barn enclosed a section of the creek. No watering problem for the keeper of this barn.

"Been riding quite a ways, I see," a man said, stepping out from the front of the barn.

Scott looked the man over. He was rather short and heavy-set, with piercing brown eyes that seemed to read Scott's history at one glance.

"Far enough," Scott said. "My horse needs some rest and feed."

"You've come to the right place for that," the man said. "Name's Eli Blessing."

The stable owner waited expectantly. Scott loosened the cinch on the saddle, then turned to face the man.

"Web Scott. Heard there was a man around here named Cole Tillotson. Know him?"

Blessing nodded. "Sure do. Owns the Tilted T about seven miles up the creek from here. Got business with him?"

Scott rubbed a finger along his chin. Blessing had an unhealthy curiosity, and Scott considered his answer carefully.

"I've got a deal simmering with Tillotson," he said. "I'd like to ride out there now. Got a horse I can rent? Mine is getting tired."

"He's worn to a frazzle, all right," Blessing said, looking over Scott's horse. "I've got a horse you can use. Not sure you'll find Cole at home, though."

Scott looked sharply at the stable owner. "Where do you think he is?"

"Probably out working around his cattle," Blessing said. "His spread covers a lot of territory. Just hate to see you ride out there and be disappointed."

"If he's on his ranch, I'll find him," Scott said grimly. "How about that horse?"

"I'll have to catch one from the corral," Blessing said, making no move to get the horse. "You might as well run up to the saloon and cut the dust loose while I get him."

"Scott shook his head. "I'll take that horse now."

Blessing shrugged and turned toward the back of the barn. "Must be powerful urgent business."

Scott waited for the man to bring a horse, uneasiness crawling through him. Blessing seemed overly anxious for Scott to kill a little time in town before riding out to the Tilted T.

Scott tagged him as one of Tillotson's men. If so, he had probably recognized the name of Scott and right now was figuring some way to get word to Tillotson that Scott was in town looking for him.

Blessing brought a horse through the back door of the barn and tied it in a stall. Then he took his time getting a blanket and saddle on it. Scott waited impatiently. If Blessing hadn't talked to anyone outside, there was no hurry. But if he had, every wasted minute was giving a rider more of a head start so he could reach Tillotson before Scott did.

"We've got a nice valley here," Blessing said as he worked with the saddle. "Some people think Tomahawk is an odd name, though. They say Old Henry Woodruff named it. He came here long before anybody else. Found a skull with a tomahawk stuck in it about a mile from where this town stands now. So he named the valley and the creek Tomahawk."

Scott shifted his feet impatiently. "I came to see Cole Tillotson, not Henry Woodruff."

"Good thing," Blessing said. "Old Henry's dead. But he's got a boy, Josh, who owns the JW Ranch, a couple of miles west of town. You'll see it on the south side of the creek as you're going out to the Tilted T. It's a question how long Josh is going to be able to hold his ranch, though. Cole Tillotson is trying to buy him out."

Blessing backed the horse out of the stall. "Here's your horse."

Scott led the horse out of the barn into the street and mounted. Then he turned to look down at the stable owner.

"Did you send word to Tillotson that I was here?"

A flash of surprise crossed Blessing's face; then he returned Scott's stare unflinchingly. "He'll find it out soon enough."

Scott reined up the street and turned west into the road that ran along the north side of the hotel. The horse was fresh and eager to run, and Scott let him pick his own pace over the flat floor of the valley.

A couple of miles from town, Scott saw the JW Ranch on the south side of the creek, just as Blessing had said he would. It was a good-looking place, with nice buildings, well kept up.

The main road stayed on the north side of the creek, and as he rode along, Scott noticed a couple of small sets of abandoned buildings. And then ahead of him, on a knoll overlooking the creek, he spotted the white buildings of what he guessed was the Tilted T.

There was only one man in the yard when Scott rode up. He stood below the porch of the house, hands on hips, staring at Scott.

"You were expecting me, weren't you, Johnny?" Scott asked, reining to a stop.

Johnny Russo glared at Scott. "Nobody invited you."

Russo had come to the Crossed S just before Mort Scott had been arrested for murdering Mike Hammond, and he had been with Tillotson ever since. Scott knew him as rather slow-witted, but willing and able to do any job Tillotson demanded; a strong man with a very fast gun and no compunctions at all against using it in any way demanded.

"Cole at home?" Scott asked, swinging down from the saddle.

Russo shifted his big frame toward the door of the house, his smoky eyes flitting toward the house and back. "He's in there," he said.

Scott flipped the reins around the hitch rack and strode across the porch into the house. Cole Tillotson was coming from a backroom, apparently attracted by the sound of voices.

Tillotson hadn't changed much. The two years since Scott had seen him had turned his graying hair to almost snow white, which made his snapping black eyes appear brighter than ever. He still carried his six-foot frame as straight as ever, and his slimness camouflaged his almost two hundred pounds.

"I wasn't expecting to see you, Web," Tillotson said affably, pretending a surprise that Scott knew he didn't feel. "You talked like you never wanted to see me again when you cut loose a couple of years ago."

"I wanted to try my luck alone," Scott said. "I made it all right till the story of Mort's prison sentence caught up with me. I've been to see Mort. He's dying, Cole. He told me some things that I had to believe."

Tillotson turned to look out the window, and Scott guessed it was to keep Scott from seeing his face. Any doubt that Scott had been harboring concerning the truth of Mort Scott's statements vanished.

"What did he tell you?" Tillotson asked finally, turning back, his face as calm as ever.

"That you stole the Crossed S."

"And you believed him?"

"Any reason why I shouldn't?"

"You didn't believe what he said at the trial."

"You made sure I didn't," Scott said, anger slowly building up in him. "You made me believe he was a hypocrite, preaching against violence but willing to murder to get what he wanted."

"That's just how it was. The courts proved it."

"You can skip the legality, Cole," Scott said. "Mort told me what really happened and why he kept still. He couldn't prove the truth, and he didn't want to hurt my mother any more than had already been done. Also, he said the ranch was in his name only. Mom couldn't have signed over any part of it to you. So you forged that deed. I figure you owe me ten thousand dollars, Cole. When do I get paid?"

"Now hold your horses, Web," Tillotson said, his voice becoming raspy with irritation. "You'll have to prove that paper was a forgery before you've got a leg to stand on. I don't care what Mort Scott says now. That ranch was part mine, and the rest was Mort's and Lily's. When Mort went to prison for life, Lily had every right to sign over their part to me so I could make the ranch pay off."

"It paid off for you, all right," Scott said hotly. "By going back to the records, I can find out whether Mort owned the Crossed S himself or whether Mom's name was also on the deed. Mort told me you were a partner in name only. I believe that, too."

Tillotson stared at Scott for a long minute, his lips pinched together. "I'll tell you what I'll do, Web. I've felt that you should have some of the proceeds of the Crossed S Ranch, even though you aren't legally entitled to any. The ranch was mine to do with as I saw fit. Let me think about it tonight, and we'll reach some kind of settlement in the morning."

"I don't need to think about it overnight," Scott said. "You owe me ten thousand dollars. I'll settle for that and nothing less."

A frown tugged at Tillotson's face. "We'll talk about it in the morning. You can bed down in the bunkhouse or, if you'd rather, you can have a room here in the house."

"I'll take a room at the hotel in town," Scott said. "Have the ten thousand ready for me when I come back in the morning. With that money, maybe I can buy a ranch without having to crawl to some banker, hoping he won't turn me down because I'm the son of a jail-bird. One more thing, Cole. How about telling the truth about what happened back there the day Mike Hammond was killed? Mort isn't going to get out of prison alive, anyway. But he ought to leave this world with a clean name."

Scott wheeled back through the door, leaving Tillotson scowling after him.

Scott noted again the empty houses along the road as he rode back to Tomahawk, and he wondered about them. How had Tillotson gained control of so much land in so short time? Ten thousand dollars would have bought some of it, but not nearly as much as was under the Tilted T brand now.

Scott returned the horse to the livery barn. He thought of asking Blessing about those empty houses but decided against it. Blessing's suspicious nature would do Scott no good in the long run.

He walked back up the street to the hotel and got a room. He went to sleep, wondering about his trip back to the Tilted T the next morning.

Scott wasn't sure what time it was when he was awakened by a sound in the room. It was so dark that the blackness was almost tangible. He lay still for a moment, sweeping the sleep from his mind and listening for the sound that had awakened him.

When he heard it again, it was right by his bed. He lunged to one side, but not soon enough. A heavy weight crashed down on him, almost smothering him. He lashed out with a fist and heard a grunt as he made contact with something that squashed like a pulpy nose.

A stream of soft curses poured from the man as a fist slammed into Scott's side. The man obviously wanted to subdue Scott without making enough noise to attract the attention of the other occupants of the hoel.

Scott rolled off the bed on the opposite side from his attacker. The man grunted as he lunged after him. Scott couldn't tell much about him except that he was big. Scott rolled to his knees, intent on meeting the next lunge of the man. And he'd make as much noise as he could.

But his quickly formulated plan died suddenly as he felt the cold steel of a gun nozzle pressed against his neck. He hadn't counted on two men.

"Just be quiet," the man behind the gun said. "We don't want to raise the whole town by shooting you here. But if that's the way you want it, you can have it."

Scott, on his hands and knees, remained quiet. The only sound in the room was the heavy breathing of the man sprawled across the bed.

"Now get up, and put on your pants and shirt. We're going for a walk."

"Have to have a light," Scott said.

"Dress in the dark or come the way you are," the man said. "Makes no difference to me."

Scott reached for the chair where he had tossed his clothes. He was sure he recognized that voice. It sounded like Johnny Russo.

He got his pants and shirt on, then pulled on his boots and moved slowly toward the door. It was so dark that he couldn't see the two men who had jumped him, but the muzzle of the gun in his back was a constant reminder of their presence.

In the hallway, there was enough light for Scott to see where he was going. He turned to look at the two men behind him and got a sharp prod in the ribs for his trouble.

"Just keep walking and go out the back door!"

Scott moved on. But he'd had his look. He had guessed right about Johnny Russo. The other man he didn't know. He was taller than Scott's six-feet-two, and bigger. Scott guessed he must weigh two hundred and forty or fifty pounds. But the thing that he'd remember best about the man was his wild blue eyes and almost bald head, although he looked to be still in his thirties.

Scott hesitated slightly before stepping into the alley behind the hotel. He could guess what was awaiting him there. But a prod from the gun drove him through the door. Fifty feet from the door, where the alley was darkest, Russo called a halt.

"Cole promised to settle with you in the morning," Russo said. "I'm going to do it now."

Scott turned to face Russo, and as he did, the big

baldheaded man clubbed a fist into his side. The breath exploded from Scott, and he reeled backward. Russo moved in quickly for a man of his size and slammed his fist into Scott's face. Russo wasn't quite as tall as Scott, but he was twenty pounds heavier.

Scott lashed out in self-defense, but it was a feeble effort at best. That surprise blow in his side had taken much of the strength from him, and his fists were puny clubs against the hammering blows of the two big men.

One fist caught him at the base of the ear, and he reeled backward against a huge box that someone had dumped in the alley. Before he could move away from the box, another blow smashed into the pit of his stomach, driving out what breath he had left. Two more fists slashed at his face as he sank to the ground.

He clung to semi-consciousness and felt a sharp stab of pain as the hard toe of a boot dug into his side. The toe made two more vicious jabs before a dim voice put an end to the punishment.

"That's about enough. Cole said not to kill him this time."

A huge hand grabbed Scott's shirt front and lifted him to his feet, then held him there on sagging legs.

"Now you listen, and you listen good!" Johnny Russo hissed in Scott's face. "You get out of town just as soon as you are able. If you ever show your face in this valley again, you'll stay here, six feet under!

Understand?"

Scott didn't even nod. The warning had registered, but at the moment he didn't care. Let Russo finish the job now; nobody was stopping him.

Russo let go, and Scott crumpled down against the big box. "Be gone from this country the next time I come looking for you," Russo said.

Heavy feet plodded up the alley, and Scott listened to them fade away. Then the night and the throbbing pain faded away, too, leaving peaceful oblivion.

III

Scott wasn't sure how long he had been unconscious when he once more became aware that he was alive and hurting. It was still dark, and nothing in the alley was discernible. He pushed himself to a sitting position, gasping at the pain that shot through his head and side.

Gingerly he tested each arm and leg. No bones broken there, although his side throbbed with pain at every move. He might have a cracked rib or two, he decided.

He pulled himself to a sitting position and rested, propped against the big box. Now that he was conscious again, what could he do? He wondered if he hadn't been better off when he couldn't think.

He wouldn't find any help in the hotel. If any help had been coming from there, it would have shown up when Russo and his giant partner had come into the hotel. Instead, someone must have told them what room he was in.

The only man Scott knew in town was the livery stable owner, Eli Blessing. And Blessing would be no help. Besides, the livery stable was more than a block away. Scott didn't feel that he could drag himself that far.

After a few minutes, he got to his feet, barely able to hold back a groan as pain stabbed through his side. He stood for a minute, then began walking slowly, fighting the pain at every step.

He turned toward the hotel and within a few feet ran into a fence. Here, away from the shadow of the hotel, the thin starlight revealed a garden on the other side of the fence.

Scott moved along the fence toward the dim outline of a house. Anyone who worked in a garden should be the kind of person who would lend a helping hand to a man in need, he reasoned. And Scott was a man in need now.

It seemed like an eternity to Scott before he reached the house. It was a neat little building, painted white, and even the back yard, which Scott came through, seemed clean and free of trash.

At the back door, Scott clutched the jamb and rested before knocking. His first knock brought no response, but he hammered harder and was rewarded by a shuffle inside.

A lamp sprang to life, and a man came to the door, opening it cautiously. The man didn't say a word but, after taking one look at Scott in the feeble light of the lamp, reached out and caught Scott's arm, leading him inside.

"Mary! Ann!" he called. "I'm going to need some help."

He set the lamp on the table, then guided Scott to a couch along the wall. Running careful fingers over the bruises on Scott's face, he squinted his eyes as he examined a lump on his jaw. Then his probing fingers came down Scott's side, and Scott winced, a small cry coming from his lips.

The man nodded. "Ribs. Who did this?"

"Doesn't make any difference, does it?" Scott said. "Will I need a doc?"

Two women came through the door, each with a robe wrapped over a nightgown. The younger one came to the cot, while the older one turned to the stove and started building a fire.

"You've got a doctor whether you want one or not," the girl said.

The man spoke then. "I'm Dr. Kinkaid. This is my daughter, Anne, and my wife, Mary. Who are you?"

"My name is Web Scott." Scott looked over the Kinkaid family. He liked the honest, sincere face of the doctor. And there was genuine concern on the faces of the women.

"Somebody certainly had a mad at you," Dr. Kinkaid said.

Scott weighed his chances. He was going to need friends now more than at any time in his life. He might find them right here. But he wouldn't if he lied to them. He reasoned that his best chance was to tell the truth and hope for the best.

"I had a business deal with Cole Tillotson," he said slowly, watching their faces. "I guess this is the way he paid me off."

The doctor nodded. "That's the way, all right. Johnny Russo did this, no doubt."

"He and help," Scott said. "A big fellow, bald-headed."

"Dan Kale," Anne Kinkaid said quickly. "Another of Tillotson's men."

"I was out at the Tilted T this afternoon," Scott said. "I didn't see him there."

"You wouldn't," Dr. Kinkaid said. "He owns the hardware store here in town. But, like Anne says, he is one of Tillotson's men."

Scott, fighting the pain in his side, detected the bitterness in the doctor's voice. "I take it you don't cater to Tillotson yourself."

The doctor nodded. "You catch on fast enough." He unbuttoned Scott's shirt. "If you'd caught on faster, you could have avoided this."

With the hot water Mrs. Kinkaid brought from the stove, Anne gently washed the bruises on Scott's face and neck. Then the doctor bound up Scott's mid-section till he felt as if he were in a cast.

"A couple of cracked ribs there," the doctor said when he finished. "But I think much of the pain is coming from bruises. They should feel better in a few days."

Scott slid his feet to the floor and sat up, wincing at the pain. "I'm obliged to you, Doc. I'll get out of your way now."

"Where do you expect to go?" the doctor asked, staring at Scott with hands on his hips.

"Back to the hotel, I reckon. I've got a room there. I don't think I'll have company again tonight."

"You're not going anywhere," Dr. Kinkaid said flatly. "I want you right here where I can watch you for a day or two. We've got an extra room."

"Now wait a minute," Scott objected. "If Cole Tillotson wants to get rid of me bad enough to order this beating I took, he'll make it hard on anyone he finds helping me."

"I'll take my chances with Tillotson," Kinkaid said, his lips pressed tightly together. "Tomorrrow I'll pick up anything you left in your room at the hotel. Anne, will you get the spare room ready?"

"It's ready," Anne said. She took Scott's arm. "Come on now. No more objections."

If Scott had had any more objections, they faded as the appeal of a day or two of rest swept over him.

Scott hardly moved during the next day. He felt that

he was one big bruise from head to foot, with a few extra bumps thrown in for good measure. Anne came into his room several times. She seemed to have taken him as her special patient.

The doctor came in just before supper time. He examined the bruises and checked the cracked ribs.

"Everything's doing fine," he said. "Now what room did you have in the hotel?"

"Room 7," Scott said. "All I left in there was my bedroll. Nothing very important in that, I guess."

"How about your horse?"

"A blaze-faced sorrel. He's down in Blessing's barn."

The doctor nodded. "Blessing will turn the horses out in the corral tonight. I can slip your horse out and bring him up here to my barn. And I'll get your bedroll from the hotel."

"What's wrong with leaving my horse down at the barn?" Scott asked, suspicion rising in him.

"I had some unusual patients at my office today," Kinkaid said. "They weren't sick; just curious. Seems they saw a horse in the corral at the barn that didn't belong there and figured his owner was still in town. If your bedroll and horse both disappear tonight, they might decide otherwise."

"You're going to do that just to hide me?" Scott asked incredulously.

"I haven't asked you anything about yourself, Scott," Kinkaid said. "But if Tillotson is enough afraid of you to have you beaten half to death to get you out of the country, you must be a real thorn in his flesh. We need more thorns for Tillotson."

"How many others hate Tillotson like you do?" Scott asked.

"Not many, I'm afraid. Josh Woodruff, maybe. But a lot of people don't like him. Ever since Tillotson came into the valley about two years ago, he's run roughshod over everybody. If he isn't stopped, the whole valley will be under his thumb in less than another year."

"I suppose you'd like to know what business I have with him?"

"I'm not asking," the doctor said. "You've got reason to fight him, and I'm hoping you'll stay and do just that."

"Cole Tillotson is my uncle by marriage," Scott said, then shook his head at the surprise on Kinkaid's face. "Not a loving relative, as you can guess. He forged a signature and stole a ranch from me. Sold it for ten thousand dollars. I came here to collect my money. That's the reason for the beating last night. I suppose he figures that pays the bill."

Kinkaid nodded. "That sounds like his way of doing things. He bought that place he built up into the Tilted T. Then he started putting pressure on every neighbor he had. Ran them out and took over their spreads. Josh Woodruff is the only other rancher left in the valley."

"Woodruff won't run?"

"He'll never run. That's why I'm afraid for him. He's about the best friend I have in the country."

"Tillotson must know you're bucking him," Scott said. "How come he hasn't run you out?"

Kinkaid looked sharply at Scott. He was a small man, only a little over five and a half feet tall and weighing about a hundred and forty pounds. But his clear blue eyes had a sharp glint in them that reminded Scott of light reflecting off steel.

"There are a couple of reasons. I'm the only doctor in Tomahawk, and even Cole Tillotson might need a doctor sometime. People here in town might not raise a fuss if another rancher was run out of the country. But it would be different if their doctor left. Tillotson would have a hornet's nest on his hands, and he knows it. I may be little, but I'll make a pretty big bump if he tries to run over me."

Scott didn't doubt that; and after listening to the doctor talk about his stand against Tillotson, he knew that he had to make a stand, too. He couldn't let this beating run him out as Tillotson hoped it would.

"You say Dan Kale is one of Tillotson's men," he said. "Is there anybody else in town that kowtows to him?"

Kinkaid nodded. "Eli Blessing down at the stable."

"I figured that," Scott said, nodding.

"And he has the deputy sheriff, Sam Hookey, in his

hip pocket. The county seat is so far from Tomahawk that the sheriff doesn't get over here more than twice a year. So he put a deputy here six months ago. Tillotson somehow got his man, Hookey, into that job. So he controls what little law we have around here."

Scott shook his head. "That could make it tough."

"It is tough," Kinkaid said, "But don't you worry about it till you get on your feet again."

It seemed to Scott that that time would never come. Anne Kinkaid made sure that Scott didn't leave his room even after he was up and pacing the floor like a caged lion.

"Dad's orders," she explained. "He says that everybody is convinced that you slipped out that night he moved your horse and bedroll. He doesn't want anybody to see you until you're ready to take care of yourself."

Scott sighed. "I suppose he's right. But I can't stay cooped up here much longer. I've got a score to settle with Johnny Russo, and I won't rest easy until it's done."

"You'll have to be careful, Web," Anne warned. "Russo is a dangerous man. And what about Dan Kale? He helped Russo beat you half to death?"

"I'll think about Kale after I've taken care of Johnny," Scott said. "I've known Johnny for a long time. I figure he took a particular delight in pounding me up."

For three more days Scott roamed around the house impatiently. Then Dr. Kinkaid agreed that Scott was ready for action. After the doctor left the house for his office that morning, Scott strapped on his gun and went outside. He wasn't eager to see anyone except Johnny Russo. Here in town, only Eli Blessing at the livery stable, Dan Kale at the hardware store and possibly the desk clerk at the hotel had gotten a good enough look at him to be able to recognize him again.

He walked the streets hopefully, watching the road leading in from the Tilted T. But it wasn't until after dinner that he saw a rider come into town on that road. His pulse quickened. It was Johnny Russo, he was sure. He couldn't get close enough for a good look at the man's face before he dodged into the saloon. But he was Russo's size and had come from the direction of the Tilted T.

Checking his gun, Scott moved up the street toward the saloon. Another rider came in on the road from the west, but Scott saw that was a woman and he promptly forgot her. His business was with Johnny Russo.

Before Scott got to the saloon, however, the man he was after came out and dodged across the street toward the hotel. But instead of going into the hotel, he ducked into the alley between the hotel and Kale's hardware.

Scott speeded up. He couldn't understand Johnny Russo dodging around like that. He was obviously afraid of someone. Surely Russo couldn't know that

Scott was after him. Even if he did, why would he dodge Scott like this? That wasn't like Russo.

Scott ducked down the alley between the hotel and hardware store. Behind the hardware, he got a glimpse of his man running toward the back of the barbershop.

Then things happened so suddenly that Scott dug in his heels and stopped in amazement. Two shots rang out, and the man seemed to stop in mid-stride, then stagger forward a step or two and collapse.

Following the amazement that struck Scott was a feeling of frustration. Someone had beaten him to his revenge. When nobody showed up to claim his victory, Scott ran forward. Only when he reached the fallen man did he realize that this wasn't Johnny Russo. This man was almost exactly Russo's size and had black hair like Russo, but his face was different.

Scott knelt beside hhim, as intent now on helping the man as he had been on destroying him a minute before. There was a faint pulse, but Scott saw the little seepage of blood on his chest. No man could live long with two bullets placed where these were. He lifted his eyes to trace the direction from which the shots had come and found himself looking at the back of the feed store which stood just beyond the barbershop.

Carefully Scott lifted the man and turned back toward Dr. Kinkaid's office, a ground floor room in the hotel with a side door. He winced as pain stabbed through his side. The man was as heavy as Johnny Russo, over two hundred pounds, and that was too much weight for Scott to be lifting before his ribs had completely healed.

People were coming from the street, but none offered to assist Scott in carrying the man. Dr. Kinkaid opened his office door and helped Scott get the man inside and on a couch.

"Who is he?" Scott asked.

"Josh Woodruff. I reckon Tillotson has finally killed him."

The doctor stooped to examine the wounds. After a minute he lifted his head with a sigh.

"Dead?" Scott asked.

Kinkaid nodded. "No man could live carrying two bullets where these are. Know who fired those shots?"

Scott shook his head. "I thought he was Johnny Russo, and I was trying to catch up with him to settle my score."

The doctor went through the dead man's pockets. From an inside pocket he brought out a long envelope. "It's here, all right," Kinkaid said. He looked up at Scott. "You're in for a big surprise."

"How come?" Scott asked.

But instead of answering, Kinkaid turned to the men jamming the door of the office. "Somebody bring Berwyn Edris in here."

"Who's Edris?" Scott asked.

"The only lawyer in town." He held up the envelope for Scott to see. "This is Josh's last will. He told me what's in it."

The lawyer came in a couple of minutes later, a tall, sandy-haired, blue-eyed man in his late twenties.

"Got a will for you to open and read," Kinkaid said, handing the envelope to the lawyer.

Edris frowned as he glanced at it. Then he turned to look at the people in the doorway. "Better make this private."

"I don't see why," Kinkaid said. "A will isn't a private affair. Let everybody know just what Josh wanted done with his property."

The lawyer's frown deepened, but he tore the envelope open. Scott watched him, wondering at his reluctance. The will was short, and Scott paid little attention to it until the last few words. "I leave to my nephew, George Ingram, one dollar. In case I meet with a violent death, I leave everything else I own, including the JW Ranch and everything in it, to the person or persons who are with me trying to help me when I die."

Dr. Kinkaid's blue eyes were twinkling as he looked at Scott. "See what I mean? You have just inherited the JW Ranch and everything on it, which must include quite a few head of cattle."

"And a barrel of trouble," Edris added, glaring at Scott.

IV

Scott was staggered by what the lawyer had read.

"Get Hookey over here," Edris shouted to one of the men standing in the doorway.

"That deputy won't be able to find the killer," Kinkaid said disgustedly. "The only thing he can find is a bottle of whiskey and a soft bed."

"This may be different," Edris said. "He may not have to hunt far for Woodruff's killer."

Scott knew then that the lawyer suspected him of killing Woodruff. "Was Woodruff a friend of yours?" he asked.

Edris shook his head. "Not particularly. But I don't like the idea of killers running loose."

Sam Hookey came into the office two minutes later, puffing, his face red. He was a heavy man, most of his weight concentrated in the middle, where his suspenders seemed to be fighting a losing battle to hold up his pants.

"Ed said Josh Woodruff had been killed," Hookey

panted.

"If you'd had your head out of that whiskey bottle, you'd have heard the shots," Edris said disgustedly. He pointed to Scott. "This stranger brought Woodruff into Doc's office."

Hookey turned to stare at Scott. "How come you got to him first?"

"I just happened to be close by," Scott said.

"Better check his gun," Edris said. "You might find Woodruff's killer without moving out of this room."

"Let's have your gun, mister," Hookey said slowly, reaching for Scott's gun.

Scott stood still while the deputy lifted the gun from its holster. Hookey broke the cylinder and squinted down the barrel. Scott watched him closely as he snapped it back in place and returned it to Scott's holster.

"Hasn't been fired since it was cleaned," he said. "He didn't have time to clean it after the shooting, did he?"

"Josh was shot only a few minutes ago," Kinkaid said. "This man had him in my office two minutes later."

"That clears him, then," Hookey said flatly. "Anybody know where the shots came from?"

"From the feed store," one man said. "I was at the blacksmith shop right across the street when it happened."

"Who did the shooting?"

"Don't know," the man said. "But I know where the shots came from, all right."

"Come on," Hookey said importantly. "Let's take a look. I'm deputizing you five men right here to go with me to look for this killer."

The deputy sheriff stamped out of the doctor's office, and the crowd followed him.

Scott turned to the lawyer. "Is that will of Woodruff's legal?"

"Of course it is," Kinkaid broke in. "Josh told me himself that he had made sure there were no loopholes in it."

The lawyer nodded slowly. "It's legal, all right. Woodruff's nephew, George Ingram, will get one dollar. Everything else goes to the man who was trying to help him when he died. I guess there is no doubt but that you're the man."

"I wasn't doing it to inherit a ranch," Scott said.

"I'm going back to my office," Edris said. "If you want to get rid of the ranch or need me for anything, you know where to find me."

After the lawyer had gone, Scott looked at Kinkaid. "Now what? I need a ranch to look after like I need a spavined horse."

Kinkaid spread a sheet over the body on the couch. "You said Tillotson stole a ranch from you. Now you have one given to you. That seems fair enough."

Scott frowned. "That's not what I came here for. I came to get the ten thousand dollars Tillotson stole from me. Woodruff's ranch isn't anything off Tillotson's nose."

"Don't be too sure about that," Kinkaid said. "Tillotson wants the JW so bad he can taste it. It's the only place in this valley that he doesn't control now. It was because of Tillotson's threats that Josh made that will."

Scott's interest quickened. "What do you know about Tillotson's threats against Woodruff?"

"I told you Josh Woodruff was a good friend of mine. He confided things to me that he wouldn't tell anyone else. He was a bachelor and he was a loner; had no close friends except me. He told me that Tillotson had threatened his life if he didn't sell to him at a dirt cheap price. Josh was stubborn as a bull. He wouldn't sell. He got the feeling some of his crew had been bribed by Tillotson. That's when he made that will."

"What good would that do?"

"Josh got suspicious of everybody. He has a foreman on the JW, Mark Sitzman, who has been with him for a good many years. Josh made a will several years ago that left the JW to Sitzman if Josh should die first. Lately Josh began getting suspicious of Sitzman, too. He made this will, leaving the ranch to the man or men who were with him at the end, fighting to help him. Josh was sure that some day Tillotson would bring his men to the JW to kill him. Josh figured that the men who stayed him in such a fight would be the loyal ones. If he got killed, he wanted them to have the ranch. If Sitzman was loyal, he'd get it. If not, he wouldn't."

"His strategy backfired," Scott said, "Sitzman wasn't in town, so he didn't have a chance to help him when he was killed."

Kinkaid nodded. "That might be. But again, maybe Sitzman wasn't with him for a reason. Josh seldom went anywhere without his foreman. But he did today. I wouldn't worry about it if I were you. I'd take the ranch."

"What about this nephew he mentioned?"

"George Ingram? I've heard Josh talk about him. Worthless as Confederate money, Josh said. He left him one dollar so he couldn't break the will, no matter how he tried."

"Just what is the JW worth?" Scott asked.

"It's a good ranch, but it has been running in trouble lately," Kinkaid said. "Josh was losing too many cattle to rustlers. I reckon Tillotson could tell something about that, too. Josh had to borrow money from me to keep going. But the ranch is worth many times what he owed."

"What about the men working on the JW? Will they stay now that Josh is dead?"

"Hard to say about that," Kinkaid said. "The men

will probably stay on if they're guaranteed their pay. After all, it's still a job for them, no matter who pays their wages. But it might be a different matter with the foreman."

"Sitzman? He was a good friend of Woodruff's, wasn't he?"

"Always had been until recently, anyway. Josh was suspicious of him lately, and maybe for good reason. Mark Sitzman is no angel. He's greedy. I wouldn't put it past him to try to get rid of Josh so he could have the JW for himself."

"If that's the way it is, he isn't going to like the idea of my taking over."

"You can be sure of that. And he's got a daughter you'd better keep an eye on, too. If I was going out there, I'd watch Sadie just as close as I would Mark."

"Is she tricky?"

"Plenty," Kinkaid said. "Her mother's dead. Died before I knew them. Her father raised her like a boy, and she's as tough as any man in the country. She can outswear and outdrink any of them."

"I think I'll go out there and see what I've inherited," Scott said.

"I wouldn't go off half-cocked," Kinkaid said. "Sitzman isn't going to like the idea of you coming out to take over. I'd take the law with me, such as it is, to make him understand this is how it's going to be."

"The deputy is out looking for Woodruff's killer."

"He won't look long," Kinkaid said. "Too much work. When he comes back, make him ride out there with you. Might save an ambush."

"Think it will be that bad?" Scott asked.

"Could be. I wouldn't put much past Sitzman if he's worked up enough. And you can bet he'll be as mad as a hen in a horse tank when he finds out you own the JW instead of him."

Scott stayed close to the doctor's office until he saw the deputy come back into town with the men he had deputized. After what had happened, there was no point in keeping it a secret that he had stayed in Tomahawk. Scott was willing to bet that Cole Tillotson had long since received the information.

"Hookey's back," Scott announced to the doctor. "I think I'll go over and see him."

"Don't ask him to go out with you," Kinkaid said. "Just tell him he's going. He'll find a thousand excuses for not riding that far if you give him half a chance."

Scott left the doctor's office and walked along the side of the hotel to the street, then turned along the front of the hotel and angled across the dusty inter-section to the deputy's office in the front of the jail building.

Hookey had just thrown his gun belt across his desk and dropped into his chair, his feet propped up in front of him. He scowled as he looked up at his visitor.

"What do you want?" he demanded. "I chased over

half the county looking for that killer and never found a trace."

"Small county," Scott said. "You've been gone only two hours. I'm going out to my new ranch. I want you to ride out with me."

The deputy's feet thumped to the floor. "Now hold on a minute! It's noon, and I haven't had my dinner. Besides, you can find your way out to the JW without me to guide you."

"I can find my way, all right," Scott admitted. "But you're going along to convince the foreman there that I really own the ranch."

"I'm not so sure you do," Hookey growled.

"You heard what the lawyer said."

"I heard him," the deputy grumbled. "But I'm going to get a bait of grub before I go. You can like that or not."

"I can wait till after dinner," Scott agreed. "But we'll go then."

Scott went back to Kinkaid's house. He knew that Anne and Mrs. Kinkaid would have dinner for him. This would probably be the last meal he'd eat there, and he was going to miss that. But it was more than just the good food that he'd miss.

"You will be careful, won't you?" Anne said as he made ready to leave after dinner.

Scott grinned easily. "I always try to finish anything I start. And I haven't got my ten thousand dollars out of Tillotson yet."

Hookey was gone when Scott got back to his office. Scott checked at the hotel, but dinner was over, and the cook there told him that Hookey had eaten and left. Remembering what Kinkaid had said about Hookey not being able to find anything but a bottle of whiskey and a soft bed, Scott headed for the saloon just across the street.

Hookey was at a table in the darkest corner, but Scott soon picked him out of the gloom. He motioned to him, and the deputy got up reluctantly and came to the door. Without a word he tramped across the side street that separated the saloon from the deputy's office and the jail.

While Hookey got his horse, Scott went back to Kinkaid's barn and got his. When he rode back to the street, Hookey was waiting, still sullen.

"No sense dragging me out to the JW," Hookey complained.

But he rode out of town with Scott. It was only two miles from town to the JW, and the two covered the distance in a short time.

The JW was a neat-appearing ranch, Scott thought as he rode into the yard with the deputy. The house was painted white, and the barn and corrals appeared in good repair. A smaller house sat behind the large one, and Scott guessed that was where Mark Sitzman and his daughter Sadie lived. There was a bunkhouse twenty yards down the slope from the big house.

"How come Woodruff had such a big house if he was a bachelor?" Scott asked.

"Josh's pappy built it," Hookey said. "The JW is the oldest spread in these parts. Old Henry Woodruff wanted an impressive mansion. In its day, that house was it."

Scott could imagine that. But he forgot the house as he saw a tall slim man with close-set eyes and thick unruly hair come from the corrals to meet them.

"Sitzman?" Scott asked softly.

Hookey nodded, then waited until the man got close. "Howdy, Mark," he said.

"What brings you out in the heat of the day, Hookey?" Sitzman demanded. "Must be something powerful important."

Hookey jerked a thumb at Scott. "He brought me. And I reckon he is a mite important. He owns the JW now."

For a long minute Sitzman simply stared, his heavy eyebrows pulled together in a dark scowl. "That's a lie!" he muttered finally. "Where's Josh?"

Scott realized that Sitzman wasn't pretending. He didn't know what had happened in town that morning.

"Ain't you heard?" Hookey asked, showing surprise himself. "Josh was killed in town this morning. Bush-whacked from the feed store. This stranger tried to help him. Carried him to the doc's office, but it was no use. Josh had a crazy will that left everything he owned to the man who was trying to help him when he died."

Sitzman started to say something, choked on the words, then tried again, "That's a lie!" he croaked finally. "If Josh is dead, I get the ranch."

Hookey leaned far over his saddle horn. "Did you know about Josh's crazy will?"

"No!" Sitzman shouted. "And I don't believe it. You'll have to show me proof."

"It's in town," Hookey said. "Edris has it. He drew up this will just a few weeks ago. And Kinkaid says Woodruff made sure there were no loopholes in it."

Sitzman looked at Scott with murder in his eyes. "He ain't going to get the JW." His hand dropped to the butt of his gun. "I'll kill him first."

"Now hold on," Hookey shouted in alarm. "Don't start any shooting, Mark. If you don't think the will is legal, check with Edris."

Sitzman glared at Scott for a moment; then his hand relaxed and came away from his gun butt. "I'll do that," he snarled. "Josh told me that this spread would be mine if anything ever happened to him. No stranger is going to walk in and take it without doing a rap for it after I've worked for Josh for ten years to get it."

A rider came charging down into the ranch yard from the west. At first, Scott thought it was one of the crew. Then he discovered that the rider was a girl. He looked at her closely. This would be Sitzman's daughter, Sadie. She could ride and swear and drink like a man, according to Kinkaid. And, looking at her in her Levi's and soiled shirt, Scott didn't doubt it. She carried a gun low on her thigh like a gunman.

"What's wrong, Pa?" she demanded.

"This jasper says he owns the JW, Sadie. Seems Josh was shot in town this morning, and he left a will, giving the ranch to whoever happened to be with him when he died. This man was there."

Sadie wheeled on Scott, her green eyes flashing fire. "You don't get this spread!" she shouted. "I don't care what any will says. You'll have to kill Pa and me to get it."

Scott jerked his head at the deputy. "Hookey here came along to see that nobody did anything foolish. Think about it, and you'll change your mind."

"My mind doesn't change that easy," Sadie said, and Scott had the feeling that Sadie's instant hatred of him would never die.

"I suppose you want us to pack up and get out," Sitzman said, his voice carrying a strong hint of the uncertainty that plagued him.

"I don't figure on making any immediate changes," Scott said. "For the time being, you can stay on as foreman if you want to."

"You're just borrowing time," Sadie observed, glaring at Scott. "The day you try to run us off the JW will be your last day on earth."

"Come on, Sadie," Sitzman said, turning toward the house behind the big white mansion. "We need to think this through."

Sadie stared at Scott for another minute before turning and leading her horse after her father.

"You'll have to watch her," Hookey warned. "She can be poison mean."

"Wonder if she ever tried being a woman," Scott said.

"She wouldn't admit it if she had," Hookey said. "Going back to town with me?"

"Why should I? This is my ranch now. I'll stay here."

Hookey shrugged. "Like you say, it's your ranch."

The deputy wheeled his horse and spurred him out of the yard as if he were glad to get away. Scott dismounted and went into the house.

He watched for the men to ride in, and when they came, he started to the corral to meet them. But the cook banged the triangle for supper, and he turned toward the cook shack and waited for the men there.

There were five men who came into the cook shack for supper. Scott introduced himself and explained what had happened. He watched their reactions. They were surprised, but there was none of the resentment that he had encountered in the Sitzmans. Though they were shocked at Josh's death, it made no difference to them for whom they worked as long as they got paid. Scott was relieved.

After supper, he returned to the big house and found a bedroom to his liking.

He was sound asleep when he heard a shot. Before his feet hit the floor, he had his gun in his hand. There were more shots, but they were some distance from the house, and Scott took time to jerk on his pants and shirt before running to the front door.

Scott guessed what it was. Tillotson had sent his Tilted T warriors to overrun the JW. Tillotson would try to wipe out all resistance to his complete control of Tomahawk Valley in one stroke.

V

Scott stood at the front door for a minute to get a bearing on what was happening outside. Guns were firing from the far side of the corral and were being answered to the bunkhouse. Scott saw a man dodging from the corrals to the bunkhouse, and the door of the bunkhouse swung open to let him in.

So far all the shots were bing concentrated on the bunkhouse. Scott wanted to be with the men.

Splitting out the door, Scott ran toward the bunkhouse, bent low. At the door, he tapped on the panel as bullets thudded into the building around the windows through which the crew was shooting.

"Who in blazes is out there?" one man asked during a lull in the shooting.

"It's me, Scott. Let me in."

The door opened, and Scott slipped inside.

"Why did you buy into this?" one man said.

"Thought it was my fight," Scott said. "Who it is—Tilted T?"

"Who else? They figure to take over now that Josh

is dead."

Scott added his gun to those already returning the fire from the corrals. "How come they didn't move in closer before starting the fireworks?"

"Good reason," one man said. "Sitzman came down after you left last night and told us to post a guard. He expected Tillotson to strike. Sam fired that first shot as a warning."

Scott frowned. Sitzman had been smarter than he had been in protecting the JW.

The shooting outside suddenly stopped. When the men in the bunkhouse stopped shooting, too, a man yelled from beyond the corrals:

"Scott, you're a dead man if you stay in Tomahawk Valley."

"How did he know you were here, Scott?" one man asked in the silence that followed.

Scott decided that somebody from town, probably Blessing or Kale, had told Tillotson that Scott had inherited the JW, and Tillotson had guessed that he would lose no time before taking over.

Suddenly a flame leaped up from a stack of hay left over from last winter. By its sudden light, Scott saw the riders heading back onto the road.

"Pulling out," one man exclaimed, emptying his gun at the riders.

"Couldn't surprise us and didn't have guts enough to fight when they found we were ready for them," another man said.

"Let's save that hay," Scott said, and broke for the door.

The men followed him as he ran toward the fire. But the dry hay was blazing fiercely, and they could do nothing to save the stack. They did manage to confine the fire to the stack and save the nearby corral fence.

Sitzman arrived at the burning stack almost as soon as the rest of the men. His close-set eyes reflected the firelight as he worked, and Scott could almost feel his rage.

"Yellow dogs!" he snapped when he stopped to catch his breath. Wouldn't stay and fight if it was an even fight. I figured they'd try to burn the house, too."

Scott knew then why Sitzman hadn't come down to the bunkhouse. He'd been back by the houses guarding them.

"Figure they'll be back?" Scott asked.

"Sure," Sitzman said. "They'll keep pecking away till they get the JW, or they're all killed. They're yellow, that's all. They've got to have every advantage or they won't fight."

With the fire out, Scott went back to the house. But he didn't sleep much the rest of the night. What would Tillotson's next move be? Scott now had something that Tillotson wanted almost as much as he wanted to get Scott out of the way. Tillotson wouldn't wait long to do something about that.

The crew stayed close to the ranch the next day. When Scott inquired about the work on the ranch, the man called Sam was quick to answer.

"Sure, there's work to be done. But Mark figures we may be needed more right here."

"Expecting Tillotson's gunmen?" Scott asked.

Sam nodded. "They tried to surprise us last night, and it didn't work. Now Mark figures they might try a raid during the daytime, figuring we'll all be out working."

Scott shook his head, remembering Cole Tillotson as he knew him. "I doubt if he'll try anything in the daylight. He might get hurt."

"He just might at that," Sam said, fondly touching the rifle beside him. "I'd like to be the one to prove that to him."

"Where's Sitzman now?" Scott asked.

"Gone somewhere. I think he's scouting the Tilted T to find out what Tillotson's got in mind."

Scott frowned. Sitzman was running the JW without any consultation with Scott. Scott didn't question the wisdom of Sitzman's moves, but he did question his motives. Was he trying to show Scott that he was boss and that Scott was just a outsider, tolerated until they could get rid of him?

Scott decided it might be wise to check the town. Tillotson had men in Tomahawk. He might learn more in town than Sitzman would at the Tilted T.

It was afternoon when Scott rode into town. Before

reaching Main Street, he reined off to his right, stopping at Dr. Kinkaid's house. Anne saw him and came to the door.

"Come in, Web," she urged. "Hurry."

Scott hitched his horse and went inside. "What's the rush?"

"Don't you know you shouldn't be exposing yourself on the street like that?"

"Why not?" Scott asked. "Doesn't everybody know now that I'm a legitimate ranch owner?"

"Don't be foolish," Anne said. "You know Cole Tillotson has men in town. Dad has heard rumors. There is a price on your head. And there are several men right here in town who would do anything for the kind of money Tillotson has put up."

"Such as Dan Kale?" Scott asked.

"He's one," Anne said. "That raid last night is surely proof enough that Tillotson will stop at nothing to get rid of you."

"I already know that," Scott said. "But how did you hear about that raid?"

"Word spreads fast in a place like Tomahawk."

"Have you any idea what Tillotson plans now?"

Anne shook her head. "We're not liable to hear any of his plans. But he's got some scheme up his sleeve, all right. Dan Kale was in Dad's office this morning, trying to find out if you really planned to stay on the JW. He dropped a hint that you'd be in for a real surprise in a day or two if you stayed on the ranch."

"That's nice," Scott said. "I like some kinds of surprises."

"You won't like this one if Tillotson has anything to do with it."

Scott felt that he was wasting time there, although talking to Anne was the most pleasant way he had ever wasted time.

"If Tomahawk is out of bounds for me, I'll head back to the JW," he said. "You can tell anybody who asks that I am staying there. I have no intention of leaving."

"I didn't think you'd run out." She followed him to the door. "Stop in whenever you can slip into town, Web. If Dad finds out anything, I'll pass the information on to you."

"I'll take that as an invitation to drop in whether there is any information or not," Scott said, grinning.

Color suffused her face. "Maybe that was what it was meant to be," she said, and shut the door.

Scott didn't see Sitzman that night. The next morning, when he ran into him down by the corral, he confronted him with a question.

"Are you planning to keep the men here at the ranch today?"

"Why not?" Sitzman asked.

"Have you checked the cattle west of here since yesterday? I saw a herd being pushed across the creek by five men. Maybe they were Tilted T critters that had strayed over here, and maybe they weren't. No JW men were out there to watch."

Sitzman swore. "Why didn't you stop them?"

"I was alone. There were five of them. That herd of cattle wouldn't do me any good if I was dead."

Sitzman swore again. "I'll check the range. If Tillotson is stealing us blind, I'll put a stop to it."

"Has he been stealing JW stock?"

"We've lost some," Sitzman admitted, "but not in wholesale lots."

Scott went on to talk to the men. Anger ran through them as he told them about the cattle.

"How about letting us go out and watch today?" Sam asked. "If they got by with running off a bunch yesterday, they'll try it again today. I'd like to catch them red-handed."

The men all seemed eager, and Scott had the feeling that they agreed more with his method of handling the situation than they did with Sitzman's.

"All right; go ahead. But ride easy and stay in pairs. If some of you run into trouble, fire a couple of shots. The others will come to help."

"Come on, boys," Sam said, and wheeled toward the corral. "Make sure your shooting irons are clean and ready."

Scott turned back to see Sitzman scowling at him.

"I've been foreman of the JW for ten years," Sitzman

said, "and I never before had to have help giving orders to the men."

"Maybe it's time somebody did help you," Scott said, and turned toward the house. Prickles ran up his back, and he knew that Sitzman had been staring at him. But the men weren't out of sight yet. Sitzman wouldn't risk a cold-blooded murder now.

The men had been gone only a few minutes when his attention was drawn by the sound of riders approaching from the direction of town. Scott wondered for a moment if he'd been wrong in letting all the men go out on the range. Then he saw that there were only two riders. This could hardly be gun trouble coming; not from the Tilted T, anyway.

Scott stepped off the veranda of the big house to meet the two riders. One was the deputy sheriff, Sam Hookey. The other man was a stranger to Scott. He was short and not very heavy, with fiery red hair and blue eyes. His skin was pale, obviously not used to the hot sun.

"What's on your mind, Hookey?" Scott asked.

"Got somebody here who wants to meet you, Scott," the deputy said. "This is George Ingram, Josh Woodruff's nephew."

Scott studied the small man. Maybe this was the surprise that Kale had hinted was coming. It would be like Tillotson to send word to Ingram that his uncle was dead if he thought it could cause a diversion for his enemies while he plotted their final downfall. And from the looks of the anger on Ingram's face, this was going to cause a rumpus, all right."

"This was my uncle's ranch, wasn't it?" Ingram asked.

"It was," Scott said. "It's mine now."

"You're a dirty liar!" Ingram shouted, his face reddening. "I'm the only living relative of Joshua Woodruff. This ranch belongs to me."

"Not according to the will," Scott said, holding his anger in check with an effort. "And I don't take kindly to being called a liar. Didn't Hookey tell you about the will?"

"Sure," Ingram said. "Hookey told me. That law spieler, Edris, told me, too. But I don't believe a word of it. If you think you can keep this ranch from me because of a litttle scrap of paper, you can just think again. I'll take it to court, and I'll put you behind bars for stealing my property."

"You're a pretty little man to be spouting off such big threats," Scott said.

"Little, am I?" Ingram shouted. "I'll show you!"

His hand dug into his pocket, and Scott guessed he had a gun there. Scott's hand shot down and brought up his own gun. Tillotson had taught him well how to do that. The little man's hand stopped halfway into his pocket. Even Hookey stared.

"Now, now," the deputy said finally. "We'll have no

guns here."

Ingram's hand came away from his pocket, and he stared for another moment at the gun that had appeared so rapidly in Scott's hand.

"Arrest him, Sheriff," he demanded.

"What for?" Hookey asked.

Scott could barely keep from smiling. Hookey wouldn't try to arrest him now even if he had a reason. He had obviously been impressed by the speed of Scott's gun hand.

"For stealing my ranch," Ingram shouted.

"According to the will I saw, he ain't stealing anything," Hookey said. "You're the one who is pushing into the wrong stall. Your uncle left you a dollar. That's all you'll get."

"I'll get more!" Ingram said. "Who's that?" He pointed to Mark Sitzman, who had just come out of his little house.

"That's Sitzman, foreman of the JW," Hookey said.

"He'll know whether there is any truth to this so-called will," Ingram said.

Ingram spurred his horse over to the JW foreman. Scott watched him as he talked to Sitzman. After a minute, he dismounted, and Sitzman invited him into the little house.

"Looks like they're going to hit it off a little better than you and him did," Hookey said.

"Looks that way," Scott agreed.

VI

Sam Hookey wasn't happy with the role he'd been handed in this affair. He hadn't wanted to make the ride out to the JW that morning. But this nephew of Josh Woodruff's, George Ingram, had come into his office right after breakfast and demanded his company.

Hookey figured there would be trouble. Ingram struck him as a trouble maker, if he'd ever seen one. So he might as well be on the spot when the trouble took place. It would save a lot of hard work investigating it all later on.

But now, as he sat on his horse and watched Ingram go into the house with Sitzman, he wondered what he should do. He might as well go on back to town. Ingram hadn't asked for an escort back to town; just out here.

Ingram didn't stay in Sitzman's house long. He came out, scowling at Scott, who had retreated to the shade of the veranda, not even inviting Hookey to get down from his horse.

"You won't stay on my ranch long, Scott," Ingram said as he swung into his saddle. "If you're smart, you'll get out now while you've still got a whole hide."

"Do you want to try to put a hole in my hide now?" Scott asked. "If you don't I'd advise you to get off my ranch and stay off."

Ingram swore loud and long as he wheeled his horse and spurred him out of the yard. Hookey had to apply his own spurs to keep up.

"Hey, hold up," he shouted when he got close enough. "You might want that horse again some day."

Ingram reined down to a trot. "I'll kill that Scott!" he snapped. "Just as sure as I'm alive, I'll kill him!"

"If you do," Hookey said, "I'll have to arrest you for murder. You sure won't kill him in a fair fight. You proved that back there a little bit ago."

"I'll kill him," Ingram repeated darkly, then rode in silence for a mile.

Hookey looked at the little man and wondered what was going on in his mind. He was tricky, Hookey decided.

"Are you in favor of Scott getting that ranch for nothing?" Ingram asked finally.

Hookey shrugged. "Can't say that I am. But there's nothing I can do about it."

"Would you do anything if you could?"

The deputy frowned. "Hadn't considered that. Don't figure the opportunity will come."

"Well, consider it," Ingram insisted. "I may need some help getting Scott off the JW. I figure you're the man to help me. That star you're wearing ought to carry a little weight."

Hookey frowned. Ingram had no idea how weightless the star really was. But maybe there was a way to use Ingram's confidence to his advantage. He could certainly use a little boost in prestige and power in Tomahawk.

"You may be right," he said. "Got something in mind?"

"Maybe," Ingram said. "All I want to know now is whether I can depend on you for official help if I need it."

"I reckon you can count on that if you stay within the law."

Ingram was silent for another long minute. "If it wasn't exactly according to Hoyle, how would you feel? Of course, I'm not expecting your services for nothing."

Hookey grinned. Ingram was starting to speak a language he understood. "I reckon you can depend on me for any help you need, as long as we can make it look legal."

"No matter how legal or illegal it really is?"

"You said it; not me," Hookey said cautiously.

Ingram grinned. "I'll remember that. I'll let you know if you can be of help."

In Tomahawk, Ingram reined in at the livery stable, left his horse and walked up the street to the hotel. Hookey rode on to the jail and dismounted. He went into his office, mulling over the ways of twisting Ingram's presence there to his advantage.

Finally, after Ingram had disappeared inside the hotel, Hookey went back outside and mounted his horse. Cole Tillotson ought to be happy to learn what Hookey knew.

Hookey stayed on the road that clung to the north bank of the creek. After passing the JW across the creek on his left, he began thinking exactly what he would say and do when he got to the Tilted T.

A lot of men in this valley hated Tillotson. But none could possibly hate him more than Hookey did.

As he jogged along, his pace slowing as his reluctance to face Tillotson grew, Hookey thought back to the reason for his being there at all. He had made a mistake back when he was still in his teens. He had loved a girl, or thought he had.

The girl hadn't been so sure. One evening he had found her taking a boat ride with another man on the little lake close to the Ohio town where he lived. He had waited until they beached the boat, his rage growing wilder by the minute. The second the man stepped on shore, Hookey had been on him.

It hadn't been much of a fight, for the other fellow was a small man, a clerk in a store in town. After

Hookey had beaten him and sent him running wildly toward town, he had turned his wrath on the girl. If she had showed fear or repentance for what she had done, his rage would have blown away. But she had been as angry as he.

His rage had exploded in his head, sending a sickening feeling washing over him. He still remembered it. He had been that angry only a few times in his life and every time it had left him sick and weak. But at that moment it had burned through him like a consuming fire.

He couldn't remember exactly what he had done. He only remembered grabbing the girl and shoving her into the water. After she was dead, he had loaded her body into the boat and rowed out to the center of the lake and shoved her overboard. Returning to town, he had spread the word that she had fallen overboard when they were out rowing and he hadn't been able to save her. He had remembered to take a dip in the lake with all his clothes on to verify his story of trying to rescue the girl.

He had thought he had covered his crime perfectly. But there had been one factor that he hadn't reckoned on. There had been a man, a bum, who had decided to spend that night sleeping in the bushes along the edge of the lake. He had heard the fight and had watched from the seclusion of his retreat. He had seen Hookey drown the girl, then take her body out into the lake and dump it.

The bum said nothing to the authorities, but had gotten in touch with Hookey a few days later and demanded enough money to make it possible for him to live at ease in society. Hookey had paid him; it had been all he could do. But it hadn't been enough. The man had come back for more money before Hookey could get it.

Hookey had left Ohio and headed west, feeling certain the former bum wouldn't follow him. But it had been a false hope. The blackmailer had found an easy living off Hookey and wasn't going to let it slip away from him.

Hookey had finally lost him in Wyoming; or at least he thought he'd lost him. He learned through an account in the paper that the man, Cole Tillotson, had just taken over a ranch down in Nebraska. Hookey at last felt that he was free of the blackmailer. But soon Tillotson had sold that ranch and moved to Tomahawk Valley. It was only a matter of weeks before Hookey had walked out into the street one day, and there was Tillotson, well dressed and prosperous-looking, but just as greedy as ever.

Tillotson had told Hookey that he needed him down at Tomahawk. At first Hookey had refused to go, but Tillotson paid no attention to Hookey's arguments. He needed him in Tomahawk. He expected him in one week; else he'd wire the authorities in Ohio what he knew about the death of that girl years ago. A week later Hookey had been in Tomahawk.

The Tilted T came in sight, and Hookey brought his thoughts back to the present. He felt like a dog crawling to the table, begging for crumbs. But if he gave Tillotson a helping hand, surely Tillotson would make life a little easier for Hookey.

Dismounting at the hitch rack, he flipped the reins over the bar and strode up the walk. He knocked and waited until Tillotson called for him to come in. It was a long wait, and Hookey did a slow burn. He had seen Tillotson's face at the window as he rode up, so he knew that the Tilted T owner was aware that he was there.

"What makes you ride out here in the sun?" Tillotson asked, scowling at the deputy.

"I had some information I thought you'd like to have."

After a long wait, Tillotson nodded. "Well, am I supposed to read your mind?"

"Josh Ingram's nephew is in town," Hookey said. "He's ready to do anything to get Web Scott off the JW."

"Tell me something I don't know," Tillotson said, settling back in his big chair.

"You know about Ingram?"

"I sent word to him about Josh's death," Tillotson said. "Why wouldn't I know about him?"

Hookey saw his chance for a good word from Tillotson go flying out the window. A surge of anger swept up in him, not so much at Tillotson as at the world in general. It was unfair that he always got the dirty end of the stick.

"I was trying to help you," Hookey snapped.

"Don't use that tone of voice when you're talking to me," Tillotson warned.

But the rage that had been building up in Hookey all the way out from town wouldn't be quieted that easily.

"I've got a right to use any tone of voice I choose. I am a man."

Tillotson got out of his chair. "No one would ever know it if you didn't say so."

"You've got no right to talk to me like that!" Hookey screamed.

"What rights do you think you have, anyway?" Tillotson demanded. "You ought to be rotting in a prison right now. Is that the right you're demanding?"

Mention of prison took the wildness out of Hookey's eyes, and he pinched his lips together, breathing hard.

"I tried to help you," he said finally, a whimpering note in his voice now. "I thought you'd appreciate it."

"Oh, sure, I appreciate it," Tillotson said disgustedly. "I appreciate your help like a horse appreciates a botfly buzzing around his chin."

Anger at Tillotson's unfairness swept over Hookey

again. "It will be a long hot day before I every try to help you again!"

Tillotson reached out his long arm and slapped Hookey so hard that he reeled back against the wall. "You'll do what I tell you, and you will do nothing else. Is that clear?"

Hookey thought of the gun at his hip. He knew that Tillotson carried a small derringer in a shoulder holster and could snatch it out in an instant. But still he couldn't keep his mind off that gun on his hip. If he only had that in his hand now, he'd put an end to Tillotson. He'd be a free man if Cole Tillotson were dead.

"Don't even consider it!" Tillotson snapped, stepping forward and slapping Hookey again. "I'd kill you before you had your gun out of the holster, and you know it. I don't want to kill you. I've got a job for you, and you can't do it if you're dead."

Hookey put a hand to his mouth, where blood was beginning to ooze. He considered striking back. He was almost as big as Tillotson. A good fight would make him feel better, even if he got licked. But Tillotson would never take part in a fight. He'd dodge back and use that derringer of his. Hookey was ready to face uneven odds, but not sure death.

He wheeled and ran out to his horse. Mounting, he spurred the horse viciously into a dead run out of the yard and down the road toward town. Some day he'd kill Cole Tillotson.

In Tomahawk, he left his lathered horse in front of his office, but he didn't go inside. Instead, he crossed the side street to the saloon.

"A shot of the usual?" the bartender asked when Hookey reached the bar.

Hookey shook his head. "Give me the whole bottle. A full one."

The bartender set a full bottle on the bar. "You must figure to hang on a good one."

Hookey merely grunted, went to a table along the wall and slouched down in the chair, pouring the glass brim full.

He didn't know how long he had been there when he heard the swinging doors open and looked up through bleary eyes to see Sadie Sitzman come in. The bottle in front of him was half empty. Sadie looked as if she needed company, and he had plenty of drinking whiskey. He'd show some people that he wasn't the worm Cole Tillotson thought he was. He could be somebody important, and those high and mighty know-it-alls like Tillotson could just go hang. He'd show them.

He waved a hand at Sadie. "Come over here, Sadie," he said thickly. "Drinks on me."

Sadie switched her course from the direction of the bar to Hookey's table. "Don't mind if I do, Sam. I need a drink, and I'm not particular where I get it."

"Got to be particular to drink with me," Hookey said. "Got to be somebody to be my equal."

"You're drunk already, Sam," Sadie said as she slid into the chair across the table from him.

"No, I ain't drunk. I'm just proving something."

"What?" Sadie poured some whiskey into the glass the bartender brought to her.

"That I'm just as important as anybody."

"Who says you're not?"

"A lot of people, a lot of people." Hookey wiped a hand over his face. He felt wonderful now, but it was getting hard to keep Sadie in focus over there across the table.

He poured himself another drink, spilling some of the whiskey on the table.

"You know, everybody thinks I'm just a pushover," he said, fighting to keep the words coming. "Well, I'm not. I could tell you of some of the things I've done that would prove that I'm no pushover."

"What things?" Sadie asked, leaning toward him.

Hookey grinned. Now here was somebody who was really interested in him. Sadie Sitzman was a woman after his own heart. She cared what had happened to him. She didn't think he was so unimportant.

Hookey poured his glass full again and lofted it high for a toast. He swore as some of the whiskey dribbled over the edge of the glass and down into his eyes. It stung. Just another of the unfair things that always happened to him. Well, he'd tell Sadie about the unfairness of the world toward him. She'd understand. And she'd help him do something about it, too.

He downed his drink and poured another one. While he was trying to get it to his lips, Sadie took it from his hand.

"You were going to tell me about the important things you'd done, Sam," Sadie prodded. "Don't forget."

He grinned. "I won't forget. And you won't, either, once I tell you." He wiped a hand over his face again. He had to tell her now right now, before he got to the point where he couldn't tell her anything. It was important that Sadie know of the things he had done in his life. Nothing had ever been so important before.

Later, Hookey couldn't remember just what had happened after that. He dimly remembered the bartender lifting him from the chair and half dragging him to the door. He had tried to talk to Sadie again, but he discovered that she was gone.

"It's closing time, you old fool," the bartender said.

Hookey ignored the fact that the bartender had called him a fool. Let him call him what he wanted to. Sadie could tell him that Sam Hookey was no fool; he was an important man.

When Hookey came to himself again, he was on the couch in his office. He blinked his eyes against the light and tried to sit up. His head felt as big as five heads ought to. What had happened? Had somebody hammered him on the noggin?

Then memory slowly came back to him. He had gone to the saloon last night to get drunk. He must have done a good job of it. He got to his feet and staggered over to the stove in the corner of the office. He fumbled around for a long time getting the fire started. Then he set the coffeepot on the stove and poured in water with a spoonful of freshly ground coffee beans. That hot black coffee would clear his head.

When the coffee was hot and he'd had three cups of it, his mind cleared and he began wishing it hadn't. He remembered talking to Sadie last night: But what had he told her? He couldn't remember that.

His head was feeling better and he was thinking about cooking something for breakfast when a rider pulled up at the hitch rack in front of his office. He glanced through the front window, and his insides seemed to freeze. Sadie Sitzman was dismounting.

Sadie came into the office, smiling at the rumpled appearance of the deputy. "Looks like you had a hard night, Sam," she said.

Hookey shook his head. "I'm not sure what kind of a night I had. My head is as big as a wagon box this morning."

"You really took on a jag last night, all right," Sadie said. "Feel like riding out to the JW this morning?"

"No," Hookey said. "I don't feel like doing anything but sitting right here."

"Mark wants to see you."

"Why didn't he come in?"

"He had work to do. He figured your time wasn't as valuable as his."

"You ride back and tell him it is," Hookey said.

"You'd better ride out and tell him yourself," Sadie said. "He wants to see you."

"What about?"

"He'll tell you that, too."

Hookey was feeling sick. Mark Sitzman had never had any business with him before. Now he had something urgent. What could that mean? Had Sadie told Mark something? Sitzman wasn't one to be squeamish if he saw a chance to take advantage of anybody.

"Can't it wait?" he asked.

Sadie shook her head. "Mark says to come now."

"I'll get my hat," he said. "I haven't had breakfast either."

"You took on enough liquid refreshment last night to last you till noon today," Sadie said. "Come on."

Hookey couldn't delay any longer. He got his hat and set it on his head. He scowled. The hat wasn't too tight, but it hurt this morning. His head had been aching so hard the roots of his hair were sore.

He walked down to the livery barn. Somebody had

taken his horse from the hitch rack in front of his office, where he had left it yesterday, and tended to it. At the barn, he waited until Eli Blessing got the horse and saddled him. Eli was usually too slow to suit Hookey, but today it seemed he was working with the swiftness of a prairie fire.

Hookey mounted and rode out to the street where Sadie was waiting for him.

At the JW, Mark Sitzman came out and motioned for Hookey and Sadie to come on back to the little house.

"Now what is so important that I had to ride out here without my breakfast?" Hookey demanded with as much confidence as he could muster.

Sitzman led them into the house and motioned to a chair for the deputy. "Better sit down and relax, Hookey," Sitzman said. "You've had a hard night."

"What do you know about that?" Hookey asked suspiciously.

"Your tongue must be tired, too," Sitzman said. "It sure waggled a lot last night."

Hookey dropped his head and groaned. He knew what Sitzman wanted. Hookey had talked too much last night, and Sadie had passed the information on to her father. Sitzman would make use of it somehow. He was that kind of man.

"What did I say that interests you?" Hookey asked finally.

"Enough to send you to the gallows in Ohio if I wanted to tell it all," Sitzman said. "But I'm not one to talk, you know."

Hookey sat with his eyes on his boots. Evidently he had told everything. How could any man be such a complete idiot as he had been last night?

"What do you want?" he asked.

"A little legal work from you, Hookey, that's all," Sitzman said. "You can rest easy. I don't tell what I know about my friends. And friends help each other out, you know."

Hookey nodded. The pattern was familiar. "What do you want me to do?"

"Just arrest Web Scott and start to jail with him. Only make sure he never gets to jail."

"Hold on," Hookey objected. "What charge will I make against Scott?"

Sitzman shrugged. "That's up to you. Surely you can think of something. It really doesn't make much difference, since he isn't going to stand trial, anyway."

"You want me to kill him?"

"I just want you to make sure he doesn't live to get to jail," Sitzman said. "Now don't tell me you can't handle a simple job like that. Any man who can deliberately drown a girl shouldn't find it too hard to shoot an unarmed prisoner. You can say the usual thing: that he tried to escape."

"I can't kill a man in cold blood."

"You can," Sitzman said. "And you'd better. It's either that or back to Ohio to stand trial for murder. Take your choice."

Hookey got up and stumbled out of the house to his office.

VII

Web Scott ate breakfast alone. Only the cook was in the cook shack, and he had just enough for Scott.

"Where are the rest of the men?" Scott asked.

The cook shrugged. "Mr. Sitzman said to tell you he had sent them out on the range to watch for rustlers."

Scott nodded. That sounded reasonable. After what Scott had seen a couple of days ago, it made sense to watch the herds both day and night.

Scott left the cook shack and went down to the corral for his horse. He wanted to look over the JW land a little more, anyway. He'd ride out and talk to the men. He knew that they weren't nearly so opposed to his taking over the JW as Mark Sitzman was. But he had to know whether they would fight with him or against him if it came to a showdown between him and the JW foreman.

He rode west from the house toward the spot where he had seen the cattle being pushed across the river a couple of days before. A rattlesnake, basking in the morning sunlight, buzzed as Scott's horse came too close. The horse snorted in fright and shied away. Scott quieted him, then shot the snake. He rode on. There were neither cattle nor riders on the south side of the creek this morning. He circled to the south until he was sure he was at the edge of the JW land or maybe beyond. He saw little bunches of cattle here and there but no riders.

After completing a big circle that he knew must have covered most of the JW range, he headed back to the ranch. Something was funny. Where could the men be?

As he approached the ranch from the east, he saw a horse leaving the yard, coming at a hard run. He reined up and waited. But the rider didn't even see him.

It was the deputy, Sam Hookey, and Scott saw the wild look in his eyes. He seemed to be frightened half to death. Nothing else could have given him that look.

Scott, shaking his head in bewilderment, rode on down into the yard and hitched his horse to the corral bars. Mark Sitzman came out of his little house and crossed the yard to him.

"Where's the crew?" Scott demanded as soon as he faced Sitzman.

"I let them go," Sitzman said easily.

"Fired them?" Scott exclaimed. "Why?"

"We've lost a lot of cattle," Sitzman said. "We don't need so many men now."

"You fired them because you were afraid they'd take my orders instead of yours," Scott accused him.

"Prove it."

"What good would it do?" Scott said disgustedly. "I'll hire more men. And I'll make sure they take my orders."

"You won't do that while I'm here," Sitzman shouted.

"How are you going to stop me?" Scott demanded. "This is my ranch, whether you like it or not."

"It won't be for long!" Sitzman yelled.

Scott sensed that this could lead to a touchy situation. But the time for caution was past. A showdown with Sitzman had to come. It might as well be now.

He started to make a sharp retort, but the words never got past his lips. Sitzman suddenly straightened up as if somebody had clapped a hand in the middle of his back. Scott saw the surprised look flash across his face a split-second before he heard the shot. Then Sitzman sagged forward and slumped to the ground.

Scott leaned over the foreman. There was a small hole in the middle of his back where a rifle bullet had struck. Scott didn't need a doctor to tell him that Mark Sitzman had been dead before he hit the ground.

Running feet brought Scott around. Sadie was coming from the little house as hard as she could run.

"What happened?" she cried.

"Somebody shot your father," Scott said.

"Who?"

Scott looked to the east and south. The shot must have come from somewhere out there. To the south the land rose in a long swell. Not much cover for a man there. But there was a knoll to the east. A man could have hidden up there. No one was in sight now. Whoever had fired the shot had managed to vanish into the prairie.

"The shot came from out there somewhere," Scott said, waving a hand to the east and south.

He turned to face Sadie and saw the suspicion and hatred in her eyes.

"You did it!" she accused him.

"I did not," he denied. "He was shot in the back."

"You were the only one who could have done it," Sadie shouted, and Scott thought for a moment she was going for her gun.

The drum of a galloping horse broke the tension in the yard, and Scott turned to see the deputy, Sam Hookey, coming down the slope. He reined his horse to a sliding halt in front of Scott and Sadie.

"I heard a shot," Hookey said. "What happened?" Then his eyes fell on Mark Sitzman sprawled in the dust. "Is he dead?"

Scott nodded. "Shot in the back."

"And he killed him," Sadie said, pointing to Scott.

Scott wheeled on Sadie. "I didn't touch my gun. Anyway Sitzman was shot in the back."

"I don't doubt that," Sadie said quickly. "He might have turned his back on you. That would be the time when you'd pull your gun. You wouldn't do it when he was facing you."

Scott looked at the deputy. There was no doubting the direction of his thoughts. Sadie was convincing him. Scott appealed to Hookey, ignoring Sadie.

"You say you heard the shot, Hookey. Was it a rifle or a six-gun?"

Hookey frowned. "I can't rightly say. I was so surprised that I didn't stop to think about it."

"I heard the shot, too," Sadie said. "I was in the house. It could have been either one. Since Scott has no rifle wth him, you can be sure it was a six-gun."

"Use your head," Scott said. "I had no reason to kill Sitzman."

"I am using my head," Hookey said with conviction. "That's why I think Sadie is right. You did have a reason for killing Mark. As long as Mark stayed on the JW, you didn't have full control of the ranch. Only with him dead could you be the real boss."

"They were quarreling just before Pa was shot," Sadie said. "I heard them yelling at each other."

Hookey turned on Scott. "How about that?"

"We were quarreling, all right," Scott said. "But we were a long way from shooting it out."

"So you shot Pa before he had any idea you were planning such a thing," Sadie accused him.

Scott stared from Sadie to the deputy. There was no doubt in either of their minds now. Scott was guilty; at least they were willing to believe it.

Once an investigation was made, Scott was positive he could clear himself. For it could be proved that Sitzman had been shot with a rifle, and even Sadie would have to admit that Scott hadn't had a rifle. But before that investigation, Hookey would take him to the jail in Tomahawk. That didn't appeal to Scott. He didn't trust Hookey. He might not live to get to jail.

And even if he did, what was there to assure him that there would be an investigation of Sitzman's murder? Too many people wanted Scott out of the way. They might just accept the easy way out. They had a man arrested for the murder; they'd convict him and let it go at that. A lot of men in Tomahawk Valley would be glad to do it that way.

Scott weighed all the possibilities and always found himself on the short end of the balances. He was convicted in the eyes of Hookey and Sadie, and the country would go along with them. Behind bars, he would never change anybody's mind. His only chance was to stay out from behind those bars.

Moving swiftly, he drew his gun, while Hookey, seeing his intention, only made a pass at his gun. The deputy brought his hands forward, safely away from his holster.

"Step down off that horse horse, Hookey," Scott

ordered.

"You'll never get away from the law, Scott," Hookey said. But he dismounted quickly.

"This will prove beyond any doubt that you're guilty," Sadie said.

"You're both sure of it now," Scott said.

"You'll never get away!" Sadie shouted. "I'll dog your trail till you're dead."

"That's your privilege," Scott said grimly. "Unsaddle your horse, Hookey."

Hookey swore loudly, but he loosened the cinch and peeled the saddle off his horse.

Scott took the guns from both Sadie and Hookey, picked the rifle out of the saddle boot on Hookey's saddle, then mounted his horse.

"I'll get you, Scott," Hookey threatened. "You know that, don't you?"

"No, I don't, Hookey. I don't figure you'll crowd me too much."

Scott rode out of the yard. Looking back, he saw that Hookey was frantically saddling his horse. Sadie had thrown herself on the ground beside her father, and he could see her shoulders shaking with sobs.

He headed straight north, splashed across the creek, crossed the trail leading to the Tilted T, and kept on going north. There were some hills and gullies there where a man and horse could disappear.

As he topped a hill, he glanced back and saw Hookey

just charging into the creek. Scott had a long lead. He didn't doubt that he could stay ahead of Hookey until the deputy got tired of riding in the hot sun. It wouldn't take a lot of exertion to dull Hookey's enthusiasm for a chase such as this.

Scott spurred his horse on to the north until he was out of sight of the deputy; then he reined sharply to the west. His horse was leaving very little trace of his passing in the short buffalo grass. If Scott could keep out of the deputy's sight, he was sure he could soon lose him. He doubted if Hookey had been given the job of deputy because of his bravery or his tracking skills.

Scott followed a swale around the crest of another knoll, and there he reined up and dismounted. Moving up to a level where he could see his back trail, he watched until Hookey came in sight. The deputy went straight on north, not even bothering to study the faint tracks in the grass that might have told him that Scott had turned west.

After Hookey was out of sight, Scott mounted and rode on. Now he had to reason out who had killed Mark Sitzman and where he would be likely to find the killer.

Sitzman had been consumed with a desire to hold onto the JW for himself. Scott reasoned that this fact would have made him a prime target for Tillotson. Cole Tillotson had his eye on the JW, the only ranch in the valley still holding out against his onslaught. So

Tillotson would have been most happy to see Sitzman dead; happy enough, perhaps, to hire someone to kill him.

Scott angled a little to the southwest toward the Tilted T. He might find the killer he was seeking on Tillotson's spread, but he'd have to ride carefully there. Tillotson wanted him dead, too. Sitzman surely must have been a thorn in the flesh of Tillotson. But Scott was even worse. Scott wondered if that bullet back at the JW might have been meant for him instead of Sitzman.

Coming in sight of the Tilted T, Scott reined up. Following a gully, he rode in as close to the ranch buildings as he dared. There he left his horse ground-reined and went on toward the house. The barn and corrals were to one side, while the gully ran within a few yards of the rear of the house. Crouching low, he scooted up the gully until he was even with the back door.

Looking around to make sure no one was in sight, he left the gully and sprinted to the rear of the house. He tried the back door and was pleased that it opened silently at his touch.

Inside the house, he stopped and let his eyes become accustomed to the gloom. The room he was in was a sort of anteroom leading into the kitchen. It was more of a catch-all, it seemed to Scott. There was a wash tub, two boxes partly filled with fuel for the stove, some old coats that looked as if they would never be worn again, a pair of old torn boots and some tools.

Scott stepped around a shovel to get to the door into the kitchen. The kitchen was empty, and he crossed it silently. He tried to remember how the front part of the house was arranged. He had been in it the first day he'd come to the country. But he'd been in only one room, and he recalled that only vaguely. He had been concentrating on Cole Tillotson that day, not on the house he lived in.

The house seemed as silent as a tomb. Scott crossed the kitchen and was about to go into the next room when he heard someone move there. Quickly he ducked back toward a door along one wall of the kitchen. If whoever had made that sound in the next room decided to come into the kitchen, Scott would have to be out of sight or face a greater danger than he had when Hookey was thinking of arresting him for the murder of Mark Sitzman.

The first door he opened led into a dark pantry. He thought of stepping in there and shutting the door. Unless the cook came for things to start dinner, he'd never be found. But he'd learn nothing there, either. He had to find a place where he could hear what went on in the big room of the house without being seen himself.

Moving along the wall, he tried another door. This led directly into a bedroom. He hadn't expected a bedroom to open off the kitchen, but he gave it only a passing thought as he stepped into the room, closing the door softly behind him.

As he moved along the bedroom wall, he discovered that he could hear the sound of heavy breathing on the other side of the wall.

He stepped back carefully. If he could hear breathing through the wall, there was nothing to keep the sound of his own breathing from reaching the ears of whoever was in the other room.

While backing away, Scott bumped into a chair. It overturned, hitting the floor with a crash that sounded to Scott like the tocsin of doom.

VIII

For an instant after the chair crashed to the floor, there was a deathly silence in the house. Then a voice on the other side of the partition bellowed an order.

"Joe, get that cat out of the house! I've told you to keep him out, or I'm going to kill him!"

Scott looked around frantically for a place to hide. He lifted his gun out of the holster. Probably there weren't more than two men in the house. He might shoot his way out. But even if he did, there would surely be other men outside. Anyway, he hadn't come there to get into a battle. He had come to learn what he could without giving away his presence.

Another voice came from a far corner of the house. "The cat isn't in the house. I put him out an hour ago."

"What fell then? Made enough noise to have been the cupboard. Sounded like it was in the bedroom, though. Come and see."

"I'm coming," the other voice said disgustedly.

Scott saw no hiding place. There were only a dresser

and bed in the room, in addition to the chair. He heard footsteps coming from the far side of the house and he knew he had only seconds to do something.

Quickly he set the chair upright, then dropped to the floor and wiggled under the bed. He still held his gun in his hand. He was in an awkward position if it should come to a fight. But it was the best he could do on such short notice.

"Look in the bedroom, too, Joe," the man in the big room said.

Scott was sure that was Cole Tillotson giving the orders. Joe, he guessed, worked around the house and probably did the cooking.

Scott heard the man go into the kitchen and move around; then he came into the bedroom. Scott knew that if the fellow searched the bedroom as he had the kitchen, he'd be sure to look under the bed to see if the cat was hiding there.

But the man only glanced around the room, then went back through the kitchen to the main room.

"That cat ain't in the house," he said. "I looked through, under and behind everything in the kitchen."

"What about the bedroom?" Tillotson asked.

"The door was shut between the kitchen and the bedroom. He couldn't have gone in there. That cat is outside. If you'll come out, I'll prove it."

"I'm not calling you a liar," Tillotson said sharply. "But something crashed. What was it?"

"Maybe a piece of wood in the woodbox shifted," Joe said. "You're just jumpy since Web Scott showed up."

"I reckon," Tillotson said. "I don't figure on resting easy till we get rid of him."

"Here comes that fat deputy," Joe said, disgust in his voice. "He's doing an awful lot of riding in the sun lately."

"Must be something important to bring him out here again."

Scott inched his way out from under the bed. There was no need to hide there now, and he didn't like the cramped quarters, not when there was the constant danger of having to fight his way out of the house.

Out in the main room, the thump of heavy boots told Scott that someone else had come in. When the sound stopped, Tillotson spoke sharply.

"What do you want, Sam?"

"Just thought you'd want to know that Mark Sitzman is dead."

"Sitzman?" Tillotson exclaimed. "What happened?"

Scott marked Cole Tillotson off his list of potential suspects. There had been genuine surprise in his voice.

"I was out at the JW this morning," Hookey said, "and after I started back to town, I heard a shot. I hurried back and found Sitzman dead. Web Scott was there with him. Sadie was accusing Scott of killing Mark. Scott admitted that he'd been quarreling with him. So I went along with Sadie. I'll spread the word that Scott killed Sitzman. Scott won't dare show his face in Tomahawk Valley."

"Why didn't you arrest him then and there?" Tillotson demanded. "If you'd taken him to jail, nobody would have doubted it."

"He got the drop on me," Hookey admitted. "Got clean away. He rode north and kept going. I figure he's clear out of the country now."

"You numbskull!" Tillotson shouted. "How could you let him get away when you had him dead to rights? We've got to get rid of him."

"I figure we are rid of him," Hookey said. "Running like he did, he proved positively to everybody that he's guilty. And like I said, he was going north when I left his trail. It didn't look like he intended to stop."

"He will stop," Tillotson snapped. "He'll be back. He came after me for swindling him out of the Crossed S Ranch. He won't stop till I get him or he gets me."

"If he comes back," Hookey suggested, "why don't you pay him off? It might be the safest way out for you."

"Paying him off wouldn't stop him," Tillotson said. "He is convinced that I double-crossed him. He won't be satisfied with anything but my hide. I taught him myself that you've got to have a gun in your hand to get what you want, and you never let anybody cross you and go free. I never figured on him turning on me. We've got to get rid of him, that's all."

"What if he doesn't come back?"

"You imbecile!" Tillotson shouted. "I told you he will be back. Now get out there on his trail and follow it till you get him."

"He's mighty fast with that gun of his," Hookey objected. "I saw him draw."

"If you're scared of him, maybe I should send you back to Ohio," Tillotson said. "Or maybe you'd like to argue the point with Russo."

"No, no, I'll go," Hookey said so fast the words fell over each other.

Scott heard Hookey's heavy boots thumping toward the door. Then Tillotson called, "Wait a minute," and the thumping stopped.

The next instant Scott realized his danger as he heard Tillotson moving toward the bedroom door. Evidently there was something in the bedroom that he wanted to give to Hookey. Too late, Scott thought of hiding. But he had no chance to make any move.

Tillotson shoved open the door and stared in disbelief at Scott. His hand started toward his hip where he usually had his gun. It wasn't there now. Scott snapped a shot a few inches above Tillotson's head. The Tilted T owner ducked and lunged backward, shouting for help.

But Scott was already almost to the partition door between the bedroom and the kitchen. He slammed into the door just as Joe hit it from the other side. Scott's momentum sent Joe sprawling full length backward into the kitchen. Scott leaped over him and dashed through the little anteroom into the open.

His first glance was toward the barn and corrals. No one was there. The bunkhouse was on the other side of the house. If men were there, they'd have to come around the house before they could see him.

Running in a zigzag pattern, Scott dashed for the safety of the gully a few yards from the kitchen door. He was almost to the gully when the first shot came from the house. It missed, snapping past him to bury itself in the far bank of the gully.

Two more shots came from the house as Scott dived headlong for the rim of the gully, rolling over it to the safety of the bottom. He was on his feet in an instant, running in a low crouch toward his horse, which still stood, ground-hitched, a hundred yards away.

More shots slammed into the gully bank behind him before the men at the house discovered that he was running. Then the shots came his way, one of them spraying dirt in his face as he ran. He knew the men were coming out of the house now, trying to get their sights on him as he ran along the ravine. He considered stopping and driving them back with a few shots. But if he stopped, he'd give them the motionless target they wanted.

Reaching his horse, he wheeled and fired twice in

rapid succession. The pursuit halted as the three men dived for the protection of the ravine. While they were recovering their balance to shoot again, Scott mounted and put the spurs to his horse.

A few shots followed him, but the distance was too great now for accuracy. He heard Tillotson shouting and knew he was ordering Hookey and Joe to get their horses and follow him.

Scott grinned. He had easily fooled Hookey before. He didn't anticipate any trouble losing him again. Joe might be a better tracker. But tracking over the buffalo grass slopes was going to be slow work even for the best trackers.

Once out of sight of the Tilted T, Scott turned his horse east and set his mind to trying to puzzle out the answer to Sitzman's murder. Tillotson hadn't done it and hadn't ordered it done. But he had men who would kill a man without orders if the opportunity presented itself and they knew it was a job that Tillotson wanted done. There had been no regret in Tillotson when he had learned that Sitzman was dead.

When he was halfway to town, he saw dust rising from the road to his right, coming from the direction of the Tilted T. He pulled his horse to a halt behind a knoll and watched. In a short time, he saw Hookey spurring his horse along the road to town. Apparently he had given up trying to trail Scott. But Hookey was alone. Where were Joe and Tillotson?

Scott reined off to the southeast, checking the road carefully before crossing it. He wouldn't go into town just yet. When Hookey got there, the town would be buzzing with excitement. Scott would have no chance to check the saloon to see if Russo was there. He'd wait until dark to move in.

He'd need a fairly safe place to hide until dark. The creek offered the best protection around there. Trees were scarce. There were a few around the JW and some around the Tilted T, planted there several years before by the owners. But there weren't many anywhere else. Even along the creek there was nothing bigger than water willows. But they would offer some protection for him now.

If Hookey brought a posse out after him, he wasn't likely to do much looking until he got quite a distance from town. Hookey must have left Scott's trail when that trail was still leading north away from the Tilted T.

It was already well along into the afternoon. Scott wouldn't have long to wait before the shadows began to creep down from the rims of the knolls and stretch along the swales.

After a two-hour wait, the deep shades of dusk settled over the valley. Scott mounted and moved along the creek bed, letting his horse wade in the shallow stream part of the time. As darkness grew deeper, he reined his horse up on the flat land and urged him into a trot. If Hookey had taken out a posse, the chances were that the town would be almost deserted. Probably Russo would be with the posse, too. But there were other incentives drawing Scott toward Tomahawk.

If the men of the town were gone, he would run little risk in visiting Dr. Kinkaid's place. He wanted to hear what Kinkaid had learned, for he knew that the doctor would be keeping his ears open every second.

The lights in town were burning brightly as Scott approached. He rode slowly now, keeping to the shadows. Behind a barn at the edge of town, he dismounted and left his horse. A horse was too easily seen. As he headed toward the main part of town, he realized that the men of the town were not gone. Lights blazed and noise echoed along the main street. There were more men than usual in town.

Passing Dr. Kinkaid's house, Scott was tempted to stop. But if Hookey was still in town, it might be because he expected Scott to come to Tomahawk. If so, Hookey would not overlook the possibility that Scott probably would go to Kinkaid's as soon as he got there.

So Scott moved on along the dark street, ducking into the alley behind the hotel. The box was still in the alley where Johnny Russo and Dan Kale had given him that beating. He turned into the little runway between the hotel and the hardware store.

Dr. Kinkaid's office opened off the alley, but the office was dark now. He moved closer to the street. then stopped while he was still in the shadows. There were men in the street, and half a dozen were shuffling around on the porch of the saloon directly across from the hotel.

Hookey came out of the saloon, and Scott could see that he'd been drinking but that he wasn't drunk. He had had just enough whiskey to make him loud and boisterous. Scott realized this was no place for him. He wasn't going to get the chance to corner Russo, even if the gunman was in town. Hookey surely had spread the word that Scott had murdered Mark Sitzman. Cole Tillotson had probably given orders to get Scott at any cost. If anybody discovered him there, he'd be the target of a dozen guns.

"How many of you boys are ready to ride in my posse?" Hookey demanded, his voice a little thick.

Scott tensed as he saw Johnny Russo push open the doors of the saloon and move out onto the porch.

"Shut up, Sam," Russo said. "Do you think you can track him through the buffalo grass in the dark?"

"There's enough men here now for a posse," Hookey argued, his foggy mind obviously not quick enough to follow Russo's simple reasoning.

"You had enough this afternoon," Russo said disgustedly. "You could have followed him then."

"We only had four men," Hookey said, rubbing his head as if to clear his thoughts. "I've seen Scott in action. We need more men to take him."

"You mean you're scared to face him without an

army," Russo snapped. "I'll take care of him alone if I find him."

Hookey turned away from Russo. "We'll ride out first thing in the morning, men. I want you all at my office at dawn."

"Count me in," one man said. "I could use that five hundred Tillotson is offering for Scott."

A drunken whoop came from another man. "I want my share of that. Dead or alive, he said. I reckon dead would be the safest way to bring him in."

A rider came into the north end of the street, rode past the deputy's office and reined up in front of the saloon. The men swarmed around him. Scott found it impossible to hear what the man was saying. He inched out into the street, trying to hear. He had little fear of detection. No one was looking his way, and the light from the saloon didn't reach that far. Judging from the excitement that centered around the newcomer, he must have some important news.

"How about that?" one man shouted to a friend just coming out of the saloon. "Mike here says he trailed Scott. That killer came toward town."

"Suppose he's here in town now?"

"Of course not," Russo said. "He's not brainless. Where did you lose his trail, Mike?"

The rider raised his voice so that all the men on the porch could hear. "About a mile west of town. Looked like he rode south. But it was getting too dark to see, so I came on into town. Thought it might save the posse a lot of riding in the morning."

"Sure will," Hookey said, sounding more sober now. "We'll cut his trail outside town and ride him down before he knows we're after him. Bet he went back to the JW."

A man stepped out of the hotel, apparently attracted by the commotion across the street. Scott froze as he realized that the man was close enough to see him clearly, even in the shadows. He wheeled and dived into the alley. The movement caught the man's attention, and his shout turned every head in the street toward him.

"Somebody just ran down the alley!"

"It must be Scott," one man shouted, and led the rush across the street from the saloon.

IX

Scott ran down the alley, the light from the street fading quickly into the deep gloom between the buildings. Scott's mind was racing ahead, trying to pick out a place where he could hide. He'd have no chance trying to fight that many men. Anyway, he had nothing against most of those men; he had no desire to fight them. But where was he going to hide?

At the end of the alley between the two buildings, he hesitated. Then he remembered the big box in the alley. It was empty, he was sure. But was it big enough for him to get inside?

The men chasing him would expect him either to head down the alley behind the hardware store or to go to Kinkaid's house. They'd remember that Kinkaid had helped him before.

Scott was almost against the box before he saw it. This was the darkest spot in the alley, and that was in Scott's favor. Quickly he felt over the box, trying to find the open side. Footsteps were pounding down the alley behind him now. He felt trapped, like a coyote caught in a corner of a barn.

He ran his hand around the top of the box. Behind him, he heard the men stop at the end of the hotel building.

"Hurry up with that torch," one man yelled.

"Coming," another yelled from the front of the building.

Scott saw the faint shadows as the torch came down the alley. He was thankful for the caution the men were showing. It gave him an extra few seconds to hide himself. But if he wasn't completely out of sight when that torch threw its light into the alley, his time would have run out. The thin sides of that box would be no protection from bullets.

His hand found the open side of the box, facing away from the hotel. Crouching, he squeezed inside the box. It was cramped, but he felt secure. He doubted if anybody would look there for him.

Scott couldn't see what the men were doing, but he could hear them. He recognized a few of the voices. Sam Hookey was not in charge now. Scott didn't hear his voice. He doubted if he was even in the group. There was an element of danger in the chase, and Hookey had probably decided against taking any part in it. Scott recognized Johnny Russo's voice dominating the others.

"Likely he went to Kinkaid's," Russo said. "I'll take

four men, and we'll go through his house, whether Kinkaid likes it or not. The rest of you head down the alley behind the stores. Check every doorway where he could hide. See if there are any open windows where he could have crawled into a building."

"What if we don't find him?" one man asked.

"It will mean that he went on to the river, I reckon," Russo said. "He may have his horse there. But I don't figure he can make it to the river without us seeing him. Even as dark as it is, we should be able to see him if he moves away from the buildings. Let's go."

Scott held his breath as the men started moving out. If he so much as breathed loudly, the men with Russo heading toward Kinkaid's might hear him. He heard the thump of their boots as they came toward him from the corner of the hotel.

Suddenly the box rocked as one man bumped into it. Scott had to shift his weight quickly to keep the box from overturning. The man swore lustily, then hurried on after Russo and the others.

When they were gone, Scott let his breath out slowly. He had his gun in his hand. But it wouldn't have done him much good if it had come to a fight with five men.

As Russo and his men approached the back door of Kinkaid's house, the light from the stars, plus the reflection of the light from Kinkaid's window, revealed them to Scott. The open side of the box was still facing Kinkaid's house.

Russo hammered loudly, and J. R. Kinkaid came to the door. The first words exchanged by the men were too soft for Scott to hear. Then Russo's voice rose in anger.

"We're going to search your house whether you like it or not," he said. "If he's here, we aim to get him. Dead or alive, it makes no difference to us."

"He's not here!" Kinkaid shouted back. "I ought to shoot you for breaking in."

"Don't try it," Russo warned. "Get out of the way. Nobody will get hurt if you behave."

Scott saw Kinkaid step back and let Russo and the four men inside. The door stayed partly open as Kinkaid looked out into the darkness. Then he disappeared, but the sliver of light still shone through the partly open door.

Scott considered leaving the box and trying to get to his horse. But he'd have to go right past Kinkaid's house to reach the place where he had left his horse. If he tried to go around Kinkaid's to get to the horse, he'd run the risk of bumping into the other men who were searching the town for him. So he waited. The search here in town would have to be given up soon.

Then Scott noticed the light from the back door of Kinkaid's house go out. In another moment it was showing again, and he realized that someone had gone through the door. In the block of light from the door, he saw a woman's figure hurrying away from the house.

That would be Anne, he knew. But what was she doing out there?

She came on toward the hotel and passed within a few feet of the box where Scott was hiding. He crawled out of the box and called softly:

"Looking for me?"

Anne gasped, then wheeled toward him. "Yes. Where were you hiding?"

"In this box," Scott said, still crouching beside the box so he wouldn't make even the faintest silhouette. "What are you figuring on doing?"

"Hiding you where they can't find you," Anne said, coming close to the box and crouching beside him.

"What made you think you could find me when Russo and his men couldn't?"

"I didn't expect you to hide from me like you did from them," Anne said simply. "But they'll come back and search this alley again. You can't stay cramped up in that small box all night."

"Reckon you're right about that," Scott said, rubbing a leg that had already begun to cramp from his confinement. "But where can you hide me?"

"I know this town well," Anne said. "You crawl back in your box for a minute or two while I check to see where the other men are. Then I'll come back and take you to a safe place."

"Why are you doing this?" Scott asked as he squeezed into the box again. "Don't you believe that I killed

Sitzman?"

"Not like they say," Anne said quickly. "You may have killed him in a fair fight. But you didn't shoot him in the back."

"I didn't kill him at all," Scott said. "Somebody with a rifle picked him off."

He heard Anne slip away. In a few minutes she came back. Scott had been watching Kinkaid's house, expecting Russo to come out. But there had been no sign of the men. They apparently were giving the house a thorough going-over.

"Come on," Anne whispered, leaning over the box. "They've already been over the lower end of town."

"Where are they looking now?" Scott asked, crawling out of the box again.

"Most of them are around the dry goods store just south of the saloon, and a couple were nosing around the harness shop south of that."

"Where are you taking me?" Scott asked as Anne led the way along the rear of the hardware store.

"To the blacksmith shop," she said. "They've already looked around it. And I happen to know that Dick Randall, the blacksmith, never locks his side door."

"Think they won't come back?"

"I doubt if they'll go over the town twice."

Scott slipped along behind Anne, both of them pressing against the buildings, where they cast no shadows in the faint light from the stars.

They crossed the open alleys between the hardware and the barbershop and the feed store, then moved along the side of the feed store until they reached the street. Scott looked at the blacksmith shop, sitting squat and dark directly across the street from them.

"I hope we can get across the street without being seen," Anne said dubiously.

"I'll go first," Scott said. "I'll walk across like I was one of the searchers. From where they are, they won't be able to tell the difference."

"Good luck," Anne said. "The door that will be unlocked is on the south side, directly across the street from the livery stable. People use it as much as they do the front door."

"Thanks for the help," Scott said, and started across the street toward the blacksmith shop, trying to act like one of the hunters instead of the hunted.

He reached the front of the shop without being challenged and moved along the side of the building. The blacksmith shop occupied the corner lot, and directly across the side street from it was the livery stable. Halfway along the side of the building, Scott found the door that Anne had told him about. He turned the knob, and it opened. He stepped inside, finding it was black as a dungeon.

He stood there in the blackness, trying to adjust his eyes, but it was too dark. Outside, he heard a man shout, and Anne called back.

The running feet sounded in the street in front of the blacksmith shop. A voice Scott didn't recognize shouted again.

"What are you doing out here, Anne? You're liable to get shot."

"You wouldn't shoot a woman, would you, Mike?" Anne said.

"Not on purpose," the man said. "But we're looking for a killer, and you can bet he'll shoot first and ask questions later. So we're not taking any chances."

"I'm glad I didn't look like your so-called killer."

"You don't know how close you came to getting shot," the man said. Then he added suspiciously, "Do you think he's down in this part of town?"

"I'm looking for him just like you are," she said. "He has probably left town. You'd have found him if he hadn't, wouldn't you?"

"We sure looked every place," the man said. "You'd better get home. The next man who sees you might not recognize you like I did."

"I'll go home right away," Anne promised.

"If you do find him, you'd better tell us," the man warned. "It will go plenty hard on your old man if we find that any of you Kinkaids has been helping him."

Scott still stood by the door, hoping to get his bearings so he could move without crashing into something. But if Randall's shop was like most blacksmith shops, there would be iron bars, plowshares, wheels, wooden handles and other pieces of wood and iron lying everywhere.

He heard nothing outside until the door behind him squeaked softly. He wheeled toward it and in the light from outside saw Anne.

"You should have gone home like that man suggested," he whispered.

"I knew you weren't familiar with the inside of this shop," she said, "and it's as black in here as the inside of a cow. I'll take you to the back where you can stay out of sight, just in case somebody looks in here again. Where is your horse?"

"Out behind that barn at the edge of town west of your place," Scott said as Anne led him by the hand to the back of the shop. His arms brushed against things on either side, but Anne guided him unerringly to the rear wall.

"They can't see you here even if they look," she said. "Now I'm going to get your horse before they find it and run it out of town. They'll think you're making a run for it and go after you, I hope."

"Don't take any more chances," Scott said.

"I'm not taking any chances," Anne told him. "They can see that I'm not you. You're a foot taller than I. If I can keep them running till morning, maybe they'll cool off enough to use some reason. Then you'll have a chance."

She was gone then, slipping away silently in the dark.

Scott crouched against the wall, grumbling to himself. He hated this sneaking and hiding. Yet that had been about all he'd done since he came to Tomahawk. He fought down the temptation to walk out there on the street and have it out with Russo and Hookey and the whole lot of them.

But what would Anne think of that? She's risked too much already to keep him safely hidden. He couldn't insult her now by throwing all that away.

Ten minutes later he heard a horse galloping down the main street outside. A moment after that yells echoed up and down the street, and then came the pounding hoofs as riders raced down the street toward the river in the direction the first horse had gone. Scott grinned in the darkness. Anne had sent the men on a wild chase, just as she had said she would.

Now was the time to get out of town, Scott decided. Right across the side street from the blacksmith shop was the livery stable. Eli Blessing had turned most of the horses out in the corral behind the barn for the night. Scott should be able to catch one. He'd have to ride bareback unless he could find a saddle. But that would be better than staying in town.

He began picking his way carefully along the aisle toward the side door. He bumped into something hanging from a rafter. It swung away from him and banged into some kind of metal. The result was a reverberating noise like the clang of a bell.

Scott stood still, wondering if the sound was really as loud as it had seemed to him. He'd been crouching there in deathly silence so long he doubted if he could judge volume. Maybe the sound hadn't carried through the walls of the shop. All the men in town might have gone off, anyway, chasing his horse that Anne had sent out of town on the run.

Then he heard running feet outside and caught a glimpse of light flashing past a crack in the wall. He sank down into a crouch again, his hand resting on an anvil in front of him.

The side door opened cautiously and a man came in, a lantern held high above his head. In his right hand, the man held a gun. Scott watched him as he carefully moved a few feet inside the door. It was Dan Kale, the hardware owner. Scott thought of the beating Kale and Russo had given him his first night in Tomahawk, and his fists balled at his sides.

Scott watched the door for more men. But none came. Maybe Kale was the only man left in town. Or maybe he had been the only one close enough to hear the clang Scott had caused.

Kale moved inside the building, looking in every direction. Scott crouched lower behind the anvil. He fingered the butt of his gun but decided against using it. He'd have the advantage, all right, if it came to guns now. But if there were other men in town, a shot would bring them on the run.

As Kale moved closer, Scott tensed, awaiting his chance. Then Kale was even with him, and as he turned his head to look in the other direction, Scott lunged at him.

Kale heard him and wheeled, bringing his gun around. But Scott hit his gun arm and sent the gun spinning. The lantern fell but somehow managed to land right side up, even the globe remaining intact.

With a wild curse, Kale lunged at Scott. But tonight Scott wasn't at the disadvantage he had been at that first night behind the hotel. He moved to one side as far as the anvil would let him and crashed a fist into Kale's face. Blood spurted, and Kale cursed loudly. He wheeled back, and again Scott weaved away from his wild swings, landing telling blows of his own.

Kale turned back again, determined to get his hands on Scott. Big as the man was, Scott didn't doubt that Kale could crush him if he got him in those big arms. Kale threw himself at Scott, arms wide to keep Scott from escaping again. But Scott ducked low and scooted away. Kale, unable to halt his lunge, hit the anvil, one knee crashing against the solid iron.

With a cry of pain, he turned back toward Scott, barely able to stand. But still he came on. Scott moved in to meet him and hammered his face with hard blows. Kale retreated until he backed into the forge and plopped down in the ashes. They were still hot from the day's work, and Kale rolled away, yelling and cursing.

He got to his knees and dived forward at Scott. Scott had to admire his courage but not his good sense. The man had no idea when to quit. Scott hammered a fist down on the back of Kale's neck with all his force, and Kale sprawled out like a dead man.

Scott turned toward the door just as Anne came running in, breathless. She took in the scene at one glance. The lantern still sat where it had fallen, throwing a weird light over the interior of the shop.

"Come on, Web," Anne said quickly. "Others heard the fight, too. You'll have to run for it."

"Where to?" Scott asked as he ran to the door.

"To our house now. They've searched it. They surely won't look there again."

Outside the blacksmith shop, Anne turned toward the rear of the building, Scott just a step behind her. They had barely turned the corner when Scott heard men pounding on the front door. Then someone came around the corner and ran for the side door.

Silently Scott and Anne ran along the rear of the buildings until they reached the side street that separated the saloon and the deputy's office. There was no sign of life at either place, and Anne led the way into the street and turned down it toward the hotel. No challenge stopped them, and they were soon at the back door of Kinkaid's place.

Anne quickly explained what she had seen in the

blacksmith shop and Dr. Kinkaid grinned happily.

"I wish I could have seen Dan Kale pounded into the dirt," he said.

"You'll likely see him tomorrow," Scott predicted. "He banged a knee into the anvil pretty hard. He'll probably need doctoring."

"I may finish breaking it if it isn't already done," Kinkaid threatened.

But Scott knew that the doctor would do what he could for Kale if the man came to him.

A knock sounded at the front door and, without waiting for anyone to answer the knock Berwyn Edris came in. Scott had ducked toward his old room the instant he heard the knock. But he doubted if he had made it in time to avoid being seen by the lawyer.

However, if Edris had seen Scott, he gave no hint of it. He talked about the excitement in town and of the sounds of battle that had come from the blacksmith shop.

"I came over to see if you were all right, Anne," he said. "Mike told me how close he came to shooting you out there in the street tonight. I wish you wouldn't go out at times like this. When they said there was trouble down at the blacksmith shop, I was afraid you might be involved again. So I came over to see."

"I'm all right," Anne said sharply. "You needn't worry about me."

"I do, anyway," Edris said tenderly. "I wish you

would stay inside till this trouble is over."

Scott couldn't see the lawyer, but he had the feeling that Edris' sharp eyes were searching the house. He wanted to know why Anne had been on the street tonight. That would make him doubly dangerous to Scott. For Edris made no pretense about his feelings for Anne. And Anne certainly had made no pretense tonight about her concern for Scott.

If, when he came in, Berwyn Edris caught a glimpse of Scott ducking into the room, Scott was willing to bet that the men who had gone after his horse a while ago would hear about it the moment they returned to town.

X

Scott stayed in his room, debating whether or not he should step out and confront Berwyn Edris. The more he thought about it, the more certain he was that the lawyer had spotted him or was convinced that he was in the house.

Still, Edris was making no hostile moves. It wasn't Scott's place to cause Kinkaid any more trouble by facing Edris with a gun. So he sat quietly in his room and waited until the lawyer had left.

When he came out of the room, Anne voiced the question that had been plaguing him.

"Did he see you, Web?"

Scott shrugged. "I don't know. I wasn't expecting him to come in without an invitation, so I wasn't out of sight yet. I saw him well enough to recognize him. It's possible that he recognized me, too."

"I think he did," Anne said. "He looked right at that door a dozen times. But he didn't say a word about it."

"I'd better get out of here now," Scott said. "If I

stay, it will bring more trouble down on you."

Kinkaid waved a hand. "Never mind that. Edris might not tell what he saw. He doesn't like Hookey, you know."

"How does he feel about Tillotson?" Scott asked. "He's the one who's offering the money for my hide."

Kinkaid nodded. "This is first time since Cole Tillotson came to this country that anybody has given him any real trouble. You've really put a burr under his saddle."

"I'm in no position to make it stick, though," Scott said. "Sooner or later I'm going to run out of luck. And once they get their hands on me, I won't last long. Not with that murder charge hanging over my head."

Kinkaid sighed. "That's right. But we'll find the skunk who shot Sitzman from ambush. Then you'll be clear. Right now you stay close to the house here. I'm already in this as deep as you are. We'll figure something out."

Kinkaid's house was too far from the main street for those inside to hear when the men came back from their fruitless chase of Scott's horse. But they found out soon that the men were back. Scott heard them first— a little slap as someone hit the picket fence in the back yard.

"I think we've got company out there," he said.

"Get away from the windows," Kinkaid said softly. He reached over and blew out the lamp. Immediately sound erupted on all sides of the house.

"You, Kinkaid," a voice shouted. "We've got your place surrounded. Send out that killer."

"That's Russo," Kinkaid said softly. "He may be the one who killed Sitzman."

"That's how I've got it figured," Scott said.

"You hear, Kinkaid?" Russo shouted louder.

"I heard," Kinkaid shouted back. "We don't have any killer in here."

"You've got Scott," Russo said. "Same thing."

"Not in my book," Kinkaid said. "If you want to come in here, get a search warrant."

"We're not fooling with that legal stuff," Russo shouted. "We want Scott. Are you going to send him out? Or do we come in and get him?"

"I'd better go out," Scott said. "There's enough men out there to tear this house apart. If they start shooting, either Anne or Mrs. Kinkaid might get hurt."

"You're not going out there," Anne said quickly. "They'd shoot you the second you stepped through the door."

"Anne's right," Kinkaid said. "Tillotson's offer of five hundred dollars said dead or alive. You can bet they'll make it dead. Especially Russo, if he gets the chance."

"I'm not going to stay here and risk having Anne or Mrs. Kinkaid shot," Scott said positively.

"I don't figure on you staying here," Kinkaid said.

"I'll give you just two more minutes," Russo shouted. "If you haven't sent Scott out here by then, we'll blast you to bits."

"I'm going out," Scott said, moving toward the door.

"You're going out, all right," Kinkaid agreed, "but not that way. Come here." He led the way to the pantry that opened off the kitchen. "See this trap door in the floor?"

Scott nodded. "Where does it go? To the cellar?"

"That's right," Kinkaid said. "There is an outside door to the cellar. But one winter that door was covered with snow most of the time. So I dug an opening here and put in a ladder so we could get into the cellar from the house without scooping all that snow."

"Can I get out of the cellar through the outside door if I go in this way?" Scott asked, getting the picture.

"Yes. We'll keep them busy from here until you have a chance to slip through their lines. Then I'll invite them in to see for themselves that you're not here."

"Hurry, Web," Anne pleaded.

"Don't wait till they start shooting to tell them I'm gone," Scott said as he pulled up the trap door. "Ill make out."

Scott climbed down the ladder, and Kinkaid lowered the trap door over his head. It was pitch dark, but Scott couldn't take time to feel his way along. He heard Kinkaid yell at Russo, asking him if he'd shoot women. Faintly he heard Russo yell back that he'd shoot anybody who stood between him and Sitzman's murderer.

Kinkaid was stalling for time, and it was up to Scott to make good use of every second Kinkaid gained for him. At the bottom of the ladder, Scott turned to his right, where he knew the big door must be. A crack of light seeped into the blackness. It was only a sliver of light, but in the pitch blackness of the cellar, it looked like a beacon.

Scott hit the steps that led up to the door and climbed until his back was pressed against the heavy door. Slowly he lifted. The door began to rise reluctantly, its hinges protesting a little. Scott, with his ears on the level of the hinges, thought the squealing of the hinges must be echoing over the yard like a siren. But there was no sound outside to indicate that the squealing had been heard by anyone else.

Finally the door was lifted enough so that Scott could slip through the opening. He caught the door and let it settle gently back in place. After the pitch blackness of the cellar, the dim light in the yard seemed very bright. Crouching, Scott surveyed the area. Russo had said that he had the house completely surrounded with men. So one direction was as good as another for Scott to try to break through.

In the dim light he crawled slowly across the yard until he reached the picket fence. He remembered that the fence didn't go all the way around the house. Using the pickets as a barrier between him and the men surrounding the house, he moved in a crouching run to the end of the fence.

Peering around the end of the fence, he saw the dim silhouette of a horse standing at the edge of the street. Scott needed a horse, and he knew what he had to do. Moving around the end of the picket fence, he crept toward the horse. He was far enough from the house now so that he knew he must be near the line of men Russo had thrown around Kinkaid's place.

"That time is about gone," Russo shouted, and Scott flattened himself on the ground. Russo was only a few yards to his left.

"He ain't coming out," a man just a few feet from Scott said. "Are you really going to open up with those two women in there?"

"They're harboring a criminal, ain't they?" Russo said. "That makes them just as guilty as the murderer. We'll blast them all if he doesn't come out."

Scott rose to a crouch. If they knew he wasn't in the house they wouldn't start shooting where Anne and Mrs. Kinkaid might be hurt. Besides, he wasn't going to get a horse without letting the men know he was out there.

Running swiftly, he reached the horse before any alarm was given. Then a man only a few feet from the horse yelled and threw himself at Scott. Scott swung the butt of his gun and flattened the man. The next instant he swung into the saddle and wheeled the horse toward open country.

"Get him!" yelled the man Scott had hit as he scrambled to his feet. "That's Scott."

Bullets ripped the night, and Scott heard their snap as they passed him. One burned a path along his ribs, but it was only a scratch. The horse under him side-stepped sharply once, and Scott guessed that the animal had been nicked.

In a few seconds the barrage was over. Scott was out of range of the short guns of the men. He could hear the shouts and the scramble behind as men ran for their horses. It would be only a matter of a minute or two until the men would be mounted and in hot pursuit.

Scott angled toward the creek west of town and raced along its banks. When he heard the noise of the men pounding out of town, he reined his horse to a slower pace and dropped down over the bank into the water willows along the edge of the creek.

Reining up, he leaned forward and put a hand over his horse's nose to prevent a nicker that would tell his pursuers what he had done. Russo's men pounded out of town, racing wildly up the road.

They wouldn't go far, Scott knew, until they would discover that Scott wasn't ahead of them. They'd come back then, looking along the river, the only place where he could have given them the slip.

As soon as the thunder of the hoofbeats had passed, Scott realized that the bullet that had stung the horse bank. The horse was limping, favoring his left back leg. Scott realized that the bullet that had stung the horse back there had gone deeper than he had thought. The horse wouldn't be much good in a chase. The closest place where he could hope to get a replacement would be the livery barn in town. But his chances of slipping back into town unseen were slight. There couldn't be a sleepy eye in town now, after all that shooting.

In the other direction was the JW. He might find a horse there. Sitzman had fired the crew, and Sitzman himself was dead. Sadie would be the only one on the ranch, unless the cook was still there. And Sadie might have gone somewhere else to spend the night. He certainly wouldn't blame her for not staying there tonight after what had happened. There might be some horses in the corral on the JW. There had been this morning.

Scott reined toward the JW, keeping well south of the creek so Russo's men, if they returned, wouldn't see him. The horse's limp grew progressively worse as Scott urged him toward the JW.

He hit the road leading from the JW to the main road into town. Turning into it, he urged his horse on.

A quarter of a mile from the ranch, the horse's limp became so bad that Scott dismounted. He could lead him the rest of the way. He ran a hand over the horse's hip and felt the spot where the blood was oozing out. The bullet must be in the muscle. Tomorrow in daylight somebody could cut out that bullet, and the horse would be all right. But the horse had done all the running he'd do tonight.

Suddenly Scott heard a distant rumble. He stopped walking, and the horse immediately halted, hanging his head. It took Scott only a second to identify that rumble. Horses.

Evidently Russo's men had discovered that Scott wasn't in front of them on the road west out of town and had doubled back. Scott listened for a minute, getting a line on the direction the horses were going now. What he discovered made him leap into action, jerking on the reins of the horse. The animal resisted the effort to get him to move, and Scott had to tug to get him out of the road.

He led the limping animal toward a swale beyond the knoll to his right. Those horses were coming that way, and they were coming fast.

Scott kept glancing back over his shoulder at the road toward town, expecting to see the bobbing forms of the riders at any moment. Off to his left he could barely see the buildings of the JW, squatting low and dark in the starlight.

He reached the shallow end of the swale and pulled his horse into it. Dragging on the reins, he led the horse along until he had him far enough from the road and deep enough into the low spot so that the men would not see him as they rode past.

The sound of the galloping horses was at Scott's back, and he turned to watch the men ride past. His horse showed no interest in the other horses. Apparently that hip wound had dulled his social instincts.

The horsemen rode into the JW yard and reined up. Even from that distance, Scott heard Russo yell. A light came on in the house, and the front door opened.

After a minute or two, the men began to mill around in the yard. Scott guessed there was a difference of opinion as to where he had gone. Some of the men apparently were ready to give up the chase and go back to town. Scott could hear Russo's voice raised in anger. Obviously Russo wanted to keep looking.

In a few minutes, the men dismounted and went from building to building, searching the entire JW yard and corrals. Scott was thankful he wasn't down there now. Then the men mounted, and most of them rode south. Three turned their horses back to the northeast on the road to town, jogging along slowly.

Scott waited until the men had been gone from the JW for a while and the light went out in the house. Then he started slowly toward the corrals, leading his reluctant horse.

There would be a horse in the corral, Scott was sure. If Sadie was in the house, she couldn't allow herself to be stranded on the ranch without a horse that she could get whenever she wanted it.

Scott led the limping horse into the corral and un-saddled him. There were four horses in the corral next to the one he was in. He hoped he could rope one without causing any commotion. He knew how Sadie felt about him. If she found him taking a horse from the corral, he had no doubt about what she would do.

As he unsaddled the horse, he noticed the brand on his hip: the Tilted T. Sadie wouldn't be too happy in the morning when she found one of Tillotson's horses in her corral.

Scott carried the saddle over to the partition fence between the corrals, took the rope off the saddle horn and crawled in with the four frisky JW horses. Swinging his loop, he made a cast and missed. It was dark and, trying not to stir up the animals, he missed twice more before he managed to get his rope on one of the horses. The horse snorted loudly as he was pulled to the fence where Scott snubbed him and started to saddle him.

"You picked a good one," someone said a few feet away.

Scott, the saddle in his hand, froze. He had no chance to reach for his gun. The fact that it was a woman's voice gave him no comfort. It had to be Sadie. And Scott was sure she would shoot him as quickly as any man would.

"I try to pick the best," he replied.

"Put the saddle down and let's talk a bit," Sadie said.

Slowly Scott turned around until he was facing her. Then he laid the saddle on the ground. "What is there to talk about?"

He expected to see Sadie with a gun in her hand. But she was standing just on the other side of the fence, her arms folded. Now she unfolded her arms and climbed over the fence.

"I figured you'd show up here as soon as Russo was gone," she said. "He told me what happened in town and how you gave them the slip. Russo was sure they had hit either you or your horse. Either way, he didn't figure you'd go too far without help."

"If you had that figured out, why didn't Russo wait for me?"

"I said that I figured it that way, not Russo," Sadie said. "He decided you'd gone on to the south. I didn't tell him what I thought. That was none of his business."

"You wanted me all to yourself. Is that it?"

"Not exactly." Sadie leaned against the fence. "I did a little thinking. You couldn't have killed Pa. He was shot with a rifle, like you said. You didn't have a rifle."

Scott relaxed a little. Maybe Sadie had a decent side to her, after all.

"Are you willing to tell Hookey that?" Scott asked.

Sadie shrugged. Why not? I want to see the right man hang."

Why don't we ride into town right now and tell him? Scott suggested.

"Sounds good to me. Catch another horse and saddle him for me."

Scott finished saddling the horse he had caught. Then he took his rope and went after another horse. He couldn't quell the uneasy feeling he had. This was too sudden a change in Sadie.

He brought the other horse to the corral fence and tied him, putting Sadie's saddle on him.

"I guess we're ready," Scott said, turning to face her.

"I think we are," she said triumphantly, her face beaming in anticipation.

It was then that Scott saw the gun in her hand, pointing straight at his middle.

XI

Scott considered making a grab for Sadie's gun before she could fire it. But he knew that he wouldn't stand a chance.

"Changed your mind?" he asked finally.

"Not about riding into town," Sadie said. "We wanted to talk to Sam Hookey. Remember?"

"We won't agree on what to tell him."

"I don't suppose we will," Sadie said, apparently relishing every moment now. "Drop your gun belt."

Carefully Scott obeyed. He didn't doubt for an instant that Sadie would put a hole through him if he showed any inclination to disobey.

"You didn't really think I'd let you have the JW, did you?" Sadie said as she picked up Scott's gun belt. "Pa and I worked hard for this, then Josh double-crossed us by making that will that let you have it. Well, you're not going to get it. With Pa dead, it's all mine. And I'm going to have it."

"Why didn't you shoot me when you first sneaked

up on me?" Scott asked, wondering what was going on in her scheming mind. "You could have."

Sadie laughed. "I wanted to see your face when you found out you'd been crossed. Anyway, shooting would have been too easy for you. You've given me nothing but trouble since you came here. You're going to pay for that. You're going to swing, and I'm going to watch it."

"You know I didn't kill your father," Scott said.

"Sure, I know it," Sadie said. "But nobody else knows that I know it. They'll believe what I tell them. And it sure won't be that you're innocent. Now get on your horse. We're going to town."

Scott opened the corral gate and led his horse outside. Sadie stayed behind him all the way, never giving him a chance to make a break. Scott knew that she wouldn't let her desire to see him hang stand in the way of shooting him if he gave her any provocation.

Once on the road away from the ranch, Sadie rode just a few feet to one side and behind Scott, her gun never wavering from him. Scott cursed himself for a fool for having let Sadie get the drop on him.

A half-mile from town, Sadie called a halt. "Sounds like we've got a welcoming committee coming," she said.

Scott nodded. There wasn't enough light to see much. But there were still some lights in town, and the sounds coming toward them were unmistakably made by a group of horses. Scott thought of Russo. But Russo had gone the other way. It wasn't likely that he had gotten back to town yet.

"Going to wait here?" Scott asked. "Those might be my friends."

Sadie snorted. "You haven't got any friends here. You ought to know that by now."

Sadie was more nearly right than Scott liked to admit. Since word had gotten around that Scott had shot Sitzman, about the only friends he had left were the Kinkaids.

The horsemen came closer. Then the leader threw a hand in the air, halting them, as he saw Scott and Sadie in the road.

"Who is it?" he shouted, and Scott recognized Hookey's voice.

"Sadie," Sadie yelled back. "And I've got your prisoner, Web Scott."

"Glory be," Hookey said. "That's sure going to save me a powerful lot of riding."

"Let's hang him now," someone behind Hookey shouted. "Save the county the expense of a trial."

"Now hold on," Sadie said. "I brought him in. I've got a little to say about what happens to him. I want to see him dead more than any of you. But I don't want it to be so easy. Let him stew in jail for a few hours; then we'll hang him."

"A few hours is too long for murderer like him!"

the man shouted.

"He goes to jail," another voice said.

Scott turned to stare at the man, not able to see him clearly in the dark. It was J. R. Kinkaid, all right. Scott wondered what he was doing in the posse.

"All right," Hookey said reluctantly. "We'll take him back to jail." He rode close to Sadie. "Don't have much of a posse," he said. "Johnny Russo took most of the best men with him. When Bill came back from the JW and said they hadn't located Scott and that Russo had gone off half-cocked to the south, I knew I had to go after this killer. I picked up what men I could."

"You've got enough," Sadie said. "I took him alone."

When they reached the end of the street, two men surged up to the front of the group, coming in on either side of Hookey.

"I say we ought to string him up right now," one said. "If we wait, something might happen so he could get away."

"No lynching," Kinkaid said sternly. "We've got to have law and order in this country."

"He's right," Hookey said with a show of authority. "It's my duty to see that my prisoner is held for trial."

"Aw, hogwash!" said the man on the other side of Hookey. "I say we should hang him."

But he looked across at Kinkaid as he said it and slowly reined his horse back into the group. Scott knew that it wasn't Hookey who was keeping them from lynching him. It was J. R. Kinkaid. A lot of men in Tomahawk opposed Kinkaid, but they all had respect for him and hesitated to defy him openly.

As they were about halfway through town, the thunder of another group of horsemen came at them from the south. Scott twisted in the saddle to look. He thought he recognized Johnny Russo in the lead. Apparently they had given up their search to the south of the JW and had come back to town.

"We'd better hurry up and get him in jail," Kinkaid said softly to Hookey. "Russo and Kale are both in that bunch. They'll cause trouble."

"Sure, sure," Hookey said, apparently undecided what he should do. If he let Russo and Kale take Scott and hang him, it would put Hookey in good with them. But Kinkaid was right there at his elbow, telling him to do his duty.

"Let's get a move on, man," Kinkaid said.

Kinkaid reached over, grabbed the reins of Scott's horse and kicked his own mount into a trot.

"Here, you can't do that," Hookey shouted.

The deputy spurred his horse after Kinkaid. They reached the front of the deputy's office and dismounted just as Russo and Kale yanked their horses to a sliding halt in front of the jail.

"We'll take him right now, Hookey," Russo shouted. "Your job is done."

"Not quite," Kinkaid said. "He's going to jail."

Scott thought of trying to escape. He had no gun, but he wasn't bound. He could run or ride. But he knew he wouldn't be able to get ten feet. Still, even that would be better than hanging. And there was no doubt what Russo would do if he had his way.

"We're taking him," Russo shouted. "Come on, Kale."

Kinkaid suddenly stepped in front of Scott, and he had a gun in his hand. "You'll stay where you belong, Russo. You, too, Kale. Hookey, go in and put Scott in jail."

Russo and Kale stopped, apparently surprised that Kinkaid would take such a strong stand. Hookey, seeing the two gunmen stop, moved quickly to obey Kinkaid's orders. Scott was pushed inside the deputy's office and on to the back, where there were two jail cells. He was shoved into one and the door locked.

He heard Russo arguing outside with Kinkaid, but the doctor wouldn't budge. Finally the voices out front stopped, and feet shuffled away. Kinkaid came into the deputy's office.

"You've got to show a little backbone, Hookey," Kinkaid said. "If you face up to those men, they'll respect you and do what they're told, too."

"Sure," Hookey said importantly. "They won't take my prisoner from me now. I've got him in jail, and he'll stay here until I can get him to the sheriff."

"See that you do that," Kinkaid said. "Russo has

gone to get the saloon keeper to open up the saloon. If he does that, you'll have trouble before morning."

"They won't take my prisoner from me," Hookey repeated.

Scott went to the tiny barred window in his cell and looked out. The saloon was right across the side street from the jail. It was dark now, but there were a dozen men standing on the porch.

As he watched, Scott saw Russo come across the street from the hotel, a man at his elbow. The front door of the saloon was opened, and the men swarmed inside. A light soon sprang up inside the saloon, and voices rose in a crescendo. Russo and Kale backed down from Kinkaid's gun a few minutes before, but if they could get some drinks in those men in the saloon, they'd have plenty of help to run over Hookey and drag Scott out of the jail.

Scott looked out to the front office where Hookey sat, toying with his gun. Courage was one thing that Hookey lacked. He hadn't even had enough to come with Russo tonight when he'd tried to get Scott out of Kinkaid's house. Only when prodded later had he taken a posse out to look for Scott. He had probably felt fairly sure then that they would never find him.

When Russo came from the saloon with a following of impatient, half drunk men, Hookey wouldn't stand up to them ten seconds. Scott knew that he was as good as stretching a rope already.

He went back to the window and listened to the shouts and curses over in the saloon. It would take the men a while to work up their courage, but a few bottles of whiskey would take away any hesitancy they might have about hanging a man without a trial.

Scott wondered if Russo wasn't acting on orders. Tillotson wanted Scott out of the way. Probably Russo had orders to get the job done any way that he could. Buying a few bottles of whiskey was a cheap way to get it done.

A stir in the front office took Scott back to the barred door. Anne Kinkaid was in the front office, facing Hookey.

"I want to talk to him," Anne said.

"Nothing doing," Hookey said firmly. "My rule is that nobody sees my prisoner. That includes you and Johnny Russo and anybody else."

"I wish you had nerve enough to enforce that rule," Anne said. "Dad says you'll cave in like a winded pup the minute Johnny Russo or Dan Kale demands that you open up and let them have your prisoner."

Hookey brandished his gun. "I'll stand them off, no matter how many there are or how mean they get. Nobody gets my prisoner."

"It wouldn't hurt to let me talk to him," Anne said.

"Nobody talks to my prisoner," Hookey repeated. "You couldn't have anything to say to him, unless you've got some scheme to help him escape." Hookey's eyes brightened. "Is that it?"

"No," Anne said disgustedly. "My father was the one who insisted he be put in jail."

"That was just to save him from hanging," Hookey said.

Scott knew that Hookey was right about that. But Kinkaid had only delayed the inevitable a short time. As soon as Russo got those men whiskied up, they'd come over. And Hookey would be brushed aside like a straw in a high wind.

"If you let those men take him out of jail and hang him, I'll kill you myself!" Anne said, tears in her voice.

"That's bad, girl," Hookey said. "You're threatening an officer of the law."

"Only if he's too big a coward to do his duty!"

Hookey scowled. "Nobody gets my prisoner," he repeated.

"Better go home, Anne," Scott called to her. "I'll be all right."

"He won't do anything," Anne shouted back.

"You can't, either, Anne," Scott said. "Come back to visit me in the morning."

For a minute, Scott thought Anne was going to refuse to leave. But then she frowned at Hookey and went back outside. Scott returned to the side window and looked across at the saloon. The noise there was increasing as the whiskey began to take effect.

"Hookey, you ought to give me a gun so I can defend myself," he shouted.

Hookey snorted. "That would be smartt, wouldn't it? Give a killer a gun and then expect him to sit in jail and wait to be hanged.

"I'm supposed to be waiting for a trail, not a hanging," Scott said.

"Same thing," Hookey said. "Everybody knows you did it."

"Sadie knows I didn't," Scott said.

Hookey came off his chair as if he'd been stung. "How do you know?"

"She told me," Scott said, surprised at the deputy's reaction. "Only she wouldn't tell you or any of the posse. She admitted to me that she knew I didn't kill him, because he was killed with a rifle and I didn't have any."

"You shut up," Hookey said, slumping down at his desk again.

Scott watched the deputy open his desk drawer and take out a bottle. That would be fine! he thought. Hookey, sober, wouldn't be much of a deterrent to Russo and Kale and their men. But Hookey, drunk, would be no good whatsoever.

He went back to the window and watched the saloon. It really didn't make much difference. Drunk or sober, Hookey wouldn't stop Russo and Kale when they came for him. And they would come.

An hour dragged by. Scott heard Hookey grunting and talking to himself out front, and the noise over in the saloon slowly deteriorated into an ominous rumble as Russo and Kale apparently whipped up tempers.

It was sometime after midnight when the front door of the saloon burst open and Dan Kale staggered out. He was followed quickly by Johnny Russo and a dozen other men. Scott decided immediately that neither Kale nor Russo was half so drunk as he was pretending to be.

The men staggered across the street to the deputy's office. Scott turned to see what Hookey was going to do about it. Hookey had left his desk, and he had his gun in his hand as he faced the door.

"That's far enough," he shouted when Kale and Russo burst through the door.

"Now you don't figure on trying to keep us from getting that murderer, do you, Hookey?" Russo demanded.

"He's my legal prisoner," Hookey said. "I can't let anybody have him."

"You ain't letting us have him," Kale said. "We're just plain taking him."

"No, you're not," Hookey said, backing to the iron bars that separated the jail from his office.

"Now just how are you going to stop us?" Russo said, advancing slowly.

"Don't come any closer," Hookey shouted.

Russo suddenly whipped out a hand and knocked Hookey's gun aside. "You're too little to be playing with guns. Give me the keys to that bird cage."

Hookey slumped down against the wall to one side of the iron door, and Scott was sure he was crying. But that was of little concern to him now. What did concern him was the haste with which Russo found the keys to the cell and opened the door.

Russo leaped into the cell, and Scott charged into him, slamming him back against the men behind him. Kale, bruised and battered and still limping from the beating Scott had given him earlier that evening, shoved in with two other men. Scott lashed out at them, but more men crowded into the cell until there wasn't room for anyone to fight.

Then somebody pinned Scott's arms to his side, and another man grabbed both his legs. The fight was over.

XII

Scott continued to struggle as he was dragged from the cell. But he knew it was no use. There were at least a dozen men there, and every one seemed determined to have a hand in hanging him.

Scott had no time to identify any of the men in the mob, other than Johnny Russo and Dan Kale. The others were probably Tilted T hands and the men in town who sympathized with Tillotson, mainly in an effort to win his good favor.

At the door to the deputy's office, they let Scott get to his feet, but two big men held onto each arm.

"Get the rope," Russo shouted.

One of the men ran to the saloon and came back, carrying a coiled rope.

"Let me have it," Russo said. "We'll fix it so he'll lead better."

He took a little time making sure the noose was tied right; then he dropped it over Scott's head. Taking a good grip on the rope, he started off toward the south end of the street.

"Now pull back if you want to die before the official hanging," Russo said.

The others laughed loudly, as though it were a huge joke. Most of the men were drunk, Scott decided. He noticed one man who wasn't laughing and took a good look at him. He was Eli Blessing, the livery stable owner. Scott had been told that he was a Tillotson man. But somehow he didn't seem to be getting much enjoyment out of the hanging.

"See that ridge pole running out from the loft of the barn?" Russo asked when they were almost to the barn. "That's going to take you to the happy hunting grounds, Scott. Look at it good."

"Going to invite Hookey down to see it?" one man asked. "Make it legal, you know."

"He can watch from his office," Kale said. "Safer for him that way."

"Want a horse?" another man asked Russo.

"Don't need it," Russo said. "Eli, bring out a barrel. Let him stand on that."

Eli Blessing nodded and disappeared inside the barn. Scott noticed again that none of the excitement and anticipation that was gripping the other men seemed to possess the livery stable owner. Somewhere along the way he had lost his enthusiasm for the chore.

Scott remembered that Blessing had been the first man he had met in Tomahawk. He had seemed ready enough then to do the will of Cole Tillotson. Scott wasn't questioning the fact that his hanging was Tillotson's will, too. But Blessing no longer seemed so eager to follow it.

One man found a short rope and came up behind Scott, jerking his hands together behind his back and tying them carelessly.

"Hurry it up," Russo shouted through the open door of the barn. "We haven't got all night."

"I don't see why not," Blessing said, coming through the door, rolling a barrel ahead of him.

"I want another drink," Kale said, laughing.

A chorus of shouts greeted Kale's statement. The drinks, Scott thought, were the main thing that held the mob together. And the promise of more free liquor would make them hurry through their grisly business now. Scott doubted if Mark Sitzman had been such a good friend to most of these men that they felt obligated to hang the man they thought had killed him.

Dan Kale helped Blessing set the barrel on end under the ridgepole. Russo lifted Scott up on the barrel, which rocked unsteadily.

"Hold that thing still," Russo snapped to a couple of the men.

Then he stepped back and threw the end of the rope toward the ridge pole. It took three efforts before the rope went over the ridge pole and came back down so Russo could grab it.

"Now then," he said in satisfaction, "any last words, Scott, before I kick this barrel?"

Scott stared at Russo. It hit him suddenly that those were probably his last seconds on earth. Somehow, up till now, it had all seemed fantastic, unreal to him. But with Russo standing there holding the end of the rope and preparing to kick the barrel out from under Scott, it became all too real.

He didn't want to die, not this way. In a battle out in the street, he would feel differently. He'd have his chance. Here he was being killed with no more concern than a man would show for a sheep-killing dog.

Scott realized dimly that these were not the thoughts that a man should have in his last moments of life. He was thinking that Johnny Russo and Cole Tillotson had plagued his life from the time he was just a youngster. They had killed Mike Hammond and laid the blame on Mort Scott, sending him to prison to waste away and die. They had stolen the Crossed S from Scott and saddled him with the stigma of being the son of a jailbird. Now, when he had come for a day of reckoning, they had stamped him with the brand of a killer as they had his father, but this time they were making sure that he died before the truth could come out.

"You know I didn't kill Mark Sitzman," Scott said, glaring at Russo. "Even if I had, it wouldn't make this much difference to you. You wanted him dead more than

I did. Why don't you tell them why you're so eager to hang me for killing your worst enemy?"

Russo scowled and drew back his foot to kick the barrel "Somebody help me hold this rope," he shouted. "I can't do it alone."

One man, not so drunk that Scott's words failed to reach him, pointed a finger at Russo. "Hey, you did hate Sitzman, didn't you?"

Russo turned toward the man, his face brick-red with anger. Then suddenly a new voice rose against him. Eli Blessing stepped up close to Russo where Scott could look directly down on him. He glared at Russo.

"You probably killed Sitzman yourself and are hanging Scott to cover up your tracks!" he shouted.

"That's a lie!" Russo screamed. "Somebody help me hold this rope."

"Just a minute!" Blessing yelled, turning to face the mob. "This is another one of Cole Tillotson's schemes to get rid of an enemy. Scott has been in Tillotson's hair from the day he got to Tomahawk. There is no proof that Scott killed Sitzman. And even if there was, how many of you men loved Sitzman enough to lay yourself open to a prison term to hang his murderer?"

A murmur ran over the men as some of those whose minds weren't completely fogged by Russo's free whiskey began to grasp the situation.

"He's a liar!" Russo screamed, aiming a fist at Blessing.

But Blessing ducked away from the fist, and Russo couldn't follow up without releasing the rope. None of the men had offered to help him hold the rope.

"Prove what you're saying," one man said, leaning toward Blessing.

Blessing nodded. "All right; I will. Tillotson brought me here and gave me the job of running the livery stable. I thought I had a chance to make a decent living. But Tillotson won't allow anybody to do anything decent. I swung a wide loop when I was younger. I got caught and served my time in prison. Tillotson knows that and holds it over me. He'll pull something to send me back to prison if I step out of line. He's told me so in plain words."

"That's what he'll do now, too," Russo shouted.

"Sure, he will if he can," Blessing said. "But I've stood back and kowtowed to him as long as I can. Hanging a man for a murder that I'll bet my soul he didn't commit is too much. It's time we stood up like men and told Cole Tillotson where to head in. He'll hold every one of you responsible for this lynching, and after tonight you'll do what he says or he'll see to it you land in jail. That's how he operates."

Men who had been carried away by the frenzy whipped up by Russo and Kale now suddenly began to sober up and look at their position in the light thrown on it by Eli Blessing. Two or three men in the rear of the mob melted away into the darkness. Several men closer to Russo began nodding their heads in agreement with Blessing.

Then Scott caught another movement out of the corner of his eye. He turned his head. Dan Kale was quietly slipping his gun out of its holster. At that instant Russo, his rage at Blessing getting the better of him, let go of the rope and reached for his gun.

With the end of the rope dangling freely over the ridgepole now, Scott suddenly felt a surge of hope. He had to do something immediately or that hope would be gone. If Russo's or Kale's bullet knocked Blessing out of the picture, the mob would swing back on Russo's side, either voluntarily or from fear.

Kale was too far away for Scott to reach. But Blessing and Russo were right in front of him. Scott launched himself from his barrel, knocking Russo sideways as he reached for Blessing. The rope slithered over the ridgepole, and Scott felt it tighten around his neck. But before it choked off his breath, it whipped over the pole and fell free.

Just as Scott knocked Blessing off his feet, Kale's gun roared. The bullet snapped through the air where Blessing had been a split-second before.

Men yelled and began milling around. Scott couldn't see whether or not anyone tried to disarm Kale. But the hardware owner was out off from the three men on the ground by the milling mob.

Scott rolled free of Blessing, and Blessing lashed

out with his gun, slamming it against the side of Russo's head. Then he rolled to his feet, grabbing Scott by the arm.

In the confusion, Blessing pulled Scott into the barn. With one hand, he reached up and flipped the noose over his head.

"Run," he whispered. "They'll be after you the second they realize you're gone."

"They believed you, didn't they?" Scott said. "They don't think I'm guilty."

"I didn't convince them you're not guilty," Blessing said. "I just made them see they were fools to lynch you. They could be sent to prison for that, and Tillotson wouldn't let them forget it."

"So they won't hang me now."

"No," Blessing said impatiently. "But they'll throw you back in that jail. They'll remember that the only two people near Sitzman when he was killed both swear that you did it. Once you're back in that jail, you know what will happen. Tillotson won't try to stir up a mob to kill you next time. He'll find a surer way."

Scott knew that Blessing was right. If he were put back in jail, he'd never walk out again. Somehow he'd be killed right there.

"What about you?" Scott asked.

"I'll take my chances. I risked my life to save yours. Don't stand here and throw it away. Get going!"

Scott turned and ducked into a stall, while Blessing

stayed by the door. Scott worked his way quickly to the far end of the barn. But before he could get out, men poured through the front door.

"Where did he go?" one man shouted.

"He slipped away," Blessing said.

"You let him go," another man shouted. "We ought to string you up."

"I just kept you from lynching a man without a trial," Blessing said. "That could keep you out of jail."

—Scott still had his hands tied behind his back and tried desperately to work free. He moved around the ink-black stall, searching for something he could use to free himself. Up in the front of the barn, he heard Blessing arguing loudly with the men, insisting that he had done what he had only because he wanted to keep the men from becoming part of a lynch mob.

Scott located a mane roacher in the feed box of the stall. Evidently Blessing used this stall to store some of his tools and gear. He fumbled around until he was holding the mane roacher open, one blade punching around his wrists.

He brought blood a couple of times before he got the scissor-like tool between the ropes holding his wrists. It took only a few strokes across the blade to cut through the ropes, and then his hands were free.

But now the men were running through the barn. Scott crouched in the deep shadows. If they searched the stalls, they'd find him. But they were running through the barn, paying no attention to the stalls. Behind them, Blessing was shouting.

"He must have gone out the back. He came into the barn ahead of me. He wouldn't stop in here."

The men poured through the rear door, and Scott slipped up to the edge of the door and peered outside. There was practically no light in the rear of the barn, but Scott could hear the men running across the street toward the blacksmith shop. Dan Kale had led them through the barn. Perhaps Kale thought that Scott would go back to the blacksmith shop to hide as he had earlier in the evening.

Scott slipped out the back door and pressed himself against the wall of the barn while he listened to the search going on across the street. When the searchers moved on, Scott started back inside. He was sure that Blessing would have a horse or two in the barn. He couldn't remember seeing or hearing any as he ran down the length of the barn. But he hadn't been thinking about horses then. Now he was. He had to have a horse to get out of town. If he stayed around there, somebody would find him. He had no gun; he'd be easy pickings.

If Johnny Russo or Dan Kale found him first, Scott knew he'd be taken in dead. Even if one of the other men found him and took him back to jail, it would amount to practically the same thing. One of Tillotson's men would shoot him through the bars.

As he reached the rear door again, he heard Russo swearing loudly up by the front door. Evidently he had recovered from the clout that Blessing had given him. Scott knew he'd have no chance to slip into the barn and get a horse while Russo was there.

While he was standing there trying to decide what his next move should be, he heard a man out in the street yell to the others:

"Get back in the barn. He may try to get a horse."

Scott heard the thump of boots out in the main street as men ran toward the barn. After listening long enough to be sure that none of the men was coming to the back of the barn, he slipped to the corner and, when the side street was clear, dodged across to the rear of the blacksmith shop.

From there, he ran along the alley to the jail. He remembered that the deputy had left his horse at the hitch rack in front of his office. He had seen it there as the mob was dragging him out of the jail. If he could reach that horse, he might get away before the mob was aware of what he had done.

The saloon was still lighted, but it was empty now. From the rear of the saloon, he looked across the street to the jail. Hookey's horse was still standing in front of his office. No one seemed to be near, so Scott dodged across the street to the rear of the jail. From there, he worked his way to the front of the building on the dark side.

Someone was inside the deputy's office. Scott could hear the voices but he couldn't make out what was being said. He had supposed that Hookey would be out helping hunt the fugitive, now that the danger of his witnessing a lynching was past.

At the window of the deputy's office, Scott stopped and raised his head enough to look inside. Hookey was standing close to the window, a scowl on his face. Scott noted that he didn't appear the least bit drunk now. Standing between him and the door was Sadie Sitzman, and she was as angry as Hookey appeared to be. Their words came clearly to Scott.

"You'll do what I say," Sadie said maliciously, "or you know what will happen to you."

"You can't bluff me with that threat," Hookey said. "Mark tried it, and it got him nowhere."

"It got him killed," Sadie said. "And I know how he was killed, too. You were the only one within a mile of the JW that morning with a rifle. How would the men in town like to know that you killed a man from ambush because he knew that you had murdered a girl years ago?"

"You dare open your mouth about that and I'll— I'll—"

Scott thought that Hookey was going to have a stroke. His face was almost purple, and the veins stood out in his neck and forehead.

"You'll what?" Sadie taunted.

"I'll tell them how you killed Josh Woodruff."

Sadie was visibly rocked by the deputy's accusation. "You can't prove a word of that."

"Can't I?" Hookey said, suddenly gloating as he saw that he had taken the advantage away from Sadie. "A lot of people know how you tried to wangle Josh into marrying you so you could get the JW legally. When he balked at marrying you, you threatened him. I sat right here in my office and saw the whole show that morning. Josh rode in, and you followed him. You rode down to the feed store and waited. Josh was shot from the back of the feed store. Everybody knows that."

"You can't prove a thing."

"I can prove just as much as you can," Hookey said. Suddenly Sadie broke into a laugh. "All right. So I killed Josh. But you won't open your mouth about it. I've got you on two murders. And don't think I won't tell everybody if you so much as get one little step out of line. You're going to do some work for me that only a lawman can do. And you're not going to make one objection."

"I'll object plenty," Hookey said.

Sadie suddenly became furious, her teeth bared in a snarl that reminded Scott of a mad dog. "You do, and I'll turn that mob on you. I guarantee they'll hang you. I'll be there to slap the horse out from under you myself."

Scott, watching, saw panic sweep over Hookey. "You can't push me around!" he shouted.

Sadie suddenly drew her gun and aimed it directly at the deputy. "Who says I can't?"

Scott looked at Hookey. The panic was still there; not even the gun could squelch it. Suddenly Hookey leaped forward. Only a couple of steps separated him from Sadie. His hand struck down, and the gun exploded as it was hit, the bullet plowing into the floor.

Hookey, fighting with a maniac's strength, wrenched the gun from Sadie's hand and stepped back. Quickly and deliberately, he fired twice. Sadie staggered back aganst the wall and slowly slid to the floor.

Shouts and running feet echoed along the street as the men who had been searching for Scott converged on the deputy's office.

Scott watched Hookey throw the gun over close to the front door and run to the door himself and stick his head outside.

"Over here, men!" he yelled. "Scott just shot Sadie Sitzman."

XIII

Scott froze in his crouch below the window. Hookey couldn't possibly know that Scott was close by. But he had certainly heard that he had escaped the lynching party and that the men were searching for him. So it had apparently struck him that he might be able to blame Sadie's murder on Scott.

But the fact that Scott was right there by the deputy's office now put Scott in the worst possible position. When the men arrived at the jail, they'd begin searching there, believing that Scott was close by. If Scott was found there, there would be no doubt as to his guilt in anybody's mind.

The urgency of getting away drove Scott into action. He turned and ran to the rear of the jail. Out front, he heard a man yell at Hookey as he came running toward him.

"Why did he shoot Sadie?"

As he ran along the rear of the jail, Scott heard Hookey's reply.

"She was the only one who actually saw him kill Mark Sitzman. I guess he figured if she was dead, nobody could prove he did it."

"Why did he kill her right in your office?"

"He tried to kill us both," Hookey said. "With both of us gone, there would have been no proof at all."

Scott heard no more. Glancing up the side street, he saw that it was empty for the moment, and he dashed across to the rear of the saloon, then he ran full speed down the alley behind the buildings. Reaching the back of the blacksmith shop, he paused to make sure the side street between the shop and the livery stable was empty.

Just as he was ready to dash across the dusty street, a rider burst out of the rear door of the barn and angled into the street only a few feet from Scott. Putting the spurs to his horse, he kicked up a fog as he charged out of town to the east.

Shouts up from the main street, and feet pounded down the boardwalk and along the dusty street again.

"He got a horse at the barn," some man yelled. "Let's catch him."

"Hold on!" another man shouted. "That couldn't be Scott. He hasn't had time to get a horse."

Scott was sure that was Cole Tillotson's voice. He hadn't known that Tillotson was in town. Apparently he had come in after Scott had been thrown in jail. Probably he had come to witness the hanging, although he had been careful not to get in the mob itself.

"He's getting away," another man yelled. "Let's get him."

Scott crouched low in the shadows at the rear of the blacksmith shop, while men ran to the livery stable and the hitch rack in front of it where some of them had their horses.

"You idiots!" shouted another voice that Scott identified as belonging to Johnny Russo. "That wasn't Scott. If he shot Sadie, he couldn't have gotten to the barn yet."

But the men were convinced that Scott had somehow gotten to the barn and taken a horse and was now riding out to the east, getting away from them.

Suddenly the whole street seemed to explode with thundering hoofs as the men reached their horses and mounted. Scott remained low in the shadows as they raced by, although he was sure they wouldn't have seen him if he'd stood right at the side of the street. They had only one purpose in mind—to catch the rider who had rushed out of town ahead of them.

When the riders were gone, Scott scanned the side street again. There was no sign of movement there, and he dashed across it to the rear of the livery stable. Going in the back door, he stopped in the shadows.

Up toward the front of the building, a lantern swung from a snap that slid along a wire running the length of the barn. From that snap, the lantern could be slid along until it shed light in any given stall. Standing close to the lantern was Eli Blessing.

Scott tried to see into the stalls along the length of the barn. Surely there would be at least one horse left. But he couldn't see any. If he could get a horse and ride to the west or south, his chances of getting out of the country would be good. Some day he'd come back and prove his innocence, but right now his only chance, the way he saw it, was to get out of Tomahawk Valley.

He moved along the stalls far enough to see that there were no horses in the barn. There were horses in the corral to the south of the barn, he knew. But he didn't dare go after one. Maybe Blessing would get one for him. He had helped Scott already tonight. He might help him some more.

Halfway along the row of stalls, Scott called a low warning to Blessing. The stable owner looked at him without any show of surprise.

"Can you get me a horse?" Scott whispered.

Blessing moved toward him. "I think so," he said softly.

Scott stepped back into the dark stall and waited for Blessing to come to him.

"We've still got company outside," Blessing said softly when he reached Scott. "Cole Tillotson is out there. And Russo and Kale didn't ride off with the other men. They figured out it wasn't you."

"Who was it?" Scott asked.

"It was George Ingram. He'd been trying to persuade the lawyer, Edris, to help him get rid of you and give him legal title to the JW. Edris couldn't do that, of course, but Ingram wouldn't believe it. From what I gathered from Ingram when he was in here getting a horse, he and Edris had a fight. Ingram hit the lawyer over the head with some kind of iron bar, and he thinks he killed him. So he's running away. Never saw anybody more scared than that fellow."

"How about getting a horse for me?" Scott asked.

"I'll do it pretty soon. You don't want to tear out of here until that posse gets well out of town. The rate Ingram was going, it will take those men at least a couple of hours to catch him. He had a good horse. Besides, if I rush out into the corral to get a horse, you can bet Tillotson or one of his two gunmen will figure out why I'm doing it."

"All right," Scott said reluctantly. "But I don't feel comfortable sitting around here. Tillotson and Russo and Kale must be pretty certain I'm still in town."

"Reckon they are," Blessing said. "But they don't have any idea where you are. If I went out to catch a horse, they'd know."

"Tillotson can just about claim this whole valley now," Scott said, "with both the Sitzmans dead."

"You're not," Blessing said. "That's the one thorn left in Tillotson's side. He owns practically everybody in this town. I told them out there what he's holding over me. Not much, maybe, but enough to make me toe the mark. At least it was until tonight. I just figured I couldn't ever live with myself if I let them lynch you, knowing that Russo probably killed Sitzman."

"Hookey did it," Scott said. "I heard Sadie accuse him of it. Seems Sitzman knew that Hookey had killed a girl back east somewhere and was blackmailing him. I didn't suspect Hookey; I had no idea he had any reason to kill Sitzman."

Blessing whistled softly. "That proves how wrong a man can be if he doesn't know all the facts. Probably the murder of that girl is the thing Tillotson holds over Hookey, too. I know he owns him, body and soul. Russo and Kale are just plain mean, the kind of killers men like Tillotson have to have around them to keep everybody else in line. I figure Tillotson pays them plenty. I hear that Russo and Kale were in prison together."

"Ought to be there now," Scott added. "What will happen to you now that you've kicked over the traces?"

Blessing was silent for a moment. "I reckon I'll have to face either Johnny Russo or Dan Kale, probably before another day is over."

"Why did you do it, when you knew what would happen?"

"I got fed up," Blessing said emphatically. "I'm filled up to here with kowtowing to Cole Tillotson."

"Maybe you'd better get two horses from the corral,"

Scott said. "Looks to me like we'd better both ride out of here."

"I'm not much on running," Blessing said. "I've done a lot of it in my time, and each time I did, I got a little sicker of it. When I took this job at Tillotson's request, I made up my mind I'd run an honest barn. When it got to the point where I couldn't do that, I'd make my stand. I reckon I've reached that point.

Silence fell between them. Scott wondered how long it would be before Blessing thought it would be safe to go out and bring a horse in from the corral. And he wondered, too, if Tillotson would let him get a horse. He didn't doubt now that Blessing was on Tillotson's list of men to be eliminated, the same as Scott was.

Scott thought he heard a sound at the rear of the barn and turned that way. Neither he nor Blessing made any noise. Scott was sure that Blessing had heard it, too. Maybe Tillotson or one of the men had decided to have a look inside the barn.

The light thrown by the lantern was almost completely absorbed by the darkness back at the rear of the barn, and it was nearly pitch black in the stall where Scott and Blessing were. Scott could see the square opening of the rear door which showed a block of dark blue sky studded wtih stars. There was nothing blotting out those stars at the moment.

Then Scott heard the sound again and wheeled as he realized he'd been looking in the wrong place. In that instant, a voice cut through the stillness. "Don't move, Scott. I've got my gun right in the middle of your backbone."

Scott saw the man then. In the darkness of the stall, he was just a dim outline. He was standing behind Blessing and apparently had mistaken Blessing for Scott. Scott recognized Hookey's voice. The deputy was the last man in town that Scott would have expected to sneak in to try to take him single-handed. Apparently Hookey hadn't seen Scott yet.

Scott moved forward silently. When he struck, he'd have to do it quickly, unerringly. Hookey played into Scott's hands then by stepping back a little from Blessing.

"Let's go outside, Scott," the deputy said. "Walk straight and easy toward that front door."

Blessing moved a step ahead, and in that instant, Scott struck. His hand came down like the edge of an iron bar across Hookey's wrist, sending his gun into the litter at his feet. His other arm came up, encircling the deputy's neck.

"Get his gun," Scott said.

Blessing had already turned. "Got it," he said a moment later. "Now what will we do with him?"

"Wish we could get him all alone at a time like this," Scott said.

"We won't catch any of the others this easy," Blessing said. "They're not as thick-headed as this one. He thought he had you. But what did he think I'd be doing all the time he was marching you out of here? He surely knew I was here in the barn, too."

"Let's make him do some talking and find out," Scott suggested.

He took Hookey's gun from Blessing and shoved it into the deputy's back, releasing his hold on his throat. "Got anything to say, Hookey?"

The deputy just stood there, saying nothing. Blessing prodded him from the other side, but still Hookey remained silent.

"Let's take him to one of the stalls where the lantern throws a little more light," Blessing said. "I figure Tillotson has some scheme afoot, and this jasper may know what it is. Maybe we can make him talk."

"I won't talk," Hookey said.

Scott prodded him up to one of the stalls toward the front of the barn where the light was stronger.

"You make quite a habit of killing people when they can't fight back, don't you?" Scott said.

"I don't know what you're talking about," Hookey said sullenly.

"First there was that woman years ago," Scott said. "Then Mark Sitzman this morning. Tonight, it was Sadie Sitzman."

"They think you killed Sadie," Hookey said, a note of triumph in his voice.

"You and I know different. You are nearer right

than you thought on one point, though. I was close to your office when Sadie was shot. I saw you shoot her."

"That's a lie!" Hookey said sharply. "Nobody saw—"

"Oh, yes, I did," Scott interrupted. "I was looking through that little window in the north side of your office. You jerked the gun away from her and deliberately shot her twice."

Realization of the truth began to seep into the deputy's face. And with it came a fear that bordered on panic.

"You might as well admit it," Blessing said. "You know that Scott is telling the truth. He saw you do it."

"All right," Hookey said. "So I killed her. She'd have killed me if I hadn't."

"Tell that to the men out there."

"They'll string you up for shooting a woman," Blessing said, "even if it is a woman they wanted out of the way. They probably would like to find an excuse to get rid of you, anyway. You know how much Tillotson loves you."

"Shut up!" Hookey shouted. "Tillotson wouldn't hurt me. I've always helped him."

"That's not the way I hear it from Cole," Blessing said.

In the dim light from the lantern, Scott could see the sweat breaking out on Hookey's forehead. The deputy obviously was deathly afraid of Cole Tillotson.

"I've done whatever Tillotson asked me to do," Hookey said.

"Like killing Sadie?" Scott asked.

"He wanted her dead, anyway," Hookey said. "He's going to own this whole valley before the week is out. I heard him say so myself."

"What's he planning to do right now?" Blessing asked.

"He's got it all figured," Hookey said. "He—"

A shot ripped through the barn. Scott and Blessing dived back deeper into the stall. Hookey dropped flat.

"I'm hit! I'm hit!" the deputy screamed.

Scott reached out and dragged Hookey deeper into the stall. The shot, he was sure, had come from the back door. Where Hookey had been sitting, he had been partially exposed to the door. Deeper in the stall, he was not.

"Let's see how bad you're hurt," Scott said.

The light from the lantern was weak that far back, but it was strong enough to show a bloody scratch across the upper arm of the deputy.

"Just a scratch," Blessing said disgustedly. "Not a deep one, either. The way you yelled, I thought you were half dead."

"They're trying to kill me," Hookey blubbered. "They're trying to kill me."

"Why, Tillotson wouldn't do that," Scott mocked.

"You help him all the time, you said."

"He tried to kill me," Hookey repeated as if dazed by the fact.

More shots ripped into the barn. Hunching down deep in the stall, the three were safe from the probing bullets. But Scott wasn't satisfied to stay there.

"They can't hit us," he said to Blessing, "but we can't shoot back, either. They might sneak inside the barn if we aren't out where we can watch."

"You're right," Blessing said. "We've got to get out of this trap."

Scott crouched, gun in his hand, as he surveyed the situation. From a stall in the center of the barn, he would be fairly well protected from either door while able to keep those doors under surveillance.

"Coming?" he said to Blessing as he prepared to make a dash.

"Right behind you," Blessing said. "Come on, Hookey."

Scott suddenly darted out of the stall and dodged around the end of the stalls till he reached the one he wanted. Guns opened up from both doors, but no bullets hit him.

Once in his stall, Scott began shooting first at one door, then at the other. Under cover of Scott's firing, Blessing made the dash to the stall without trouble.

"Now what?" Blessing asked after he caught his breath. "We're in a fairly safe spot. But we still can't do much damage to them."

"It will be just a lucky shot if either of us hits anything. Looks to me like a stand-off."

"It will be unless they decide to smoke us out," Blessing said.

Scott nodded. That was the big advantage that Tillotson and his men held now. One match in the dry hay, and the livery barn would go up like a tinderbox.

XIV

The shooting continued spasmodically for an hour. Scott noticed after a time that there was no longer any shooting from the rear door. He called Blessing's attention to that.

"Could be a trap," Blessing said. "Maybe they think we'll try to make a run for it through that back door. They'd be waiting for us."

Scott nodded. "Could be. Where's Hookey?"

"I've been wondering about that. I told him to follow me. Maybe he's still crouching back there under the manger in the front of that stall. He'd be safe there, you know."

Scott nodded. "Maybe. One thing sure: he won't take a hand in the shooting if he can help it."

"Only two things can make Hookey fight," Blessing said. "One is to give him an advantage so he runs no risk of geting hurt, the way it was when he killed Mark Sitzman. The other is to corner him. Any rat will fight when he's cornered."

"Like he did when Sadie threw her gun on him?"

"I reckon," Blessing said. "Once he got the advantage, he killed her without turning a hair. He's not the kind of man I'd want to call a friend."

Scott agreed with Blessing on that. "What do you figure Tillotson will do now?"

"Hard to say," Blessing returned. "It will be daylight soon. The men who rode out after Ingram should figure out their mistake when they see him, if they don't catch him or lose his trail before then."

"Do you think Tillotson will just sit tight till they get back? Or will he burn us out?"

"I doubt if he'll do that if he can find any other way," Blessing said. "He owns this barn, you know. I just worked for him. He won't destroy any of his own property if he can help it."

Scott decided that Tillotson would probably wait until the men returned. Then he'd have a force strong enough to run roughshod over Blessing and Scott. An occasional bullet slapped into the heavy wood of the stall, more of a reminder that they were not forgotten, Scott thought, than an attempt to inflict any damage.

Once, during the darkest hour just before dawn, Scott heard a yell at the front of the barn. It was a weird, panic-stricken yell and defied any attempt to identify the man who gave it. It was followed a couple of minutes later by two shots. But no bullets slammed into the barn.

"Something funny is going on out there," Blessing said.

"Maybe they're fighting among themselves," Scott suggested.

"That would be too good to be true," Blessing said. "But I sure can't figure out that yell and those shots."

After that dark hour, the eastern sky began to lighten. The gray fingers of dawn crept slowly through the rear door of the barn and stretched across the littered floor.

The lantern, which had given what light there had been inside the barn through the night, seemed to fade until the yellow flame behind the round globe was only a tiny slice of color lost in a brightening world.

"I don't want to spend the day here," Scott said. "I'm going to try to get out the back door while it is still pretty dark."

"Be careful," Blessing warned. "They may be waiting for us to try that very thing."

"I can see well enough now to get a good look out there."

"I'll stay here and put up a cover for you," Blessing said.

Scott clutched his gun in one hand, picked his course before leaving the protection of the stall, then dived into the alley of the barn. A bullet dug up litter behind him as a surprised gunman at the front door snapped a shot at him. Blessing opened up from the safety of the stall, driving back the man at the front door.

Scott reached the back door and stopped, peering around the corner. The light wasn't very strong out there, but it was strong enough to assure Scott that nobody was in sight.

Dodging outside, he paused, his gun ready. In spite of the fact that he knew someone might be waiting in ambush, he felt safer there than he had at the door, knowing the man at the far end of the barn might brave Blessing's marksmanship to get a shot at Scott's back.

There was no sound in the alley, and Scott ran to the corner of the barn. The man at the front of the barn knew that Scott had gone out the back way. Someone would be around to get him. They couldn't let him get away from the barn where he could become the hunter instead of the hunted.

There was no one in the side street between the barn and the blacksmith shop, and Scott ran along the side of the barn. He was halfway to the front when a man charged around the corner in front of him.

Both Scott and the man stopped as though they had hit an invisible wall. Johnny Russo stood there in front of Scott, his gun in his hand.

Scott brought up his gun at the same instant that Russo did his. The two shots blended into one. But Scott was already falling as he shot, a trick that Cole

Tillotson had taught him during the days when Scott's father had objected to Scott learning so much about handling a gun.

Scott's bullet went straight into Russo's chest, while Russo's bullet merely tugged at the sleeve of Scott's shirt as it snapped past. There were no more shots from either gun. Russo staggered a step forward and sprawled in the dust, while Scott waited, his gun ready.

Scott got to his feet and walked forward carefully. He had to be sure the danger frrom Johnny Russo was past. Even if it was, there was still danger from the other guns. Dan Kale and Tillotson were somewhere in town. And he had no idea where Sam Hookey was.

Scott approached the spot where Russo had fallen and saw from the way Russo was crumpled in the dust that he had no more to fear from him. As he looked down at Russo, something slammed into the side of the barn only inches from Scott's head. Instinctively Scott dropped to the ground as the report of a rifle echoed along the street.

Rolling over once, Scott took a quick look up the street. Not much of it was visible to him from there. The corner of the blacksmith shop shut off much of his view of the main street. He could see the feed store and barbershop across the street and one corner of the hardware store. There was a little puff of smoke coming from the doorway of the hardware store.

Scott rolled toward the blacksmith shop as two more

bullets dug into the dirt in his wake. Then he was out
of sight of the hardware store and got to his feet. The
man at the hardware must be either Kale or Tillotson.
Scott had to get closer or he'd be no match for a man
with a six-gun. Not only that, but whoever was in the
store had the building for protection. Scott had nothing.

Scott thought of dodging across the street, taking his
chances on moving fast enough so that the man
couldn't hit him. From over there he could come up
on a side of the hardware building that had no windows. But he discarded that plan. Somewhere in town
was at least one more man waiting for him. Chances
were he was in front of the livery barn. If Scott dodged
into the street, trying to escape the bullets of the man
in the hardware, he'd be easy picking for the other
man.

Dodging around behind the blacksmith shop, he
ran along the alley. He stopped to catch his breath behind the harness shop, directly across from the hardware. But still there was a street between him and the
store, and Scott knew he could never get across it from
there.

There had been no sound from the rifleman in the
hardware store since he had shot at Scott down by the
barn and Scott began to wonder if the man might have
decided to abandon his position. If he did, all of Scott's
maneuvering would be wasted. Even worse, the man
might move to a place where he could get a clear shot

at Scott.

All Scott could do was hope the man stayed in his protected position in the store. It would be hard to rout him out, but that would be safer for Scott than having to hunt for him.

Scott ran on up the alley, crossing behind the dry goods store and the saloon. In the street between the saloon and the deputy's office, he turned toward the main street. At the corner of the saloon, he paused to scan the front of the hardware store. The rifle was still there at the open door, although Scott couldn't see the man behind it.

The light wasn't strong yet. That had probably saved his life back there by the livery barn. But, close as he was to the store now, it wouldn't save him again. From the angle of the rifle barrel, Scott guessed that the man still thought he was down by the barn. That would give Scott an extra second in his dash across the street. And he had to cross the street before he could hope to meet the rifleman on anything resembling even terms.

Drawing a deep breath, Scott launched himself into a zigzag run across the street toward the hotel. He was more than halfway across before the rifle opened up. But the man had been in too big a hurry to switch directions with the rifle, and the bullet struck five feet behind Scott. Scott threw himself in a headlong dive behind the north end of the hotel veranda. The rifle roared again, but the bullet hit the veranda, and Scott breathed a relieved sigh.

Getting to his feet, he ran along the side of the hotel and around the back. The hardware was next to the hotel, with a wide alley between. Dr. Kinkaid's office in the corner of the hotel opened into the alley.

There was no window in the north side of the hardware store, and Scott didn't hesitate a second as he came to the alley. The man in the store would be hurrying toward the back door now, knowing that Scott planned to come that way. Scott had to beat him to it.

As he ran across the alley, Scott noted that there was a light in the Kinkaid house to the west. A light wasn't needed outside now but inside a house it would be. Apparently Dr. Kinkaid was up; maybe his whole family. With so much shooting going on, it would be odd if everyone in town wasn't awake and watching.

Reaching the rear of the hardware store, Scott paused. The rifleman had had time to get to the back door. But everything was quiet there. Scott wondered if the door was locked. Moving cautiously to it, he stood to one side and tried the knob. The door slowly swung open.

Scott knew that the man must be waiting to blast him the instant he appeared in that doorway. Still, he had to get inside.

Scott found a small box at his feet and picked it up. He tossed it through the doorway, and the rifle roared. The box was splintered in mid-flight. The instant the rifle fired, Scott dived through the door, hitting the floor and rolling. The rifle roared again, but the bullet was off target.

Scott came to his knees, his eyes on the spot where he had seen the flash of the rifle in the deep gloom inside the store. Scott fired twice. Then he dived behind some cases that were stacked at one side of the door.

The rifle fired again, then was quiet. The next bullet that slammed into the cases came from a hand gun. Scott found some satisfaction in the realization that the fight was on even terms at last.

He dodged to another pile of boxes, getting a better view of the place where the man was hidden. He was in the main part of the store, crouched behind a counter. On the counter almost directly above the man's head was a glass-bowled lamp half full of kerosene. Apparently the man had had it lit; then the shooting down at the barn when Scott had met Russo had drawn his attention. He had taken a hand in the fight and had blown out the lamp to keep the interior of the store dark.

Scott fired again, this time aiming at the big bowl of the lamp. Glass shattered and kerosene splashed over everything close to it. The man behind the counter suddenly leaped up, howling, as glass and kerosene showered over him.

Scott moved out from behind the boxes, gun in hand, as Dan Kale came over the counter, rubbing his eyes.

"Stop right there, Kale," Scott ordered. "Drop that gun."

The gun clattered to the floor. "I can't see!" Kale howled.

"That's fine," Scott said. "What were you doing here instead of being down at the barn?"

"I came after more shells for my rifle," Kale said sullenly.

Scott nodded. "Were you guarding the back door of the barn?"

"For a while," Kale said. "Let me wash this kerosene out of my eyes."

"Where's Hookey?" Scott demanded. "Have you seen him?"

Kale swore. "Get me some water."

Scott directed Kale to a water bucket he had spotted on a stool by another counter. Kale plunged his hands and face into the bucket, rubbing his eyes.

"Have you seen Hookey?" Scott repeated.

"Yes," Kale said. "He sneaked out of the barn a while after we started shooting. We let him come out, and he swore he was going to kill Tillotson before Cole killed him. Tried it, too. Got on top of the barn and tried to drop that rope around Cole's neck; the one Russo planned to hang you with."

"I suppose Hookey missed," Scott said. "He never did anything right in his life."

"He did worse than miss," Kale said, rubbing his

face with a rag he found by the bucket. "He got tangled up in that rope somehow and hung himself by the foot. He's still hanging from that ridgepole, head down."

"Alive?"

"No. Johnny shot him. Tillotson's orders."

The back door opened cautiously, and Kinkaid stuck his head inside.

"All clear in here?" he asked.

"All quiet," Scott said. "Come on in. Can you lock Kale up in the jail? Seems we don't have a deputy any longer."

"Be glad to," Kinkaid said, moving quickly inside the store. "I've been doctoring Berwyn Edris. He got a nasty crack on the head, but he'll be all right."

Anne came in the back door. "Are you all right, Web?" she asked.

"Sure," Scott said. "But you'd better get back home. This isn't over yet."

"Why not? It—"

Her words were cut off by a burst of gunfire coming from the livery barn. Scott ran to the front of the store and out on the porch. He stopped there, trying to see what was happening. The sun wasn't yet up, but the dusk in the street was rapidly melting away.

Eli Blessing stumbled out the door of the barn as another shot echoed along the street from the direction of the feed store. Blessing jerked around and went down. But immediately he began to crawl toward the corner of the barn.

Scott ran into the street, firing at the feed store to draw the attention of the man there. It had to be Tillotson. The men who had ridden out after Ingram were not back yet. All the others who had remained in town were accounted for.

Tillotson turned his gun on Scott, and Scott dived back into the protection of the alley between the hardware store and the barbershop. The feed store was just beyond the barbershop.

"Come on out, Cole," Scott yelled. "Russo's dead and Kale's headed for jail. You're finished."

"Come and get me!" Tillotson yelled back.

Scott looked across the street. If he were over there, he might be able to blast Tillotson out of the feed store. But Tillotson would pick him off if he tried to dodge across. He might come in the back door of the feed store as he had come in on Dan Kale. But facing Kale's gun was one thing; facing Cole Tillotson's was another.

Still, going in the back door was the only way, and Scott knew it. He moved along the side of the barbershop to the rear corner and stepped around it. Just as he did, the rear door of the feed store burst open and Tillotson leaped out, firing as he came. He evidently had been waiting for Scott to make that very move. Having taught Scott how to fight that kind of battle, he knew what to expect from him.

Although Scott was caught by surprise, his reaction was instantaneous. He threw himself sideways, bringing his gun to bear as he went down. Tillotson's bullet dug into Scott's arm, while Scott's bullet missed its target completely.

Scott rolled twice. When he stopped, he saw the Tilted T owner steadying himself on one knee to make sure of his aim. Scott threw himself sideways again, firing as he did so. Tillotson's shot missed completely this time, but Scott's bullet knocked Tillotson backward.

Tillotson rolled over, bringing his gun up hastily. Scott fired again, his bullet driving into Tillotson's shoulder. Tillotson dropped his gun and flopped back on the ground. But he was up in an instant, reaching for the gun with his left hand.

Scott was on his feet then, running toward Tillotson. "Don't do it, Cole!" he shouted. "I'll kill you."

"Why not?" Tillotson hesitated only for a moment to glare up at Scott. "Go ahead and shoot."

Just as Tillotson's left hand closed on the gun, Scott put a foot on his wrist.

"Drop it!"

Only after Scott put heavy pressure on the wrist did Tillotson let his fingers relax. The gun dropped back to the ground.

"Why couldn't you kill me and be done with it?" Tillotson asked, pinching his lips together against his pain.

"That would be too easy," Scott said. "You've got a lot to pay for. Come on. The doc can fix you up."

Kinkaid was just opening his office after taking Kale to the jail and motioned for Scott to bring his prisoner there. While Kinkaid worked on Tillotson, Scott went back to the barn and got Eli Blessing. Blessing wasn't hurt as badly as Scott had feared and was able to walk to the doctor's office without help.

"What are you going to do with me now?" Tillotson demanded weakly when Scott got back to the office.

"I'm going to give you a choice, Cole. When those men get back from chasing Ingram, they're going to be plenty sore, but sober. They'll be ready to listen to the truth. You can clear the Scott name of the murder for which Mort was convicted, or I'll tell those men exactly how you've been using them and let them pass judgment on you."

Tillotson paled. "They'd hang me," he croaked.

"If they decide that's what you deserve, why not?" Scott said.

Tillotson debated only for a minute, then nodded. "All right," he said wearily. "I'll tell the authorities what really happened. It was Johnny Russo who killed Hammond; not Mort Scott. We framed Mort so I could get the Crossed S. I figured at first that I'd take you along with me, almost as my son. That's why I taught you how to handle a gun so well. But you were too stubborn; you had to go on your own. Together we could have owned a half-dozen counties, Web, and controlled everything in this end of the state, from cattle to politics."

"What about that ten thousand dollars you stole from me?" Scott asked as if he hadn't heard what Tillotson had said.

Tillotson sighed. "I'll sign over the Tilted T. That will pay you back with interest. I'll have no more use for it."

"I'll put Tillotson in jail with Kale," Kinkaid said. "Then I'll fix up you and Eli. You'll have to ride to the county seat and bring the sheriff. I don't want the responsibility of these prisoners any longer than necessary."

Scott nodded. He wasn't surprised that Kinkaid could take over authority so easily. He had been the one pillar of strength opposing Tillotson.

Kinkaid finished bandaging Tillotson, then guided him across the street to the jail. Scott turned to see Anne staring steadily at him.

"Now you'll own the whole valley," Anne said. "You already own the JW."

Scott sensed her resentment. "The JW belongs to your father," he said. "He owns the mortgage. As for the Tilted T, most of the land controlled by Tillotson doesn't belong to the ranch at all. Homesteaders will soon file on that. I won't have a very big ranch; maybe not big enough for a doctor's daughter."

Anne flushed. "A soddy on a homestead will be big enough for me," she said, all her resentment gone, "providing I have the right man with me."

"And who is that going to be?" he asked.

"You guess," she said softly, ignoring Eli Blessing lying on the couch as she came to Scott's arms.

She left no room for guessing. And that was the way Scott liked it.